2023

ADVANCES IN
SMALL ANIMAL CARE

EDITOR-IN-CHIEF
Philip H. Kass

SECTION EDITORS
Joseph Hahn
David Levine
Denis J. Marcellin-Little
Elisa M. Mazzaferro
Jason W. Stull

ELSEVIER

Publishing Director, Medical Reference: Dolores Meloni
Editor: Stacy Eastman
Developmental Editor: Jessica Cañaberal

Editorial Office:
Elsevier, Inc.
1600 John F. Kennedy Blvd,
Suite 1800
Philadelphia, PA 19103-2899

International Standard Serial Number: 2666-450X
International Standard Book Number: 978-0-443-18417-8

ADVANCES IN SMALL ANIMAL CARE

EDITOR-IN-CHIEF

PHILIP H. KASS, BS, DVM, MPVM, MS, PhD
Diplomate, American College of
Veterinary Preventive Medicine
(Specialty in Epidemiology)
Vice Provost for Academic Affairs
Distinguished Professor of Analytic Epidemiology
Department of Population Health and Reproduction,
School of Veterinary Medicine
Department of Public Health Sciences,
School of Medicine
University of California,
Davis, California, USA
phkass@ucdavis.edu

SECTION EDITORS

JOSEPH HAHN, DVM
Executive Director, Companion Animal and Equine
Professional Services
Merck Animal Health
Rahway, NJ
joseph.hahn@merck.com

DAVID LEVINE, PT, PhD, DPT, MPH, FAPTA
Board-Certified Clinical Specialist in Orthopaedic
Physical Therapy
Professor and Walter M. Cline Chair of Excellence in
Physical Therapy
Department of Physical Therapy
The University of Tennessee at Chattanooga
615 McCallie Ave Dept #3253
Chattanooga, TN 37403
David-Levine@utc.edu

DENIS J. MARCELLIN-LITTLE, DEDV
Diplomate, American College of Veterinary Surgeons
Diplomate, American College of Veterinary Sports
Medicine and Rehabilitation (Charter)
Professor, Small Animal Orthopedic Surgery
University of California, Davis
djmarcel@ucdavis.edu

ELISA M. MAZZAFERRO, MS, DVM, PhD,
DACVECC
Staff Criticalist, Cornell University Veterinary
Specialists
Adjunct Associate Clinical Professor of
Emergency-Critical Care
Cornell University College of Veterinary Medicine
President, American College of Veterinary
Emergency & Critical Care
880 Canal St
Stamford, CT 06902
emazzaferro@hotmail.com

JASON W. STULL, VMD, MPVM, PhD, DACVPM
Assistant Professor, The Ohio State University
College of Veterinary Medicine, Department of
Veterinary Preventive Medicine
Columbus, OH
stull.82@osu.edu

CONTRIBUTORS

EDITOR

PHILIP H. KASS, BS, DVM, MPVM, MS, PhD
Diplomate, American College of Veterinary Preventive Medicine (Specialty in Epidemiology); Vice Provost for Academic Affairs, Distinguished Professor of Analytic Epidemiology, University of California, Davis, Davis, California, USA

AUTHORS

ELIZABETH ARMITAGE-CHAN, VetMB, PhD
Diplomate, American College of Veterinary Anaesthesia and Analgesia; Member of the Royal College of Veterinary Surgeons, Professor, LIVE Centre, Royal Veterinary College, North Mymms, Hatfield, United Kingdom

HEIDI BANSE, DVM, PhD
Diplomate, American College of Veterinary Internal Medicine (Large Animal); School of Veterinary Medicine, Louisiana State University, Baton Rouge, Louisiana, USA

JENNIFER A. BARNHARD, BVetMed (Hons), MS, MRCVS
Veterinary Surgical Centers, Vienna, Virginia, USA

MICHAEL J. BLACKWELL, DVM, MPH
Director, Program for Pet Health Equity, College of Social Work, Center for Behavioral Health Research, University of Tennessee, Knoxville, Tennessee, USA

GARY BLOCK, DVM, MS
Diplomate, American College of Veterinary Internal Medicine; Ocean State Veterinary Specialists, East Greenwich, Rhode Island, USA

MATTHEW W. BRUNKE, DVM
Diplomate, American College of Veterinary Sports Medicine and Rehabilitation; Veterinary Surgical Centers, Vienna, Virginia, USA

YEKATERINA BURIKO, DVM
Diplomate, American College of Veterinary Emergency and Critical Care; Department of Clinical Sciences and Advanced Medicine, University of Pennsylvania School of Veterinary Medicine, Philadelphia, Pennsylvania, USA

BRITTANY JEAN CARR, DVM, CCRT
Diplomate, American College of Veterinary Sports Medicine and Rehabilitation; The Veterinary Sports Medicine and Rehabilitation Center, Anderson, South Carolina, USA

ROBERT GOGGS, BVSC, PhD, MRCVS
Diplomate, American College of Veterinary Emergency Critical Care; Diplomate, European College of Veterinary Emergency and Critical Care; Associate Professor, Emergency and Critical Care, Department of Clinical Sciences, Cornell University College of Veterinary Medicine, Ithaca, New York, USA

HELI K. HYYTIÄINEN, PT, MSc, PhD
Department of Equine and Small Animal Medicine, Faculty of Veterinary Medicine, University of Helsinki, Helsinki, Finland

DEEP K. KHOSA, BSc, BVMS, PhD
Member of the Australian and New Zealand College of Veterinary Scientists (Small Animal Medicine), Associate Professor, Ontario Veterinary College, University of Guelph, Guelph, Ontario, Canada

NINA R. KIEVES, DVM
Diplomate, American College of Veterinary Surgeons; Diplomate, American College of Veterinary Sports Medicine and Rehabilitation; Department of Clinical Sciences, The Ohio State University College of Veterinary Medicine, Columbus, Ohio, USA

DAVID LEVINE, PT, PhD, DPT, MPH, CCRP, FAPTA
Department of Physical Therapy, University of Tennessee at Chattanooga, Chattanooga, Tennessee, USA

LEONEL LONDOÑO, DVM
Diplomate, American College of Veterinary Emergency and Critical Care; Capital Veterinary Specialists, Jacksonville, Florida, USA

DENIS J. MARCELLIN-LITTLE, DEDV
Diplomate, American College of Veterinary Surgeons; Diplomate, American College of Veterinary Sports Medicine and Rehabilitation; Veterinary Orthopedic Research Laboratory, School of Veterinary Medicine, University of California, Davis, Davis, California, USA

JULIE A. NOYES, DVM, PhD, MS, MA
American Association of Veterinary Medical Colleges, Washington, DC, USA

AUGUSTA O'REILLY, MSSW, LCSW, VSW
Director of Veterinary Social Work, Program for Pet Health Equity, College of Social Work, Center for Behavioral Health Research, University of Tennessee, Knoxville, Tennessee, USA

KIRSTEN E. OLIVER, RVT, CCRP, VTS (Physical Rehabilitation)
Veterinary Surgical Centers, Vienna, Virginia, USA

ARIELLE PECHETTE MARKLEY, DVM, cVMA, CVPP, CCRT
Diplomate, Academy of Integrative Pain Management; Diplomate, American College of Veterinary Sports Medicine and Rehabilitation; Department of Clinical Sciences, The Ohio State University College of Veterinary Medicine, Columbus, Ohio, USA

EMMA K. READ, DVM, Master of Veterinary Science
Diplomate, American College of Veterinary Surgeons - Large Animal; Associate Dean for Professional Programs, The Ohio State University College of Veterinary Medicine, Columbus, Ohio, USA

ADDIE R. REINHARD, DVM, MS
CEO, MentorVet, Lexington, Kentucky, USA; Adjunct Instructor, Lincoln Memorial University College of Veterinary Medicine, Harrogate, Tennessee, USA

ULRICH SCHIMMACK, PhD
Department of Psychology, University of Toronto, Mississauga, Ontario, Canada

ELIZABETH STRAND, PhD, LCSW
The University of Tennessee, Knoxville, Tennessee, USA

ASHLEI TINSLEY, VMD
Department of Clinical Sciences and Advanced Medicine, University of Pennsylvania School of Veterinary Medicine, Philadelphia, Pennsylvania, USA

ASHLEY A. TRINGALI, BS
Veterinary Surgical Centers, Vienna, Virginia, USA

JOSH VAISMAN, MAPPCP (PgD)
Flourish Veterinary Consulting, Firestone, Colorado, USA

ALESSIO VIGANI, Dr med vet, PhD
Diplomate, American College of Veterinary Emergency and Critical Care; Diplomate, European College of Veterinary Emergency and Critical Care; Diplomate, American College of Veterinary Anesthesia and Analgesia; Clinic for Small Animal Internal Medicine, Vetsuisse Faculty, Zurich, Switzerland

JOHN VOLK, BS
Brakke Consulting, Greensboro, North Carolina, USA

SHEENA M. WARMAN, BSc, BVMS
Diploma in Small Animal Medicine, Diplomate, European Diploma in Small Animal Medicine (Companion Animal); EdD, Senior Fellow of the Higher Education Academy, FRCVS, Professor of Veterinary Education, Bristol Veterinary School, University of Bristol, Langford, Bristol, United Kingdom

MELANIE WERNER, Dr med vet
Clinic for Small Animal Internal Medicine, Vetsuisse Faculty, Zurich, Switzerland

CONTENTS

VOLUME 4 • 2023

SECTION I: REHABILITATION

Gait analysis is a tool used to collect objective information in a research setting and when managing clinical patients to assess limb use and lameness in dogs and cats. Gait changes resulting from orthopedic and neurologic problems can be monitored over time to assess the progression of disease and/or response to therapy. Objective gait analysis measurements most commonly reflect the use of the whole limb but may not always represent joint-specific dysfunction or overall patient function. Subjective and objective gait evaluations include the comparison of findings from the left and right sides of the body and the comparison of findings from the patient to normal values.

Patient-centered care is increasingly advocated in human physical therapy and musculoskeletal rehabilitation to improve quality care and patient outcomes. Veterinary physical rehabilitation is an essential aspect of veterinary care and is inherently multidimensional. Historically, rehabilitation focused on physical aspects and omitted components critical to success, including the owner of the patient, the behavioral status of the patient, and anticipated future activities. These other components need to be considered to create genuine patient-centered care plans, which are needed to improve quality of care and patient outcomes. This article will outline a framework for veterinary patient-centered care focused on physical rehabilitation.

Clinical Instruments for the Evaluation of Orthopedic Problems in Dogs and Human Patients, a Review, *37*

Heli K. Hyytläinen, David Levine, and Denis J. Marcellin-Little

Like in humans, measurements of musculoskeletal function in dogs collected by clinicians or owners can be grouped into specific instruments describing the level of disability of a joint or a limb. The repeatability of these instruments among clinicians and over time can be evaluated to confirm their reliability. Comparison to other methods will describe validity. Several outcome measure questionnaires such as the Comprehensive Brief Pain Inventory, the Canine Orthopedic Index, the Helsinki Chronic Pain Index, and the Liverpool Osteoarthritis in Dogs questionnaires have sufficient validation for use in many clinical situations.

Musculoskeletal Problems in Sporting Dogs, *53*

Matthew W. Brunke, David Levine, Denis J. Marcellin-Little, Kirsten E. Oliver, Jennifer A. Barnhard, and Ashley A. Tringali

Many dogs compete in sports. The most popular sports include conformation, agility, disc dogs, dock diving, flyball, herding, tracking, rally obedience, canine freestyle, and racing short and long distances (eg, lure coursing, dog sledding). The purpose of this article is to review common dog sports, discuss the physical requirements of these sports, review common

SECTION II: EMERGENCY AND CRITICAL CARE

Extracorporeal Therapies in the Emergency Room and Intensive Care Unit, *61*
Leonel Londoño

The use of extracorporeal blood purification has become an important therapeutic tool in tertiary hospitals due to the spectrum of clinical applications that go beyond the need for renal replacement therapy. In the emergency room, extracorporeal therapies can be used for the treatment of acute intoxications to remove the circulating toxins before they cause clinical signs or organ failure. In the intensive care unit, extracorporeal therapies are being used more frequently to manage immune-mediated disease that fails conventional treatment with immunosuppressive therapy.

The Use of Biomarkers to Track and Treat Critical Illness, *71*
Robert Goggs

Biomarkers are objectively measurable parameters that provide clinicians with timely information to guide diagnosis and patient management beyond that which can be obtained from routinely available data. The literature contains thousands of articles on biomarkers in veterinary medicine. Specifically reviewed are the acute kidney injury markers neutrophil gelatinase-associated lipocalin, cystatin, clusterin, and kidney-injury molecule-1; the cardiac troponins and natriuretic peptides as biomarkers of heart disease; the acute phase protein C-reactive protein; procalcitonin; inflammatory cytokines; the markers of neutrophil extracellular trap formation cell-free DNA and nucleosomes; and markers of injury to the endothelium and endothelial glycocalyx including hyaluronan.

Controversies of and Indications for Use of Glucocorticoids in the Intensive Care Unit and the Emergency Room, 89

Yekaterina Buriko and Ashlei Tinsley

Corticosteroids are ubiquitous endogenous compounds that are essential for most body functions. Exogenous steroids are routinely used for a plethora of conditions associated with substantial and sometimes detrimental inflammation or immune-mediated tissue destruction. In this article, we will review the relevant physiology of steroids, pharmacology of the common exogenously administered steroids, common side effects of glucocorticoid administration, as well as some of the more controversial and less researched indications for steroid therapy in veterinary medicine. Relevant human literature as well as available information on veterinary species will be presented to augment the discussion.

The Microbiome in Critical Illness, 101

Melanie Werner and Alessio Vigani

Evidence suggests that the intestinal microbiome may play an important role in the pathogenesis and progression of acute critical illness in humans and other mammals, although evidence in small animal medicine is sparse. Moreover, the intestinal microbiota plays many important metabolic roles (production of short-chain fatty acids, trimethylamine-N-oxide, and normal bile acid metabolism) and is crucial for immunity as well as defense against enteropathogens. The use of probiotics and fecal microbiota transplantation as instruments to modulate the intestinal microbiota seems to be safe and effective in studies on critically ill dogs with acute gastrointestinal diseases.

SECTION III: VETERINARIAN WELLNESS

Early Career Veterinary Well-being and Solutions to Help Young Veterinarians Thrive, 113

Addie R. Reinhard

The early career is one of the most challenging times for the veterinary professional. Research shows that burnout, stress, and psychological distress seem to be highest among younger veterinarians. This article will focus on defining this issue as well as providing actionable solutions to support young veterinarians in the transition to practice. A multifaceted approach using individual, organizational, workplace, and veterinary school strategies will be proposed. By providing a network of support, we can make an impact on improving overall mental health and well-being of early-career professionals.

Veterinarians' Personality, Job Satisfaction, and Wellbeing, 123

John Volk, Ulrich Schimmack, and Elizabeth Strand

Aside from obvious physical characteristics, people also differ in their psychological aspects. Personality psychology is the science of these personality traits and their correlates and consequences for individuals' feelings, behaviors, and life outcomes. The dominant view of personality rejects the notion of personality types. Rather, personality differences are described in terms of differences along quantitative dimensions. While there are many personality dimensions, they are related to 5 broad dimensions called the Big Five. The Big Five are named Neuroticism, Extraversion, Openness, Agreeableness, and Conscientiousness. Meta-analysis suggests that Neuroticism is the strongest negative predictor of wellbeing, However, relatively little research has examined how neuroticism influences job satisfaction and wellbeing, and it is not clear whether results from other populations generalize to veterinarians. We report results from 2 national representative studies of veterinarians' personality, job satisfaction, and well-being. We found that neuroticism is the only Big Five factor with notable effects on job satisfaction that contributes to veterinarians' wellbeing. The second study showed that neuroticism had different relationships with various job aspects. The strongest relationship was found for work-life balance. Our discussion focuses on strategies that might help veterinarians high in neuroticism to improve their work-life balance and to increase their wellbeing.

Practice Culture: The Golden Ticket to Increasing Well-Being in Practice, 133

Josh Vaisman

Recent research suggests that many veterinarians and veterinary support staff struggle with burnout, psychological distress, and low well-being. Workplace climate can impact veterinary professionals' experience of burnout, psychological distress, and well-being.Veterinary leaders can develop and employ specific behaviors to encourage and enable the four workplace climate qualities that appear to support veterinary well-being.

SECTION IV: ACCESS TO VETERINARY CARE

Access to Veterinary Care–A National Family Crisis and Case for One Health, *145*
Michael J. Blackwell and Augusta O'Reilly

Access to veterinary care influences the well-being of all community members, both human and nonhuman. Thus, societal harm is inflicted when human-related barriers impede access to veterinary care. When communities network to maximize the utilization of resources and activities and welcome partnerships with professions such as veterinary social work, barriers to care can be reduced. It is important for veterinarians to advocate for a One Health system and consider participation as a provider of services to families with limited means. Veterinarians who treat nonhuman family members are providers of family health care, the new paradigm.

Competency and Controversies Along the Spectrum of Care, *159*
Gary Block

Declining access to veterinary care is a critical issue facing the veterinary profession. Understanding the concept of standard of care and utilizing the spectrum of care as a way to address this issue will benefit pet owners and their pets. Evidence-based medicine should play a larger role in creating as wide a spectrum as possible and will create greater value for the resources expended. Until broadly accepted clinical practice guidelines are created, white papers, consensus statements, and specialty organization disease monographs should be better utilized by practitioners. Financial limitations will continue to play an important role in limiting access to veterinary care.

Preparing Veterinarians to Practice Across the Spectrum of Care: An Integrated Educational Approach, 171

Sheena M. Warman, Elizabeth Armitage-Chan, Heidi Banse, Deep K. Khosa, Julie A. Noyes, and Emma K. Read

All veterinarians need to practice across a spectrum of care (SoC), and it is essential that our veterinary students are trained to provide care options that consider factors relating to each patient, client, veterinarian, and practice. This article discusses the role of different clinical settings in workplace-based training and highlights the importance of a collaborative approach to optimize students' preparedness for practice. The authors then use a "bricks and mortar" analogy to describe the emerging pedagogy around SoC.

Advances in Small Animal Care 4 (2023) xv–xvi

ADVANCES IN SMALL ANIMAL CARE

Preface

Year Four of This Journal: More Insights into What the Future Portends for Veterinarians in Small Animal Practice

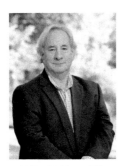

Philip H. Kass, BS,
DVM, MPVM, MS, PhD
Editor

With each ensuing year and subsequent issue of this journal, it is hoped that the boundaries of clinical small animal veterinary medicine continue to expand to encompass new developments on the cusp of becoming accessible to tertiary care facilities, if not eventually mainstream practices. This issue continues to push this frontier forward, while recognizing that veterinary medicine cannot exist without veterinarians, and hence, their own well-being is not being overlooked and is also an important focus here.

My aspiration for this journal is to bring the future closer to reality and expose veterinarians to not only what soon lies ahead but also what is present in the here and now, and but for lack of awareness could encroach as a new part of our standards of practice. This can only be successfully done through the creative scholarship of a distinguished roster of authors, both national and international. The time between receipt of the initial drafts of these manuscripts and the publication date is less than 1 year, guaranteeing that this new knowledge is truly cutting-edge veterinary medicine. Whether they

are opinion pieces or review articles, all are extensively documented to ensure that they adhere to the highest scientific standards.

The first part of this issue, comprising the first four articles, addresses physical health, well-being, and novel treatments. The article, "Gait Changes Resulting from Orthopedic and Neurologic Problems in Companion Animals: A Review," by Carr and colleagues addresses a problem routinely seen in companion animal practice: a limping pet, or more formally, a pet with a gait abnormality, the causes of which can be approximately divided into musculoskeletal joint problems and neurologic conditions. "Patient-centered Physical Rehabilitation in Companion Animals" by Pechette Markley and colleagues explores the underutilized realm of physical therapy focused on patient's needs, while working in partnership with owners. The article, "Clinical Instruments for the Evaluation of Orthopedic Problems in Dogs and Human Patients: A Review," by Hyytiäinen and colleagues addresses the utilization of diagnostic instruments and surveys to evaluate orthopedic problems in dogs. "Musculoskeletal Problems in

https://doi.org/10.1016/j.yasa.2023.07.002
2666-450X/23/ © 2023 Published by Elsevier Inc.

Sporting Dogs" by Brunke and colleagues speaks to musculoskeletal injuries that are particularly diagnosed in sporting breeds of dogs.

The second part of this issue addresses novel approaches to diagnosing and treating certain intractable and vexing clinical diseases or syndromes. "Extracorporeal Therapies in the Emergency Room and Intensive Care Unit" by Londoño provides a comprehensive overview of the different types of extracorporeal therapies used in tertiary care hospitals, including hemodialysis, hemoperfusion, and therapeutic plasma exchange. The uses of these procedures are many, although have not yet seen extensive adoption, including removal of toxins, management of septic patients, and treatment of immune-mediated diseases. "The Use of Biomarkers to Track and Treat Critical Illness" by Goggs reviews newer biomarkers that have clinical value, focusing on those of particular importance to emergency and critical care practice. The article, "Controversies of and Indications for Use of Glucocorticoids in the Intensive Care Unit and Emergency Room," by Buriko and Tinsley provides a valuable overview of a topic that continues to be controversial: the administration of glucocorticoids in an emergency setting and for critically ill patients. It underscores the need for additional evidence to validate this particular immediate need use in small animals. "The Microbiome in Critical Illness" by Werner and Vigani introduces another rapidly emerging area: the importance of the intestinal microbiome both in maintaining health and immunity and in how it can be affected in the presence of illness.

The next three articles depart from the clinical realm and turn to focus on veterinarians themselves. No one doubts the emotional strain, psychological issues, and psychosomatic symptoms that veterinarians experience, with their genesis often early on in their veterinary medical education, not to mention the looming financial strains confronted after graduating. "Early Career Veterinary Well-Being and Solutions to Help Young Veterinarians Thrive" by Reinhard takes a holistic look at the stresses that new veterinarians experience and proposes interventions that can make their careers more rewarding and successful. The article, "Veterinarians' Personality, Job Satisfaction, and Well-Being," by Volk and colleagues is also focused on veterinarians as individuals that exist in a highly charged profession and proposes strategies that might help veterinarians high in neuroticism (a disposition to have negative thoughts and experiences) improve their work-life balance and increase their well-being. "Practice Culture: The Golden Ticket to Increasing Well-Being in Practice" by Vaisman emphasizes that the culture modeled and practiced in a hospital setting with a team of complementary employees has a profound influence on their (including veterinarians) satisfaction and can establish a positive climate that promotes psychological safety and success.

The final three articles address an emerging area of societal importance: one that concerns promoting far wider access to veterinary care, especially to pet owners from economically disadvantaged populations. "Access to Veterinary Care: A National Family Crisis and Case for One Health" by Blackwell and colleagues posits that lack of access can lead to a public health threat and proposes a one-health paradigm that envisions owners and pets as a cohesive unit of family members. The lack of access to care is envisioned as a challenge that must be confronted as a moral imperative, best addressed by a One Health health care model. "Competency and Controversies Along the Spectrum of Care" by Block introduces the principle of "spectrum of care" as a continuum of diagnostic and treatment options to enhance health care access and stands in contrast to "standard of care" and "gold-standard care" that remains out of the reach of many pet owners. The following article, "Preparing Veterinarians to Practice Across the Spectrum of Care: An Integrated Educational Approach," by Warman and colleagues builds upon this "spectrum-of-care" paradigm by advocating for its instruction in educational institutions and promoting it in the workplace. In particular, it advocates for its support of faculty from all clinical specialties as "essential to support the transformational change required to broaden the spectrum of care where graduates are confident and competent to practice."

As this journal continues to flourish, it is imperative that we provide the most up-to-date and accessible resources for practitioners that bridge the gap between peer-reviewed scientific journals, publishing the discovery of new knowledge, and the textbooks that can be years in the making. I welcome your feedback about the contents of this journal and invite you to propose topic areas for forthcoming issues on emerging and new prospects that have the potential to revolutionize veterinary medicine.

Philip H. Kass, BS, DVM, MPVM, MS, PhD
Diplomate, American College of
Veterinary Preventive Medicine
Epidemiology Subspecialty
University of California, Davis
One Shields Avenue
Davis, CA 95616, USA

E-mail address: phkass@ucdavis.edu

SECTION I: REHABILITATION

Advances in Small Animal Care 4 (2023) 1–20

ADVANCES IN SMALL ANIMAL CARE

Gait Changes Resulting from Orthopedic and Neurologic Problems in Companion Animals

A Review

Brittany Jean Carr, DVM, DACVSMR, CCRT[a],*, David Levine, PT, PhD, MPH, DPT, CCRP, FAPTA[b], Denis J. Marcellin-Little, DEDV, DACVS, DACVSMR[c]

[a]The Veterinary Sports Medicine and Rehabilitation Center, 4104 Liberty Highway, Anderson, SC 29621, USA; [b]Department of Physical Therapy, University of Tennessee at Chattanooga, 615 McCallie Avenue, Chattanooga, TN 37403, USA; [c]Veterinary Orthopedic Research Laboratory, School of Veterinary Medicine, University of California, 1285 Veterinary Medicine DR, VM3A rm 4206, Davis, CA 95616, USA

KEYWORDS
- Gait • Lameness • Weight distribution • Gait analysis • Force plate • Pressure-sensitive walkway
- Kinematic gait analysis • Ground reaction force

KEY POINTS
- Gait analysis is a tool used to collect objective information in a research setting and when managing clinical patients to assess limb use and lameness in dogs and cats.
- Dogs and cats with orthopedic problems most often shift weight away from affected limbs. Dogs and cats with neurologic problems may develop an unsteady gait or decreased mobility.
- Gait changes resulting from orthopedic and neurologic problems can be monitored over time to assess the progression of disease and/or response to therapy.
- Objective gait analysis measurements most commonly reflect the use of the whole limb but may not always represent joint-specific dysfunction or overall patient function.

GENERAL FEATURES OF GAIT

Walk

The walk is the slowest gait and the only gait with a phase where three feet can contact the ground simultaneously, in contrast with faster gaits, where no more than two feet contact the ground simultaneously. In the walk, there are alternately two feet or three feet on the ground. The order of footfall is as follows: left rear foot (LR), left fore foot (LF), right rear foot (RR), right fore foot (RF), repeat. A hind limb always makes the first move, followed by the forelimb on the same side. The rear foot is placed down on the ground just ahead of where the ipsilateral front foot (which has now been lifted and moved forward) had been located.

Trot

In the trot, contralateral forelimb and hind limbs (eg, RF and LR, followed by LF and RR) move diagonally forward and land on the ground at the same time. In most dog breeds, there is a characteristic suspension period after each pair of diagonal legs lifts off and before the other pair contacts the ground [1]. When trotting, the foot of the hind limb that is moving forward steps into the spot where the ipsilateral front

---

*Corresponding author, *E-mail address:* Dr.brittcarrbenson@gmail.com

https://doi.org/10.1016/j.yasa.2023.05.001
2666-450X/23/

foot left the ground a moment before. When viewing a trotting patient from the side, the front foot should be seen lifting just before the rear foot lands.

The trot is an efficient, ground-covering gait. For maximal efficacy, the patient should use all muscular energy to drive the body forward and its center of mass should not shift from side to side [1]. The trot is the gait that is often used to detect lameness as it is the only gait for which each limb is not assisted by simultaneous weight bearing by its contralateral limb, since it is an alternating diagonal gait. Thus, when a patient is experiencing pain or functional impairment in one limb, it is often revealed by a head nod (also named head bob) most obvious when a forelimb lameness is present or asymmetrical motion of the pelvis (hind limb lameness). In addition, the trot is symmetrical and slow enough for the trained human eye to detect aberrations in stride length and foot placement.

Pace

For the pace, ipsilateral forelimbs and hind limbs move forward together, and simultaneously contact the ground. Similar to the trot, there is a suspension period, which occurs before the contralateral forelimb and hind limbs strike the ground. The order of footfall is LR and LF, followed by a short period of suspension, then RR and RF. From an energy expenditure viewpoint, the pace is an inefficient gait in that the center of gravity shifts from side to side, requiring the patient to expend energy centering the body rather than driving forward. Further, it is challenging to change speed and turn effectively when pacing. Thus, the pace has been considered to be a gait potentially used to cope with orthopedic problems. Dogs that routinely pace have either been inadvertently trained to gait this way by consistently walking on leash at speeds that are between their ideal walk and trot speeds or they have a physical problem that prevents them from feeling comfortable at a trot [1].

Canter

The canter is a three-beat gait and somewhat complex in that there are two different styles of canter, the transverse and the rotary canter. The order of footfall for the transverse canter is as follows: RR, LR and RF together (the forelimb actually strikes the ground slightly later than the hind limb), then LF. When cantering or galloping, the second of either the forelimbs or hind limbs to contact the ground is referred to as the front or rear lead leg, respectively, because the second leg contacts the ground in front of the first leg to strike the ground. In the case of the transverse canter, the

patient uses the same lead leg for both the forelimbs and hind limbs.

The order of footfall for the rotary canter is: RR, LR and LF, then RF. Note that while, on the second step, the forelimbs and hind limbs are considered to strike the ground together, the forelimb actually strikes the ground just after the hind limb. In the rotary canter, the patient uses opposite leads on the hind limb (in this example, the left lead) and the forelimb (in this example, the right lead).

Dogs and cats preferentially use the rotary canter rather than the transverse canter. The rotary canter gives the patient a rolling appearance, particularly when the patient is viewed from the rear, as the two ipsilateral legs abduct as they move cranially together. This motion should not be mistaken for a lameness. The rotary canter provides dogs and cats with a distinct advantage when turning. When turning the patient uses the forelimb that on the side to which the patient is turning as the lead leg. By using the front lead leg that is on the side to which the patient is turning, the patient is able to abduct that forelimb and pull itself in the direction of the turn. Because there is a point at which both hind limbs are on the ground, when using the rotary canter, the patient is also able to effectively push itself with both hind limbs in the direction of the turn.

Gallop

At the gallop, there are two suspension periods, a short one after the forelimbs leave the ground and a longer one after the hind limbs leave the ground. Once the forelimbs have left the ground, the patient flexes the entire spine to bring the hind limbs forward under its body. The two hind limbs strike the ground with one foot slightly before the other. The patient then pushes off with the rear limbs and extends the rear limbs and spine while reaching forward with the two forelimbs. There is a suspension period as the patient is driven through the air with its body in full extension, then the forelimbs contact the ground, one slightly ahead of the other. The patient then pulls the forelimbs under the body and pushes off from the ground with the hind limbs, experiencing the second suspension period as it flexes the spine and brings the hind limbs forward to initiate the next stride. As in the canter, dogs and cats most often use different lead legs on the forelimb and hind limbs when galloping. The pattern of footfall for the rotary gallop using the RF leg as lead would be RR and LR, then LF and RF.

Amble

When a dog is walking and begins to speed up, the forelimb moves forward very soon after the hind limb moves forward, and it appears as if ipsilateral limbs are moving forward together. As long as three feet remain on the ground for a brief period of time, this gait is still considered a walk. However, this fast walk is often referred to as an amble. The amble is a normal but not typically preferred. Patients use this gait when they are tired but want to move quickly, to use a different set of muscles from the trot, or when they are not fit enough or have not been trained to trot at a slower speed [1].

GAIT EVALUATION
Visual Observation of Gait
In clinical practice, gait is often visually evaluated first. A flat and even surface is optimal for the visual evaluation of the gait at the walk and trot. While the walk is often the easiest gait to observe abnormalities because it is the slowest gait, a mild lameness may not be detectable. The trot is the optimal gait to use for detecting lameness as it is the only gait in which the forelimbs and hind limbs do not receive assistance from their respective contralateral limbs when bearing weight. One should observe the patient from multiple vantage points, moving away, coming toward, from both sides, and while circling. If the patient is a performance animal, evaluating the patient while performing specific tasks related to their job or sport is also helpful.

A systematic and disciplined approach should always be used to clinically evaluate a patient's gait. Findings should be included in the medical record and may be semi-quantified using a numerical rating scale (Table 1) or visual analog scale.

While visual gait observation is often easily implemented in most clinical settings and helpful in

identifying a lameness, the gold standard for quantifying lameness is the quantification of gait characteristics using objective gait analysis. For example, one recent study compared the visual observation of gait to force plate analysis in 17 normal, sound Labrador Retrievers and 131 Labrador Retrievers that were evaluated 6 months after surgery done to manage unilateral cranial cruciate ligament injury [2]. The observer only identified 11% of the 131 dogs as being abnormal, whereas force plate analysis indicated that 75% of the 131 dogs failed to achieve ground reaction forces (GRF) consistent with sound Labrador retrievers. No statistical agreement between the visual observation of gait and force plate analysis was present when patients with severe lameness were excluded from the analyses. Despite that, the visual observation of gait remains a practical and important tool used in clinical practice.

Kinetic Gait Analysis
Kinetic gait analysis measures the GRF that are the result of a step. The most widely used method for kinetic gait analysis is force plate analysis, in which metal plates are mounted within a floor or walkway to measure GRF (Table 2). The forces are measured in 3 dimensions: vertical, craniocaudal (acceleration and breaking), and mediolateral.

These forces are presented graphically as force–time curves (Fig. 1). Peak forces are the maximum forces generated during a step. Impulses are the area under the force–time curve. Peak vertical force (PvF) is the single largest force during the stance phase Vertical impulse (VI) can be derived by calculating the area under the vertical force curve over time. Both PvF and VI are used to evaluate limb use. In general, a dog with lameness has a lower PvF and VI in that limb [5–7]. Braking force, braking impulse, propulsive force, propulsive impulse, and mediolateral force are also able to be calculated and can be helpful in evaluating mechanisms of locomotion (see Table 2) [6].

Force plate measurements have been the most widely used and validated quantitative gait application in veterinary medicine to date [5]. Thus, force plate analysis is viewed as the "gold standard" for the quantification of gait characteristics by objective gait analysis.

However, as with any form of gait analysis, there are disadvantages to force plate gait analysis, which include the inability to measure stride and step length, the need for consistent patient velocity and multiple trials, the need for space for a long, dedicated walkway, the cost and complicity of software and equipment, and difficulty in setting up, breaking down, and moving

TABLE 1
Numerical Rating Scale for the Visual Assessment of any Specific Gait Pattern

Lameness Grade	Description
Grade 0	Clinically sound
Grade 1	Barely detectable lameness
Grade 2	Mild lameness
Grade 3	Moderate lameness
Grade 4	Weight bearing when standing or walking, but non-weight bearing when trotting
Grade 5	Non-weight-bearing lameness

Data from Refs. [3,4].

TABLE 2
Types of Ground Reaction Forces

Ground Reaction Force	Definition
Peak Vertical Force (PvF)	The maximum force exerted perpendicular to the surface during stance phase and represents only a single data point on the force–time curve
Vertical Impulse (VI)	Derived by calculating the area under the vertical force curve using time
Rising slope	Slope of the line where force is 0 at the start of stance phase to the maximum force
Falling slope	Slope of a line from the maximal force to the end of stance time where force is 0
Braking Force	The force that causes the object to slow down
Braking Impulse	Corresponds to the deceleration period of the stance phase and is calculated as the area under the force-time curve
Propulsive Force	Force imparted causing object to increase velocity
Propulsive Impulse	Corresponds to the acceleration phase of the stance phase and is calculated as the area under the force-time curve
Mediolateral force	The force exerted horizontally to the surface during stance phase

equipment. The analysis of force place findings is challenging when dogs are affected in both forelimbs or both hind limbs [8]. Also, while force plate analysis provide information on the use of each limb, it does not provide information on a function of a specific joint. When only one joint is abnormal in a limb, limb disuse detected using force plate analysis is attributed to that abnormal joint. However, when multiple joints are abnormal in a limb, it is generally not possible to know the impact of each abnormality on limb use. It is also unclear how force plate changes translate to functional changes in dogs with cats with chronic pain. In one study, there was a low correlation between force place measurements and owner-reported

disability [9]. These disadvantages make force plate gait analysis impractical and/or impossible for many clinical settings.

Kinematic Gait Analysis

Kinematic gait analysis quantifies the positions, velocities, acceleration/deceleration, and angles of various anatomic structures in space. It is most often used to measure joint angles throughout gait (Fig. 2). Most kinematic gait analysis systems use colored, retroreflective, or light-emitting diode (LED) markers that identify specific anatomic landmarks. When the dog is in gait, the movement of the markers is tracked by a series of cameras. The locations of the markers over time are then used to create a 2-D or 3-D model of the dog's gait with calculations of bone and joint excursions (Table 3). Some kinematic analysis systems are markerless. Data analysis can be automated or may rely on the manual processing of video images [10,11].

While a large amount of information can be gathered from kinematic analysis, one major limitation is the variation of structures between breeds, as well as within breeds [5]. Additional limitations include the potential for skin movement and accuracy and repeatability of marker placement. Also, 3-D kinematic analysis system are costly and complex and gait analysis is often technically challenging. As a consequence, the use of 3-D kinematic analysis is clinical practice is limited.

Temporospatial Gait Analysis with Pressure-Sensing Walkways

Temporospatial parameters refer to measurements of time (temporal) and distance (spatial). The use of pressure-sensing walkways to analyze normal and abnormal gait in dogs and cats has been validated [12–24]. Temporospatial gait analysis uses a pressure-sensing mat or walkway and computer software to calculate velocity, stance time, swing time, stride length, step length, and total pressure index (Fig. 3, Table 4).

Forces exerted to change speed, change direction, or maintain balance can interfere and complicate the interpretation of measurements [13,25]. The side the handler is on can influence the results of gait analysis, particularly when evaluating the forelimbs; thus, it is recommended to perform multiple passes with the handler switching sides between passes [14]. Typically, patients are kept on a loose leash with their heads oriented forward in the direction of travel while moving at a constant velocity down the center of the mat. As with any other gait analysis system, there are advantages and disadvantages to using a pressure-sensing walkway (Table 5). However, given their practicality and ease of

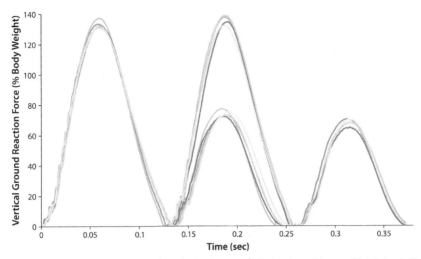

FIG. 1 Force-time curves of five passes (trials) of a 7-year-old Labrador retriever with bilateral elbow dysplasia trotting on two force plates. Each pass is represented with a different color. The peak vertical ground reaction forces are approximately 1.35 times body weight for each forelimb and 0.70 times body weight for each pelvic limb. The area under each curve represents the vertical impulse.

use relative to force plates and kinematic analysis, pressure-sensing walkway systems are becoming more commonly used in clinical practice.

Weight Distribution Analysis

Weight distribution analyzers measure the distribution of body weight on each limb during stance. Dogs bear approximately 60% of their weight on their forelimbs and 40% of their weight on their hind limbs [26]. Devices have become commercially available for small animal use and have been validated to detect subtle changes in weight bearing and monitor change during rehabilitation therapy programs for various orthopedic and neurologic conditions [27–32]. The advantage of this type of analyzer when compared to other forms of gait analysis includes the need for less space and time, lower cost, ease of use, and ease of data acquisition. Disadvantages include the inability to save individual measurement data and the potential for results to be influenced by positioning of the handler, proximity of the closest wall, positioning within an enclosed space, and the effect of local environmental factors during testing (Phelps 2007). However, recent studies have shown in spite of these challenges, when used appropriately, these systems allow for the repeatable measurement of body weight and weight distribution in dogs [27–31].

Instrumented Treadmills

Instrumented treadmills have become available for use in small animal medicine as an alternative to other traditional forms of gait analysis as they require less space, are typically less expensive, and rely on user-friendly software. Instrumented treadmills use either force or pressure sensors and are able to rapidly capture many steady-state gait cycles at a consistent speed [33–35]. There has been concern that gait patterns on a treadmill and overground differ, but several studies did not detect significant differences between overground gait patterns and those assessed on an instrumented treadmill [33,36,37]. Recent studies have found that instrumented treadmills can be used to reliably record data with patient habituation and an appropriate statistical model [33–35,37–43].

GAIT CHANGES SECONDARY TO ORTHOPEDIC AND NEUROLOGIC PROBLEMS

Gait Changes in Response to Joint Disease

Canine hip dysplasia

Dogs with canine hip dysplasia (CHD) can present with a wide range of lameness that can be minimal to quite significant when observed with a trained eye [44]. Objective gait analysis has made it easier to quantify subtle gait changes characteristic to CHD. Kinetic force plate studies have shown that dogs with CHD have reduced vertical peak and vertical impulse measurements as well as decreased hind limb propulsion force [45–47]. However, a recent study found that the severity

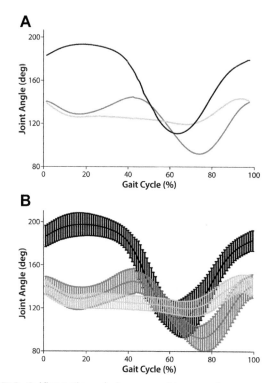

FIG. 2 Kinematic analysis was used to generate a curve showing mean shoulder (light gray), elbow (gray), and carpal (dark gray) joint angles in the sagittal plane during a gait cycle in 10 normal dogs at a walk. Mean joint angles can be shown as simple curves (**A**) or can be shown with the standard error of the mean (**B**), a representation of the variability among dogs.

of hip dysplasia or hip osteoarthritis was not associated with the amount of static or dynamic weight bearing [48]. Fourier analysis has been performed and shown subtle yet significant gait aberrations in the forelimbs of dogs with CHD that are undetected via conventional

TABLE 3 Kinematic Parameters	
Kinematic Parameter	**Definition**
Range of Motion	Calculated from the displacement at a specific joint
Displacement	Distance recorded when a marker changes position
Angular Velocity	Speed at which change in distance occurs

analysis [49]. Several kinematic studies have further described the gait characteristics of dogs with CHD [50–52]. Dogs with CHD have been shown to have subtle increases in coxofemoral extension at the end of the stance phase and in flexion of the femorotibial joint throughout the stance and early swing phases of the stride [50]. Dysplastic dogs have also been shown to have a longer stride length, decreased distance between the rear feet, increased lateral pelvic motion, described as swaying gait or pelvic waddle, greater coxofemoral joint adduction, and mediolateral movement of the rear feet [50,51]. Further, coxofemoral joint angular acceleration in dogs with hip dysplasia has been shown to be greater in the middle to end of stance phase, whereas deceleration was greater in the late stance to early swing phase and middle to end of the swing phase when compared to healthy dogs [50,51]. Finally, dogs with CHD have kinematic alterations in their forelimbs, specifically significantly decreased maximum angular velocity of the carpal joint [52]. Kinematic gait aberrations in dogs with CHD are thought to be compensation, because of pain or biomechanical effects attributable to hip dysplasia and degenerative joint diseas [52].

Cranial cruciate ligament injury

Most dogs with CCL injury have a weight-bearing to non-weight bearing lameness that is easily detected and subjectively quantified during visual lameness evaluation [53,54]. Multiple types of objective gait analysis have been used to characterize gait abnormalities found with cranial cruciate ligament (CCL) injury and study patient response to surgical therapy. Dogs with CCL rupture have significantly reduced peak vertical force and vertical impulse and significantly reduced braking and propulsion impulse [2,55–74]. Multiple studies have been done using force plate gait analysis to assess changes in GRF after the surgical management of CCL injury [2,55,56,62–74].

Initial studies were performed in dogs with CCL rupture that were treated with intra- or extra-capsular management techniques [55,56]. Peak vertical force and vertical impulse increased significantly 4 to 6 months after surgery compared to untreated controls. Significant differences between stabilization methods were identified and more normal GRF were observed after extracapsular stabilization than intraarticular stabilization [55,56].

More recent studies have also investigated GRF following osteotomy procedures. Voss and colleagues evaluated GRF in dogs with unilateral CCL rupture who underwent tibial tuberosity advancement (TTA)

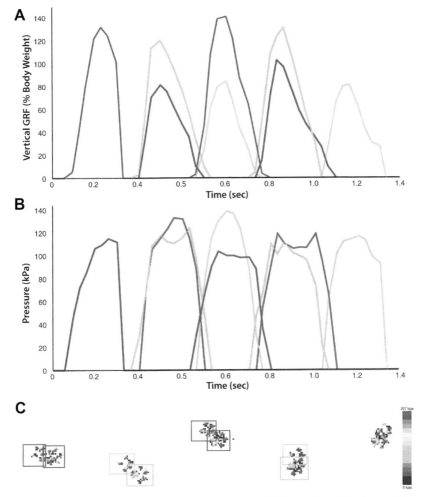

FIG. 3 A pressure sensitive walkway was used to measure vertical ground reaction forces (**A**) and peak pressure (**B**) generated by each limb during a pass across the walkway. The footprints of the pass used to generate these curves and pressure scale are shown (**C**). Each footfall can be selected (colored squares) to analyze forces and peak pressure generated by each limb.

and found that vertical GRF were significantly higher at 4 four to 16 weeks after surgery, but remained significantly lower than those of control dogs [62]. TTA significantly improved limb function in dogs with CCLR; however, it did not result in full return to function 16 weeks after surgery. The authors concluded that a return to a function of approximately 90% of normal can be expected in dogs with CCLR undergoing TTA [62]. Another study investigated the association of radiographic changes and functional outcome after TTA in dogs with CCL rupture and found that GRFs improved after surgery, however, GRFs were not correlated with radiographic OA scores [63]. GRF after the Modified

Maquet Procedure (MMP) was evaluated in 35 dogs with unilateral CCL rupture. in GRF significantly improved in all treated limbs over time [64]. The median increase in GRF was constant from 15 to 90 days, with 54% of patients achieving normal gait symmetry.

One study assessed GRF in dogs with the unilateral transection of the CCL and a tibial plateau leveling osteotomy (TPLO) and found a significant decrease in PvF and VI of the treated hind limb 8 8 weeks after surgery, compared with baseline and 18-week measurements [65]. However, when compared with baseline values, no significant difference was found between

TABLE 4
Measurements Calculated with Temporospatial Gait Analysis

Term	Definition
Stance time	Stance phase of gait cycle and time paw is in contact with ground
Swing time	Swing phase of gait cycle and time paw is in air
Stride length	Distance from one footfall to the next footfall of same limb
Step length	Distance between heel point of one foot to heel point of contralateral foot
Total pressure index	Sum of peak pressure values recorded from each activated sensor by a paw during mat contact; related but not equal to the PvF measured using force plates

the 18-week PvF and VI in dogs that had unilateral transection of the CCL and TPLO. Another recent study evaluated GRF in dogs with unilateral CCLR who had a TPLO. GRF had significantly improved by two2 months

TABLE 5
Advantages and Disadvantages of Temporospatial Gait Analysis Relative to Force Plates

Advantages	Disadvantages
Fewer body size restrictions	Ability limited to the measure total ground reaction forces
Multiple readings from a single pass	Inability to separate vertical, horizontal, and transverse data, as with force plate analysis
Transportability	High cost
Data analysis is user-friendly	
Determination of stride and step length	
Can be used with patients with more unsteady gait, including neurologic patients, patients in ambulation carts	

after TPLO and normalized seven7 months after TPLO [67]. Further, this study demonstrated that forelimb GRF was altered in dogs with CCL rupture as the PvF in the ipsilateral forelimb was significantly higher than in the contralateral forelimb before TPLO. Forelimb PvF asymmetry was identified after the TPLO and was statistically significant 46 to 90 days after surgery. GRF have also been studied in small breed dogs with CCLR who underwent TPLO. Symmetry indices were significantly higher (a sign of clinical improvement) 1 month after surgery compared to preoperative values and at 8 8 weeks symmetry indices had normalized [66].

Superiority of one surgical technique over another has not been clearly established in the literature; however, comparative studies have identified subtle differences in GRF between techniques [68–74]. One study compared the outcome of dogs with unilateral CCL rupture with TPLO versus lateral fabellar suture (LFS) and found that PvF of affected hind limbs at a walk and trot was 5 five to 11% higher for dogs in the TPLO group compared to those in the LFS group during the 12-month-period after surgery [68]. This study failed to identify a significant improvement in the Canine Brief Pain Inventory, a client questionnaire reflecting functional impairment, in goniometry, and in thigh circumference results; however, owner satisfaction 12 months after surgery were significantly different between groups, with 93% and 75% of owners of dogs in the TPLO and LFS groups reporting a satisfaction score of 9 nine or greater on a scale of one1 to 10, respectively [68]. The long-term functional outcome of dogs with unilateral CCL rupture after TPLO or LFS was compared using PvF and VI in another study. Eight weeks after surgery, the TPLO group had more symmetric limb loading than the LFS group at the walk and trot [69]. The SI of TPLO patients did not differ from the control group 6 months to 1 year after surgery. By comparison, SI for the LFS group were less symmetrical than the control group at all time periods. Finally, median time to normal function did not differ at a walk between groups, but was shorter for the TPLO group for VI and PvF. Another study assessed the outcome after the management of CCL rupture with TPLO or capsular fascial imbrication (CFI) in small breed dogs. 91% of limbs treated with TPLO and 29% of limbs treated with the CFI showed absolute values comparable to healthy dogs when evaluated using PvF, VI, and symmetry indices 6 months or more after surgery [70]. TPLO led to a significantly faster recovery and a higher degree of owner satisfaction than CFI. One study compared outcomes of dogs with unilateral CCL rupture managed using TPLO or TTA Rapid and found that, while the SI between healthy and affected limbs for the relative stance time during the gait cycle was significantly higher for the TTA Rapid group than the TPLO group 1 month after surgery, no significant differences in gait parameters between the two groups were detected 6 months after surgery [71]. Krotscheck and colleagues compared the GRF of dogs with unilateral CCL rupture treated with LFS, TTA, and TPLO, to each other and to controls [72]. The mean SI for the TPLO group did not differ from the normal control group 6 to 12 months after surgery and TPLO resulted in operated limb function at a walk and at a trot similar to the control population 6 to 12 months after surgery. Conversely, while walk SI for dogs with TTA patients did not differ significantly from the control group 12 months after surgery, trot SI for TTA and LFS did not return to normal and did not differ between TTA and LFS. One study compared the outcome of the management of CCL rupture after TPLO and MMP [73]. A significant improvement in GRF was reached in all dogs and significant differences among dogs treated with either method were not found at any postoperative reexamination. When compared with the control group, mean values 6 months after surgery were 94% for PvF and 86% for VI for the TPLO group and were 89% for PvF and 80% for VI for the MMP group. The long-term functional outcomes of dogs with CCL rupture treated with an intracapsular stabilization or a tibial osteotomy were compared in another study [74]. At a mean of 2.8 ± 0.9 years after surgery, no significant differences were found between mean GRF and static weight bearing between surgically treated and control dog limbs. However, in surgically treated limbs, approximately 30% of the dogs had decreased static or dynamic weight bearing when the symmetry of weight bearing was evaluated, 40% to 50% of dogs showed limitations of active range of motion in sitting position, and 67% of dogs had weakness in thrust from the ground. The distribution percentage per limb of PvF in dogs treated using the intracapsular technique was significantly lower than in dogs treated with an osteotomy. In summary, regardless of the surgical technique performed, most studies using force plate gait analysis have reported that GRF return to normal within 5 to 7 months after surgical repair of CCL rupture [55,56,59,62–74].

Kinematic gait analysis has also been used to quantify gait alterations in dogs with CCL rupture and is thus thought to be a more sensitive tool to characterize joint-specific dysfunction [53,54,60,61,75–82]. Several studies have quantified changes in joint-specific alterations that result from CCL rupture. The evaluation of lameness at the trot in chronic research models of CCL rupture has shown that the stifle joint remains more flexed throughout the stride, especially in late stance and early swing, when limb propulsion occurs [54,76]. Compared with normal stifle dynamic range of motion, little or no extension of the stifle joint develops in late stance [54,60,76,77]. Evaluation of dynamic angular velocity of the stifle joint has also shown that flexion and extension joint angular velocity is decreased in the stance phase, which is thought to be secondary to pain [54,60,77,83]. Also, the coxofemoral and tarsal joints respond to femorotibial flexion by extending more throughout the stance phase [54,60,77]. Similar kinematic findings and alterations in hind limb joint range of motion have also been documented in dogs that are predisposed to cranial cruciate ligament injury [61].

The kinematics of the stifle joint after CCL transection and in the absence of surgical stabilization has been described in a 2-year study [84]. Peak anterior tibial translation (ATT) and coronal-plane instability increased immediately after CCL loss and did not improve over time. ATT immediately before paw strike and mean stifle adduction throughout stance became increasingly abnormal over time, with the greatest changes occurring 6 to 12 months after CCL transection. The authors concluded that overload failure of secondary restraints such as the medial meniscus, which has been reported to fail in a similar timeframe in CCL-deficient dogs, was the likely cause of these progressive changes. Another recent kinematic study confirmed that CCL rupture causes profound craniocaudal translational and axial rotational instability, which is most pronounced during the stance phase of gait. The authors concluded that surgical stabilization techniques should aim to resolve both craniocaudal subluxation and axial rotational instability [85].

Kinematic gait analysis has also been used to asses and compare outcome following surgical interventions [53,78–82]. In a chronic research model of extracapsular repair of CCLR, kinematic quantifications of lameness improved 6 months after repair but did not return to preinjury levels, suggesting that the kinematic description of lameness is more sensitive to describe joint dysfunction that is not detected by subjective observers or by force plate gait analysis [53].

Early kinematic outcome after the treatment of CCL rupture by TPLO was assessed in one study [78]. Hind limb stance duration significantly increased during the 12-week study period and recovered near-normal values at 12 weeks. However, while the range of hind limb paw velocity significantly increased, it did not reach normal values by 12 weeks after surgery, suggesting persistent alteration in hind limb kinematics 12 weeks after surgery [78]. Another recent study assessed femorotibial kinematics during walking in 16 dogs with unilateral CCL rupture that were managed with TPLO at 6 months following surgery [79]. In the dogs studied, CCL rupture resulted in a mean ($\pm$SD) 10 ± 2.2 mm cranial tibial translation at midstance phase, which was converted to 2.1 ± 4.3 mm caudal tibial translation 6 months after TPLO. However, this study found that five of 16 TPLO-treated stifles had 4.1 ± 0.3 mm of persistent cranial tibial subluxation during mid-to-late stance phase 6 months after surgery and 10 of 16 TPLO-treated stifles had 4.3 ± 0.4 mm of caudal tibial subluxation throughout the gait cycle 6 months after surgery. The authors concluded that postoperative axial rotational and flexion/extension patterns were not different from control, but stifles with caudal tibial subluxation had more external tibial rotation during mid-to-late stance phase than stifles with cranial tibial subluxation.

One study compared GRF of dogs with CCLR who had a capsular-fascial imbrication and dogs with CCL rupture who underwent TPLO [80]. Four months after surgery, the severity of lameness expressed as symmetry index for peak vertical force for the TPLO group (5.8%) did not differ significantly from the capsular-fascial imbrication group (19.1%). However, a significantly increased ability to extend the stifle joint was present in the TPLO group 4 months after surgery. One study assessed kinematic gait analysis of the hind limb in 10 dogs with unilateral CCL rupture after TPLO or cranial tibial wedge osteotomy (CTWO) [81]. Stifle and tibiotarsal joint functions were not affected by TPLO surgery, but stifle and tibiotarsal joint angles were altered, following CTWO surgery when compared with preoperative values. More specifically, the angular velocity patterns of CTWO were characterized by increased stifle joint extension velocity from the middle to end swing phase and decrease in peak velocities toward flexion during the swing phase. This study concluded that dogs that underwent a CTWO procedure were more likely to have significantly hyperextended gait patterns of the swing phase after surgery than the dogs that underwent TPLO.

Another study assessed the kinematics of the hind limb during swimming and walking in 13 healthy dogs and 7 dogs with CCL rupture that underwent LFS [82]. Stifle joint ROM was significantly lower in dogs with CCL rupture than in healthy dogs, regardless of whether dogs were swimming or walking. In healthy dogs, swimming resulted in a significantly greater ROM in the hip joint than did walking, but in dogs with CCL

rupture, ROM of the hip joint did not vary with swimming versus walking. For dogs in both groups, swimming resulted in significantly greater ROM of the stifle and tarsal joints than did walking, primarily because of greater joint flexion. Results suggested that in dogs with CCLR that underwent ECR, swimming resulted in greater ROM of the stifle and tarsal joints than did walking. The authors concluded that, if ROM is a factor in the rate or extent of return to function in dogs with CCLR that undergo LFS, aquatic rehabilitation with swimming could result in a better overall outcome than walking alone.

Canine elbow dysplasia

Elbow dysplasia (ED) is a common developmental disorder of the elbow that often refers to several pathologies that result from abnormal development, including the fragmentation of the medial coronoid process, osteochrondrosis or osteochondritis dissecans of the medial aspect of the humeral condyle, joint incongruity, and ununited anconeal process [86,87]. Many dogs with ED present with a mild to severe forelimb lameness. Progression of osteoarthritis is reportedly inevitable, regardless of whether the patient is conservatively or surgically managed [86]. In a study of English bulldogs, an increase in the severity of radiographic elbow osteoarthritis was associated with a caudal shift of the center of mass when standing and when trotting.

Multiple studies have characterized GRF as well as temporospatial gait changes commonly found in dogs with ED and elbow OA [88–90]. Force plate data have confirmed that dogs with ED and OA have reduced PvF and impulse when compared to normal dogs [88–90]. Temporospatial gait changes include a reduction in total pressure index, stride length, step length, and gait cycle [91].

Kinematic studies have been performed to quantify joint-specific dysfunction in dogs with ED [92,93]. One study evaluated elbow kinematics in normal Labrador Retrievers and in Labrador Retrievers with medial coronoid process disease [92]. Dogs with medial coronoid disease were 9° more extended between 43% and 55% of the gait cycle and 16° more supinated prior, early during, and after foot strike. The antebrachium was 9° more supinated during foot strike and 3° more abducted during early stance. Increased supination and extension during weight bearing may be a response to pain and allow the patient to offload the medial compartment. Another kinematic study assessed radio-ulnar translation in healthy dogs and dogs with ED [93]. Healthy elbow joints exhibited a mean

($\pm$SD) relative radio-ulnar translation of 0.70 ± 0.31 mm, while dysplastic joints showed a translation of 0.50 ± 0.30 mm. No significant difference between groups was detected. The authors concluded that while dynamic radioulnar incongruency (dRUI) is present in every canine elbow joint as part of the physiological kinematic pattern, dysplastic elbow joints do not show increased radio-ulnar translation, therefore, dRUI should not be considered causative for medial coronoid disease.

Objective gait analysis is commonly used to assess ED patient response to therapy. One study evaluated both kinetic and kinematic gait variables in dogs with ED before and after the arthroscopic management of unilateral medial coronoid process disease [90]. While kinetic variables improved after arthroscopy, kinematic variables did not change significantly after 180 days, suggesting that full function was not recovered. Further, osteoarthritis and goniometric measurements in affected joint worsened over the 180-day study period. Functional variables did not correlate with morphologic findings.

Patellar luxation

Patellar luxation is most commonly a result of a congenital or developmental disorder; however, it can be secondary to trauma causing tearing or stretching of the joint capsule and fascia and leading to patellofemoral (PF) instability [94]. On rare occasions, patellar luxation is found as a complication secondary to the treatment of CCL disease or fractures of the femur or tibia [95]. Dogs with subclinical patellar luxation can develop acute severe lameness due to concomitant CCL injury as the result of degenerative joint changes or joint instability [96]. A study found that concurrent CCL rupture was reported in 41% of the stifle joints of dogs with medial patellar luxation. Risk factors included age, increased luxation grade, and advanced degenerative joint disease (DJD) [97].

Clinical signs and presentation of patients with patellar luxation vary, and lameness may be intermittent or continuous and usually is a mild-to-moderate weightbearing lameness, with occasional lifting of the limb. A common observation during gait evaluation is that the patient extends the leg backward to allow the patella to seat back in the groove after luxation. This is often described as a "skip." Patellar luxations are graded from I to IV, based on severity. Patients with grade I patellar luxation are typically asymptomatic, and owners may not report an observable lameness. Dogs with grade II patellar luxation commonly present with an occasional "skip" with a mild-to-moderate

weightbearing lameness. While patients with grade III and IV patellar luxation usually have a persistent lameness and an abnormal posture. Patients with medial patellar luxation may have a crouched posture, hold the hind limb in constant semiflexion with internal rotation, and have a varus deformity of the affected stifle [96,98]. Patients with lateral patellar luxation may appear to hold the stifles closer to each other with the lower limbs abducted.

A kinematic study assessed PF kinematics during daily activities in normal dogs [99]. As the stifle joint flexed, the PF joint also flexed and the patella moved caudally and distally within the femoral trochlea during each activity. Patellar flexion and distal translation during walk and sit were linearly coupled with the femorotibial flexion angle. Offset was evident while trotting, where patellar positions differed significantly between early and late swing phase. Patellar flexion ranged from 6° to 51° while trotting. The largest flexion angle (92°) occurred when sitting. In that study, the patella was found to contact the entire proximodistal length of the femoral trochlea during daily activities. PF kinematics in dogs with CCL rupture have been analyzed during walking [100]. Craniocaudal PF translation was similar between CCL-deficient and control stifles throughout the gait cycle. The patella was more distal and positioned in greater flexion throughout the gait cycle in CCL-deficient stifles when compared to the control stifle at equivalent time points. There was no significant difference in PF position between CCL-deficient and control stifles at equivalent femorotibial flexion angles; however, common femorotibial flexion angles were only found over a small range during the swing phase of gait. This study concluded that CCL rupture altered PF kinematics during walking, where the changes were predominately attributable to the femorotibial joint being held in more flexion. This study was restricted to 2D-motion. Thus, the results cannot be applied to abnormal motions that occur mediolaterally, as in the case of patellar luxation.

Limited research is available to asses PF kinematics in patients with patellar luxation. One recent study assessed PF 3-D kinematics in French bulldogs with and without medial patellar luxation (MPL) [101]. From the seven dogs analyzed, three exhibited medial patellar subluxation and one exhibited medial patellar permanent luxation during the gait cycle. MPL occurred mostly around toe-off in both the walk and trot. Patellar position was generally not gait-related at the analyzed timepoints. In dogs with MPL, the patella was placed significantly more distally at touch-down and at mid-swing, and significantly more medial at mid-swing compared to dogs without MPL. To date, kinematic studies have not been performed to assess PF kinematics in patients with lateral patellar luxation.

In summary, orthopedic problems lead to a decrease in vertical forces and impulses. Quantifying such alterations is useful to monitor disease progression and the response to therapy. However, it is important to realize that these changes are only one part of the clinical picture and may not always be fully representative of limb function or correlate with morphologic findings. Kinematic and temporospatial gait attributes may aide in further characterizing patient function. Furthermore, it is equally important to consider the orthopedic disease process prior to selecting which form objective gait analysis to best characterize and monitor the lameness. Not all conditions are well documented in literature; however, in the authors' experience, some conditions, such as supraspinatus tendinopathy or medial shoulder syndrome, may present with a subtle shortening of stride and/or gait cycle rather than a significant reduction in PvF, VI, or TPI, in which case temporospatial or kinematic may better quantitate the lameness. Thus, it is important that the clinician prudently select the form of objective gait analysis and interpret gait alterations within the clinical context of the data.

Gait Changes in Response to Neurologic Disease
Cervical spondylomyelopathy
Kinetic and kinematic gait alterations associated with cervical spondylomyelopathy (CSM) in dogs have been reported [102–104]. Peak mediolateral force (PMLF), VI, and peak propulsive force (PPF) have been found to be significantly lower in CSM-affected dogs compared with normal dogs [102]. Also, significantly more variability in PvF in CSM-affected dogs has been found, with the largest difference in the CV of PvF in the forelimbs of CSM-affected dogs compared to forelimbs of normal dogs. Kinematically, the minimum and maximum distances between forelimbs increases and the forelimb stride has a shorter duration in CSM-affected dogs. For the hind limbs, a significant reduction in stifle flexion and extension as well as the number of strides were found in CSM affected dogs, compared to normal dogs [103]. Kinetic and kinematic follow-up gait analysis in Doberman Pinschers with CSM treated medically and surgically has also been reported. Kinematic analysis showed that there was a reduction in truncal sway and an increase in stifle flexion after medical or surgical treatment. Force plate analysis also showed improvement in PvF. However,

there was no correlation with either method of gait analysis and clinical recovery.

Spinal cord injury
With spinal cord injury, dogs can present with great variation in their gait and ambulatory status depending on the location and degree of injury. With more mild injury dogs often are still ambulatory but have weakness in the affected limbs while dogs with more severe injury may be non-ambulatory or paralyzed. A recent study evaluated the center of pressure of dogs with chronic thoracolumbar spinal cord injury and found that dogs with spinal cord injury shifted their center of pressure cranially and, when given more support while walking, had a higher stepping score, defined as hind limb steps/forelimb steps x 100 [38].

Though somewhat challenging to perform in dogs with spinal cord injury, objective gait analysis has been successfully used to quantitate gait changes. Kinetic and kinematic gait analysis in the hind limbs of normal and post-hemilaminectomy Dachshunds has been performed [105]. No significant differences were identified between tarsal, stifle, hip, and tail ROM between the control Dachshunds and post hemilaminectomy (PHL) Dachshunds. Although PvF between controls and PHL Dachshunds did not differ significantly, mean PvF varied on average by 14% between the hind limbs of PHL Dachshunds. Also mean horizontal and vertical components of pelvic ROM were 51% and 36% greater in PHL Dachshunds than to controls, respectively.

Temporospatial gait analysis has also been validated for use in ambulatory dogs with spinal cord injury [16]. Velocity, acceleration, height, and weight did not significantly affect any of the coefficients of variation (CV). The model with the highest accuracy (89%) was a multivariate model using the CV calculated by combining feet of each dog of stride length, stride time, and swing time. This study concluded that the combination of CV (combined feet) of stride length, stride time, and swing time was accurate and had great potential as an outcome measure in dogs with SCI.

Degenerative lumbosacral stenosis
Dogs with degenerative lumbosacral stenosis (DLS) often present with pain on hind limb extension, intermittent to progressively worsening lameness induced by exercise, and, in severe cases, with sciatic nerve deficits. Force plate analysis has been used to further quantitate gait alterations in German shepherd dogs with DLS. Studies have shown that dogs with DLS have decreased propulsive forces of the hind limbs

[106,107]. Even if it is unclear whether dorsal decompression fully restores propulsive forces, surgical management partially restores propulsive forces and most owners are satisfied with the outcome after surgery [106,107].

In summary, when neurological disease results in limb weakness or paralysis, objective gait analysis is challenging. Data are difficult to record, process, and interpret. If one is to attempt collecting objective gait data, multiple passes are often required. When foot pattern is irregular, as seen with severe ataxia, temporospatial gait analysis software may find it challenging to correctly identify the foot pattern. Thus, manual correction and processing may be required. While this can take additional time and effort, quantifying gait characteristics can be helpful in monitoring disease progression and response to therapy.

Gait Changes in Response to Amputation

Multiple studies have documented stance and gait alterations in canine amputees [28,108–112]. At a stance, in dogs with a previous forelimb amputation and also in dogs with a previous hind limb amputation, the largest mean increase in weight bearing is in the contralateral forelimb [28,109]. While walking, GRF, impulses, stride times, and stance times have been shown to be significantly different in patients with a previous amputation when compared to quadruped dogs with the greatest amount of change in dogs who had a previous forelimb amputation [108,109]. One study in dogs where a hind limb amputation was artificially recreated found that the observed changes in the craniocaudal forces and the vertical impulse ratio between the fore- and hind limbs suggest that a nose-up pitching moment occurs during the affected limb pair's functional step and to regain pitch balance for a given stride cycle, a nose-down pitching moment is exerted when the intact limb pair supports the body [109]. These kinetic changes were attributed to a compensatory mechanism in which the unaffected diagonal limb pair is involved. The authors concluded that, in canine hind limb amputees, the intact pair of support limbs should be monitored closely.

Hogy and colleagues quantitated kinematic and kinetic gait characteristics of dogs during trotting after the amputation of a hind limb [110]. Hind limb amputees had increased peak braking forces in the contralateral forelimb and increased propulsive forces and impulses in both the ipsilateral forelimb and remaining hind limb. Compared to control dogs, amputees were also found to have an increase in range of motion at the tarsal joint of the remaining hind limb, increased range of motion in the cervicothoracic and thoracolumbar vertebral

regions, and extension of the lumbosacral vertebral region. Amputees were also found to have increased lateral bending toward the remaining hind limb, which resulted in a laterally deviated gait pattern. Hence, amputees alternated between a laterally deviated gait when the h limb was in propulsion and a regular cranially oriented gait pattern when either forelimb was in propulsion with horizontal rotation around L7.

Kinematic and kinetic gait characteristics of dogs during trotting after the amputation of a forelimb have also been documented [111]. In amputees, weight increased significantly by 14% on the remaining forelimb and by a combined 17% on hind limbs. Compared to values for control dogs, amputees also had significant increases in stance duration and vertical impulse in all limbs, a significant increase in braking GRF in the remaining forelimb and hind limb ipsilateral to the amputated limb, and significant increase in propulsive GRF the ipsilateral hind limb. The remaining carpus and ipsilateral hip and stifle joints had significantly greater flexion during the stance phase. The vertebral column was also found to have significant changes in the range of motion in the cervicothoracic, thoracolumbar, and lumbosacral regions; however, these changes varied based on the vertebral region. The ipsilateral hind limb assumed dual fore- and hind limb roles, because the gait of a forelimb amputee during trotting appeared to be a mixture of various gait patterns.

One study quantitated stance and weight distribution after TPLO in forelimb and hind limb amputee dogs (AmpTPLO) and found that joint angles, hind limb abduction, and pelvic tilt of AmpTPLO and control amputee dogs did not differ statistically [112]. Mean weight bearing of the hind limb of AmpTPLO and control amputee dogs did not differ statistically nor did the position of center of mass and posture of AmpTPLO and control amputee dogs. The authors concluded that weight distribution and posture of amputee dogs is not negatively impacted by TPLO.

Gait Changes in Response to Onychectomy in Cats

Gait characteristics have been recently studied and similarly to dogs, cats exert greater forces on their forelimbs than their hind limbs [21,22,24,113,114]. However, cats have significant differences in force-time waveforms as well as mediolateral GRFs when compared to dogs, which is thought to be explained by the more crouched position of cats as well as differences in paw supination-pronation [113].

Several studies have assessed forelimb GRFs in cats who have undergone onychectomy [115,116]. PvF and VI were significantly lower in the immediate post-operative period following onychectomy. One study compared postoperative analgesic protocols on limb function following onychectomy in cats and found that values for PvF, VI, and the ratio of PvF of 1 operated forelimb/3 other limbs increased over time after surgery. However, for all groups, values were still significantly decreased compared with baseline values 12 days after surgery. The authors concluded that analgesic treatment should be considered for several weeks after onychectomy in cats [116]. Another study assessed GRFs in cats with bilateral onychectomy that had occurred more than 6 months prior [117]. No significant difference was found for PvF or VI between cats that had an onychectomy and controls. The authors concluded that the absence of differences in PvF and VI between the 2 groups of cats suggests that bilateral forelimb onychectomy did not result in altered vertical forces more than 6 months after surgery. Overall and unfortunately, kinematic data assessing limb function and movement after onychectomy in cats are limited.

FACTORS INFLUENCING GAIT ANALYSIS

Gait characteristics can also be influenced by patient variables or external and environmental variables. It is important to be aware of these variables to ensure data quality and repeatability when collecting data.

Velocity

Variation in velocity is commonly implicated as affecting gait characteristics and GRFs [118–122]. Even within the walk or trot, there can be variation in patient velocity. It is recommended that velocity and acceleration are maintained within ±0.3 m/s and ±0.5 m/s², respectively, whether the patient is walking or trotting [5]. Thus, it is important to ensure that the patient is traveling at constant speed when performing multiple passes and when collecting follow-up data. In clinical research environments, this is most often achieved by placing a photocell timing system along the force plates and kinematic walkway.

Acclimation, Handler, and Leash Side

Acclimation of the patient to the setting and equipment is important when acquiring accurate and repeatable gait data [5,37,39,123–126]. When using an instrumented treadmill, habituation has been documented to decrease variation and alterations in gait that may be caused by the treadmill [37,39,123]. Both handler and leash side also have been shown to affect gait variables [18,127]. In one recent study, changing handlers

influenced the TPI of the forelimbs up to 8%, while changing leash side accounted for 12% and 14% of the variation in symmetry indices of TPI and number of sensors activated between forelimbs, respectively, however changing handlers and leash side did not influence hind limb variables [18]. To maximize success, it is important to allow for a patient to acclimate to the setting and equipment and to have the same handler. To avoid alterations due to the leash side, it is recommended to have an equal number of passes with the leash on the left and on the right, whenever possible.

Harnesses

Many dogs wear harnesses either for recreation or as part of their occupational role. Harnesses have been thought to affect gait and have recently been studied [128,129]. The effect of commercially available restrictive and non-restrictive harnesses on temporospatial gait characteristics in ten healthy dogs has been investigated. Restrictive harnesses were defined as harnesses that fit across the shoulder joint, whereas non-restrictive harnesses were defined as harnesses that did not contact the shoulder. Regardless of the harness type, when wearing a harness, a longer forelimb stride length, shorter forelimb step length, shorter forelimb gait cycle, and greater forelimb TPI% were observed. This study also found that regardless of harness type, some dogs were highly reactive to wearing a harness. This study concluded that objective gait analysis should always be performed without wearing a harness. Another study also assessed the effects of restrictive and non-restrictive harnesses on shoulder extension in dogs at walk and trot and found that shoulder extension was 2.6° and 4.4° less in dogs wearing a non-restrictive harness than in dogs wearing a restrictive harness, at walk and trot, respectively [128]. Harnesses limit shoulder extension, but perhaps not in the way that was originally anticipated, since extension is significantly reduced under non-restrictive harnesses compared with restrictive harnesses. Finally, a recent study assessed the effect of two types of Guide Harnesses on GRF and stride length of Guide Dogs for the Blind [129]. Compared to walking with a collar and leash, none of the harnesses when used with a leash had an effect on GRF or stride length. However, both harnesses when used with a handle and under the re-enactment of the lead work, altered vertical impulse. Additionally, stride length was shortened if the Y-harness when a handle was used. The authors concluded that future studies should focus on the type of attachment of the harness and the angle of attachment, that is influenced by the size of the handler.

Ground Surface

The effects of surface type on gait have been assessed [130,131]. While no significant differences in GRF have been found between linoleum and carpet when performing force plate gait analysis, significant differences have been found between various pressure-sensing walkway covers [130,131]. Thus, when using a pressure-sensing walkway, the same cover type should be used during follow-up visits to evaluate clinical outcomes, for the duration of research studies, and at all locations for multi-institutional studies [131].

Dog Breed

Studies have compared the gait of the Labrador Retriever to the Rottweiler, the Greyhound, the Border Collie, and the German Shepherd Dog and found differences in gait characteristics [132–136]. Gait characteristic differences were attributed to variation in conformation, function, and body weight, and these studies have suggested that each breed should have a breed-specific database and reference ranges for gait variables. Differences in gait characteristics among breeds should be contemplated when considering the function of each dog in a performance setting and their susceptibility to orthopedic injury. Additional research is needed determine the extent to which these reference values differ in dogs with various orthopedic disorders.

Obesity

Obesity has also been shown to affect gait characteristics in dogs [137]. Mean stride lengths for forelimbs and hind limbs at both velocities were shorter in obese than in lean dogs. Stance phase range of motion (ROM) was greater in obese dogs than in lean dogs for shoulder, elbow, hip, and tarsal joints at both velocities, whereas swing phase ROM was greater in obese dogs than in lean dogs for elbow and hip joints. Overall, obese dogs exerted greater peak vertical and horizontal GRF than did lean dogs, and body mass and peak vertical GRF were significantly correlated. The authors concluded that greater ROM detected during the stance phase and greater GRF in the gait of obese dogs, compared with lean dogs, may cause greater compressive forces within joints and could influence the development of osteoarthritis.

GAIT ANALYSIS IN A CLINICAL SETTING

Objective gait analysis is a useful tool in both clinical and research settings to assess lameness in canine and feline. A systematic and disciplined approach should always be used to clinically evaluate a patient's gait. It is important to understand normal and abnormal gait as well as how each mode of gait analysis quantifies gait.

Gait characteristics can also be influenced by patient variables or external and environmental variables. It is important to be aware of this to create an optimal environment for gait analysis and ensure data quality and repeatability. A quiet setting that is void of distractions with flat, level footing is preferred. Allowing time for patient acclimation to the setting and equipment will also help optimize data collection.

Finally, it is imperative to realize that changes in gait are only one part of the clinical picture. While objective gait analysis measurements are often reflective of the entire limb, they may not represent joint-specific dysfunction, correlate with morphologic findings, or correlate with patient function. Having a comprehensive understanding of the underlying disease process will also aid the clinician in deciding which form of objective gait analysis is best for quantifying the specific lameness and monitoring disease progress and patient response to interventions.

CLINICS CARE POINTS

- Subjective gait analysis is used when evaluating all dogs with a suspected orthopedic problem.
- Objective gait analysis is most often used to collect data for clinical trials, generally using force plates or pressure-sensitive walkways.
- When conducting objective gait analysis, handler behavior, patient behavior, patient control, speed, and acceleration must be highly consistent.
- Subjective and objective gait evaluations include the comparison of findings from the left and right sides of the body (left/right asymmetry) and the comparison of findings from the patient to normal values (difference from reference gait or reference values).

REFERENCES

[1] Zink MC, Carr BJ. Locomotion and athletic performance. In: Zink MC, Van Dyke JB, editors. Canine sports medicine and rehabilitation. Hoboken (NJ): John Wiley & Sons; 2018. p. 23–42.

[2] Evans R, Horstman C, Conzemius M. Accuracy and optimization of force platform gait analysis in Labradors with cranial cruciate disease evaluated at a walking gait. Vet Surg 2005;34:445–9.

[3] Impellizeri JA, Tetrick MA, Muir P. Effect of weight reduction on clinical signs of lameness in dogs with hip osteoarthritis. J Am Vet Med Assoc 2000;216: 1089–91.

[4] Quinn MM, Keuler NS, Lu Y, et al. Evaluation of agreement between numerical rating scales, visual analogue scoring scales, and force plate gait analysis in dogs. Vet Surg 2007;36:360–7.

[5] Gordon-Evans WJ. Gait analysis. In: Tobias KM, Johnston SA, editors. Veterinary surgery: small animal. St Louis (MO): Elsevier; 2012. p. 1190–6.

[6] Gillette RL, Angle TC. Recent developments in canine locomotor analysis: a review. Vet J 2008;178:165–76.

[7] Nunamaker DM, Blauner PD. Normal and abnormal gait. In: Newton CD, Nunamaker DM, editors. Textbook of small animal Orthopaedics. Philadelphia: JB Lippincott; 1985. p. 1084–5.

[8] Sharkey M. The challenges of assessing osteoarthritis and postoperative pain in dogs. AAPS J 2013;15: 598–607.

[9] Brown DC, Boston RC, Farrar JT. Comparison of force plate gait analysis and owner assessment of pain using the Canine Brief Pain Inventory in dogs with osteoarthritis. J Vet Intern Med 2013;27:22–30.

[10] Corazza S, Mundermann L, Chaudhari AM, et al. A markerless motion capture system to study musculoskeletal biomechanics: visual hull and simulated annealing approach. Ann Biomed Eng 2006;34:1019–29.

[11] Feeney LC, Lin CF, Marcellin-Little DJ, et al. Validation of two-dimensional kinematic analysis of walk and sit-to-stand motions in dogs. Am J Vet Res 2007;68: 277–82.

[12] Light VA, Steiss JE, Montgomery RD, et al. Temporal-spatial gait analysis by use of a portable walkway system in healthy Labrador Retrievers at a walk. Am J Vet Res 2010;71:997–1002.

[13] Besancon MF, Conzemius MG, Derrick TR, et al. Comparison of vertical forces in normal Greyhounds between force platform and pressure walkway measurement systems. Vet Comp Orthop Traumatol 2003;16:153–7.

[14] Lascelles BD, Roe SC, Smith E, et al. Evaluation of a pressure walkway system for measurement of vertical limb forces in clinically normal dogs. Am J Vet Res 2006;67:277–82.

[15] Webster KE, Wittwer JE, Feller JA. Validity of the GAITRite walkway system for the measurement of averaged and individual step parameters of gait. Gait Posture 2005;22:317–21.

[16] Gordon-Evans WJ, Evans RB, Conzemius MG. Accuracy of spatiotemporal variables in gait analysis of neurologic dogs. J Neurotrauma 2009;26:1055–60.

[17] Lequang T, Maitre P, Roger T, et al. Is a pressure walkway system able to highlight a lameness in dog? J Anim Vet Adv 2009;8:1936–44.

[18] Keebaugh AE, Redman-Bentley D, Griffon DJ. Influence of leash side and handlers on pressure mat analysis of gait characteristics in small-breed dogs. J Am Vet Med Assoc 2015;246:1215–21.

[19] Carr BJ, Canapp SO Jr, Zink MC. Quantitative comparison of the walk and trot of Border Collies and Labrador Retrievers, breeds with different performance requirements. PLoS One 2015;10:e0145396.

[20] Fahie MA, Cortez JC, Ledesma M, et al. Pressure mat analysis of walk and trot gait characteristics in 66 normal small, medium, large, and giant breed dogs. Front Vet Sci 2018;5:256.

[21] Lascelles BD, Findley K, Correa M, et al. Kinetic evaluation of normal walking and jumping in cats, using a pressure-sensitive walkway. Vet Rec 2007;160:512–6.

[22] Schnabl-Feichter E, Tichy A, Bockstahler B. Coefficients of variation of ground reaction force measurement in cats. PLoS One 2017;12:e0171946.

[23] Schnabl-Feichter E, Tichy A, Gumpenberger M, et al. Comparison of ground reaction force measurements in a population of Domestic Shorthair and Maine Coon cats. PLoS One 2018;13:e0208085.

[24] Stadig SM, Bergh AK. Gait and jump analysis in healthy cats using a pressure mat system. J Feline Med Surg 2015;17:523–9.

[25] Voss K, Galeandro L, Wiestner T, et al. Relationships of body weight, body size, subject velocity, and vertical ground reaction forces in trotting dogs. Vet Surg 2010; 39:863–9.

[26] Levine D, Marcellin-Little DJ, Millis DL, et al. Effects of partial immersion in water on vertical ground reaction forces and weight distribution in dogs. Am J Vet Res 2010;71:1413–6.

[27] Wilson ML, Roush JK, Renberg WC. Single-day and multiday repeatability of stance analysis results for dogs with hind limb lameness. Am J Vet Res 2019;80: 403–9.

[28] Cole GL, Millis D. The effect of limb amputation on standing weight distribution in the remaining three limbs in dogs. Vet Comp Orthop Traumatol 2017;30: 59–61.

[29] Bosscher G, Tomas A, Roe SC, et al. Repeatability and accuracy testing of a weight distribution platform and comparison to a pressure sensitive walkway to assess static weight distribution. Vet Comp Orthop Traumatol 2017;30:160–4.

[30] Alves JC, Santos A, Jorge P, et al. Characterization of weight-bearing compensation in dogs with bilateral hip osteoarthritis. Top Companion Anim Med 2022; 49:100655.

[31] Clough WT, Canapp SO Jr, Taboada L, et al. Sensitivity and specificity of a weight distribution platform for the detection of objective lameness and orthopaedic disease. Vet Comp Orthop Traumatol 2018;31: 391–5.

[32] Phelps HA, Ramos V, Shires PK, et al. The effect of measurement method on static weight distribution to all legs in dogs using the Quadruped Biofeedback System. Vet Comp Orthop Traumatol 2007;20:108–12.

[33] Brebner NS, Moens NM, Runciman JR. Evaluation of a treadmill with integrated force plates for kinetic gait analysis of sound and lame dogs at a trot. Vet Comp Orthop Traumatol 2006;19:205–12.

[34] Häusler KA, Braun D, Liu NC, et al. Evaluation of the repeatability of kinetic and temporospatial gait variables measured with a pressure-sensitive treadmill for dogs. Am J Vet Res 2020;81:922–9.

[35] Söhnel K, Fischer MS, Häusler K. Treadmill vs. overground trotting - a comparison of two kinetic measurement systems. Res Vet Sci 2022;150:149–55.

[36] Torres BT, Moëns NM, Al-Nadaf S, et al. Comparison of overground and treadmill-based gaits of dogs. Am J Vet Res 2013;74:535–41.

[37] Bockstahler BA, Skalicky M, Peham C, et al. Reliability of ground reaction forces measured on a treadmill system in healthy dogs. Vet J 2007;173:373–8.

[38] Lewis MJ, Williams KD, Langley T, et al. Development of a novel gait analysis tool measuring center of pressure for evaluation of canine chronic thoracolumbar spinal cord injury. J Neurotrauma 2019;36:3018–25.

[39] Fanchon L, Grandjean D. Habituation of healthy dogs to treadmill trotting: repeatability assessment of vertical ground reaction force. Res Vet Sci 2009;87:135–9.

[40] Fanchon L, Valette JP, Sanaa M, et al. The measurement of ground reaction force in dogs trotting on a treadmill: an investigation of habituation. Vet Comp Orthop Traumatol 2006;19:81–6.

[41] Abdelhadi J, Wefstaedt P, Galindo-Zamora V, et al. Load redistribution in walking and trotting Beagles with induced forelimb lameness. Am J Vet Res 2013; 74:34–9.

[42] Assaf ND, Rahal SC, Mesquita LR, et al. Evaluation of parameters obtained from two systems of gait analysis. Aust Vet J 2019;97:414–7.

[43] Drüen S, Böddeker J, Nolte I, et al. Bodenreaktionskrafte der caninen Hintergliedmasse: Gibt es Unterschiede beim Gang auf Laufband und Kraftmessplatte? Berl Munch Tierarztl Wochenschr 2010;123:339–45.

[44] Greene LM, Marcellin-Little DJ, Lascelles BD. Associations among exercise duration, lameness severity, and hip joint range of motion in Labrador Retrievers with hip dysplasia. J Am Vet Med Assoc 2013;242:1528–33.

[45] McLaughlin RM Jr, Miller CW, Taves CL, et al. Force plate analysis of triple pelvic osteotomy for the treatment of canine hip dysplasia. Vet Surg 1991;20:291–7.

[46] Budsberg SC, Chambers JN, Lue SL, et al. Prospective evaluation of ground reaction forces in dogs undergoing unilateral total hip replacement. Am J Vet Res 1996;57:1781–5.

[47] Anderson GI, Hem T, Tanes C. Force plate gait analysis in normal and dysplastic dogs before and after total hip replacement surgery: An experimental study. Vet Surg 1988;17:22–7.

[48] Mölsä SH, Hyytiäinen HK, Morelius KM, et al. Radiographic findings have an association with weight bearing and locomotion in English bulldogs. Acta Vet Scand 2020;62:19.

[49] Katic N, Bockstahler BA, Mueller M, et al. Fourier analysis of vertical ground reaction forces in dogs with unilateral hind limb lameness caused by degenerative disease of the hip joint and in dogs without lameness. Am J Vet Res 2009;70:118–26.

[50] Bennett RL, DeCamp CE, Flo GL, et al. Kinematic gait analysis in dogs with hip dysplasia. Am J Vet Res 1996;57:966–71.

[51] Poy NS, DeCamp CE, Bennett RL, et al. Additional kinematic variables to describe differences in the trot between clinically normal dogs and dogs with hip dysplasia. Am J Vet Res 2000;61:974–8.

[52] Miqueleto NS, Rahal SC, Agostinho FS, et al. Kinematic analysis in healthy and hip-dysplastic German Shepherd dogs. Vet J 2013;195:210–5.

[53] DeCamp CE. Kinetic and kinematic gait analysis and the assessment of lameness in the dog. Vet Clin North Am Small Anim Pract 1997;27:825–40.

[54] DeCamp CE, Riggs CM, Olivier NB, et al. Kinematic evaluation of gait in dogs with cranial cruciate ligament rupture. Am J Vet Res 1996;57:120–6.

[55] Budsberg SC, Verstraete MC, Soutas-Little RW, et al. Force plate analyses before and after stabilization of canine stifles for cruciate injury. Am J Vet Res 1988; 49:1522–4.

[56] Jevens DJ, DeCamp CE, Hauptman J, et al. Use of force-plate analysis of gait to compare two surgical techniques for treatment of cranial cruciate ligament rupture in dogs. Am J Vet Res 1996;57:389–93.

[57] Ferrigno CRA, de Souza ANA, Ferreira MP, et al. Comparative analysis of vertical forces in dogs affected with cranial cruciate ligament disease and tibial plateau angles greater or less than 25 degrees. Vet Comp Orthop Traumatol 2020;33:387–90.

[58] Wustefeld-Janssens BG, Pettitt RA, Cowderoy EC, et al. Peak vertical force and vertical impulse in dogs with cranial cruciate ligament rupture and meniscal injury. Vet Surg 2016;45:60–5.

[59] O'Connor BL, Visco DM, Heck DA, et al. Gait alterations in dogs after transection of the anterior cruciate ligament. Arthritis Rheum 1989;32:1142–7.

[60] Ragetly CA, Griffon DJ, Mostafa AA, et al. Inverse dynamics analysis of the pelvic limbs in Labrador Retrievers with and without cranial cruciate ligament disease. Vet Surg 2010;39:513–22.

[61] Ragetly CA, Griffon DJ, Hsu MK, et al. Kinetic and kinematic analysis of the right hind limb during trotting on a treadmill in Labrador Retrievers presumed predisposed or not predisposed to cranial cruciate ligament disease. Am J Vet Res 2012;73:1171–7.

[62] Voss K, Damur DM, Guerrero T, et al. Force plate gait analysis to assess limb function after tibial tuberosity advancement in dogs with cranial cruciate ligament disease. Vet Comp Orthop Traumatol 2008;21:243–9.

[63] Morgan JP, Voss K, Damur DM, et al. Correlation of radiographic changes after tibial tuberosity advancement in dogs with cranial cruciate-deficient stifles with functional outcome. Vet Surg 2010;39:425–32.

[64] Della Valle G, Caterino C, Aragosa F, et al. Outcome after modified Maquet procedure in dogs with unilateral cranial cruciate ligament rupture: Evaluation of recovery limb function by use of force plate gait analysis. PLoS One 2021;16:e0256011.

[65] Ballagas AJ, Montgomery RD, Henderson RA, et al. Pre- and postoperative force plate analysis of dogs with experimentally transected cranial cruciate ligaments treated using tibial plateau leveling osteotomy. Vet Surg 2004;33:187–90.

[66] Amimoto H, Koreeda T, Ochi Y, et al. Force plate gait analysis and clinical results after tibial plateau levelling osteotomy for cranial cruciate ligament rupture in small breed dogs. Vet Comp Orthop Traumatol 2020;33:183–8.

[67] Amimoto H, Koreeda T, Wada N. Evaluation of recovery of limb function by use of force plate gait analysis after tibial plateau leveling osteotomy for management of dogs with unilateral cranial cruciate ligament rupture. Am J Vet Res 2019;80:461–8.

[68] Gordon-Evans WJ, Griffon DJ, Bubb C, et al. Comparison of lateral fabellar suture and tibial plateau leveling osteotomy techniques for treatment of dogs with cranial cruciate ligament disease. J Am Vet Med Assoc 2013;243:675–80.

[69] Nelson SA, Krotscheck U, Rawlinson J, et al. Long-term functional outcome of tibial plateau leveling osteotomy versus extracapsular repair in a heterogeneous population of dogs. Vet Surg 2013;42:38–50.

[70] Berger B, Knebel J, Steigmeier-Raith S, et al. Long-term outcome after surgical treatment of cranial cruciate ligament rupture in small breed dogs. Comparison of tibial plateau leveling osteotomy and extra-articular stifle stabilization. Tierarztl Prax Ausg K Kleintiere Heimtiere 2015;43:373–80.

[71] Livet V, Baldinger A, Viguier E, et al. Comparison of outcomes associated with tibial plateau levelling osteotomy and a modified technique for tibial tuberosity advancement for the treatment of cranial cruciate ligament disease in dogs: A randomized clinical study. Vet Comp Orthop Traumatol 2019;32:314–23.

[72] Krotscheck U, Nelson SA, Todhunter RJ, et al. Long term functional outcome of tibial tuberosity advancement vs. tibial plateau leveling osteotomy and extracapsular repair in a heterogeneous population of dogs. Vet Surg 2016;45:261–8.

[73] Knebel J, Eberle D, Steigmeier-Raith S, et al. Outcome after tibial plateau levelling osteotomy and modified Maquet procedure in dogs with cranial cruciate ligament rupture. Vet Comp Orthop Traumatol 2020;33:189–97.

[74] Mölsä SH, Hyytiäinen HK, Hielm-Bjorkman AK, et al. Long-term functional outcome after surgical repair of cranial cruciate ligament disease in dogs. BMC Vet Res 2014;10:266.

[75] Korvick DL, Pijanowski GJ, Schaeffer DJ. Three-dimensional kinematics of the intact and cranial cruciate ligament-deficient stifle of dogs. J Biomech 1994;27:77–87.

[76] Vilensky JA, O'Connor BL, Brandt KD, et al. Serial kinematic analysis of the trunk and limb joints after anterior cruciate ligament transection: Temporal, spatial, and angular changes in a canine model of osteoarthritis. J Electromyogr Kinesiol 1994;4:181–92.

[77] Adrian CP, Haussler KK, Kawcak CE, et al. Gait and electromyographic alterations due to early onset of injury and eventual rupture of the cranial cruciate ligament in dogs: A pilot study. Vet Surg 2019;48:388–400.

[78] de Medeiros M, Sanchez Bustinduy M, Radke H, et al. Early kinematic outcome after treatment of cranial cruciate ligament rupture by tibial plateau levelling osteotomy in the dog. Vet Comp Orthop Traumatol 2011;24:178–84.

[79] Tinga S, Kim SE, Banks SA, et al. Femorotibial kinematics in dogs treated with tibial plateau leveling osteotomy for cranial cruciate ligament insufficiency: An in vivo fluoroscopic analysis during walking. Vet Surg 2020;49:187–99.

[80] Böddeker J, Drüen S, Meyer-Lindenberg A, et al. Computer-assisted gait analysis of the dog: comparison of two surgical techniques for the ruptured cranial cruciate ligament. Vet Comp Orthop Traumatol 2012;25:11–21.

[81] Lee JY, Kim G, Kim JH, et al. Kinematic gait analysis of the hind limb after tibial plateau levelling osteotomy and cranial tibial wedge osteotomy in ten dogs. J Vet Med A Physiol Pathol Clin Med 2007;54:579–84.

[82] Marsolais GS, McLean S, Derrick T, et al. Kinematic analysis of the hind limb during swimming and walking in healthy dogs and dogs with surgically corrected cranial cruciate ligament rupture. J Am Vet Med Assoc 2003;222:739–43.

[83] Sanchez-Bustinduy M, de Medeiros MA, Radke H, et al. Comparison of kinematic variables in defining lameness caused by naturally occurring rupture of the cranial cruciate ligament in dogs. Vet Surg 2010;39:523–30.

[84] Tashman S, Anderst W, Kolowich P, et al. Kinematics of the ACL-deficient canine knee during gait: serial changes over two years. J Orthop Res 2004;22:931–41.

[85] Tinga S, Kim SE, Banks SA, et al. Femorotibial kinematics in dogs with cranial cruciate ligament insufficiency: a three-dimensional in-vivo fluoroscopic analysis during walking. BMC Vet Res 2018;14:85.

[86] Bruecker KA, Benjamino K, Vezzoni A, et al. Canine elbow dysplasia: Medial compartment disease and osteoarthritis. Vet Clin North Am Small Anim Pract 2021;51:475–515.

[87] Michelsen J. Canine elbow dysplasia: aetiopathogenesis and current treatment recommendations. Vet J 2013;196:12–9.

[88] Kapatkin AS, Tomasic M, Beech J, et al. Effects of electrostimulated acupuncture on ground reaction forces and pain scores in dogs with chronic elbow joint arthritis. J Am Vet Med Assoc 2006;228:1350–4.

[89] Carrillo JM, Manera ME, Rubio M, et al. Posturography and dynamic pedobarography in lame dogs with elbow dysplasia and cranial cruciate ligament rupture. BMC Vet Res 2018;14:108.

[90] Galindo-Zamora V, Dziallas P, Wolf DC, et al. Evaluation of thoracic limb loads, elbow movement, and morphology in dogs before and after arthroscopic management of unilateral medial coronoid process disease. Vet Surg 2014;43:819–28.

[91] Preston T, Wills AP. A single hydrotherapy session increases range of motion and stride length in Labrador retrievers diagnosed with elbow dysplasia. Vet J 2018; 234:105–10.

[92] Caron A, Caley A, Farrell M, et al. Kinematic gait analysis of the canine thoracic limb using a six degrees of freedom marker set. Study in normal Labrador Retrievers and Labrador Retrievers with medial coronoid process disease. Vet Comp Orthop Traumatol 2014; 27:461–9.

[93] Rohwedder T, Fischer M, Böttcher P. In vivo fluoroscopic kinematography of dynamic radio-ulnar incongruence in dogs. Open Vet J 2017;7:221–8.

[94] Roush JK. Canine patellar luxation. Vet Clin North Am Small Anim Pract 1993;23:855–68.

[95] Arthurs GI, Langley-Hobbs SJ. Complications associated with corrective surgery for patellar luxation in 109 dogs. Vet Surg 2006;35:559–66.

[96] Di Dona F, Della Valle G, Fatone G. Patellar luxation in dogs. Vet Med (Auckl) 2018;9:23–32.

[97] Campbell CA, Horstman CL, Mason DR, et al. Severity of patellar luxation and frequency of concomitant cranial cruciate ligament rupture in dogs: 162 cases (2004-2007). J Am Vet Med Assoc 2010;236:887–91.

[98] Kowaleski MP, Boudrieau RJ, Pozzi A. Stifle joint. In: Johnston SA, Tobias KM, editors. Veterinary surgery small animal. 2nd edition. St Louis (MO): Elsevier Saunders; 2017. p. 1071–168.

[99] Moore EJ, Kim SE, Banks SA, et al. Normal patellofemoral kinematic patterns during daily activities in dogs. BMC Vet Res 2016;12:262.

[100] Kim SE, Zann GJ, Tinga S, et al. Patellofemoral kinematics in dogs with cranial cruciate ligament insufficiency: an in-vivo fluoroscopic analysis during walking. BMC Vet Res 2017;13:250.

[101] Lehmann SV, Andrada E, Taszus R, et al. Three-dimensional motion of the patella in French bulldogs with and without medial patellar luxation. BMC Vet Res 2021;17:76.

[102] Foss K, da Costa RC, Rajala-Schuttz PJ, et al. Force plate gait analysis in Doberman Pinschers with and without cervical spondylomyelopathy. J Vet Intern Med 2013; 27:106–11.

[103] Foss K, da Costa RC, Moore S. Three-dimensional kinematic gait analysis of Doberman Pinschers with and without cervical spondylomyelopathy. J Vet Intern Med 2013;27:112–9.

[104] Foss KD, Smith RL, da Costa RC. Kinetic and kinematic follow-up gait analysis in Doberman Pinschers with cervical spondylomyelopathy treated medically and surgically. J Vet Intern Med 2018;32:1126–32.

[105] Sutton JS, Garcia TC, Stover SM, et al. Kinetic and kinematic gait analysis in the pelvic limbs of normal and post-hemilaminectomy Dachshunds. Vet Comp Orthop Traumatol 2016;29:202–8.

[106] van Klaveren NJ, Suwankong N, De Boer S, et al. Force plate analysis before and after dorsal decompression for treatment of degenerative lumbosacral stenosis in dogs. Vet Surg 2005;34:450–6.

[107] Suwankong N, Meij BP, Van Klaveren NJ, et al. Assessment of decompressive surgery in dogs with degenerative lumbosacral stenosis using force plate analysis and questionnaires. Vet Surg 2007;36:423–31.

[108] Kirpensteijn J, van den Bos R, van den Brom WE, et al. Ground reaction force analysis of large breed dogs when walking after the amputation of a limb. Vet Rec 2000;146:155–9.

[109] Fuchs A, Goldner B, Nolte I, et al. Ground reaction force adaptations to tripedal locomotion in dogs. Vet J 2014; 201:307–15.

[110] Hogy SM, Worley DR, Jarvis SL, et al. Kinematic and kinetic analysis of dogs during trotting after amputation of a pelvic limb. Am J Vet Res 2013;74:1164–71.

[111] Jarvis SL, Worley DR, Hogy SM, et al. Kinematic and kinetic analysis of dogs during trotting after amputation of a thoracic limb. Am J Vet Res 2013;74:1155–63.

[112] Ben-Amotz R, Dycus D, Levine D, et al. Stance and weight distribution after tibial plateau leveling osteotomy in fore limb and hind limb amputee dogs. BMC Vet Res 2020;16:188.

[113] Corbee RJ, Maas H, Doornenbal A, et al. Forelimb and hindlimb ground reaction forces of walking cats: assessment and comparison with walking dogs. Vet J 2014; 202:116–27.

[114] Schnabl E, Bockstahler B. Systematic review of ground reaction force measurements in cats. Vet J 2015;206: 83–90.

[115] Robinson DA, Romans CW, Gordon-Evans WJ, et al. Evaluation of short-term limb function following unilateral carbon dioxide laser or scalpel onychectomy in cats. J Am Vet Med Assoc 2007;230:353–8.

[116] Romans CW, Gordon WJ, Robinson DA, et al. Effect of postoperative analgesic protocol on limb function following onychectomy in cats. J Am Vet Med Assoc 2005;227:89–93.

[117] Romans CW, Conzemius MG, Horstman CL, et al. Use of pressure platform gait analysis in cats with and without bilateral onychectomy. Am J Vet Res 2004;65: 1276–8.

[118] Riggs CM, DeCamp CE, Soutas-Little RW, et al. Effects of subject velocity on force plate-measured ground reaction forces in healthy greyhounds at the trot. Am J Vet Res 1993;54:1523–6.

[119] Roush JK, McLaughlin RM Jr. Effects of subject stance time and velocity on ground reaction forces in clinically normal greyhounds at the walk. Am J Vet Res 1994;55:1672–6.

[120] McLaughlin R Jr, Roush JK. Effects of increasing velocity on braking and propulsion times during force plate gait analysis in greyhounds. Am J Vet Res 1995;56:159–61.

[121] Renberg WC, Johnston SA, Ye K, et al. Comparison of stance time and velocity as control variables in force plate analysis of dogs. Am J Vet Res 1999;60:814–9.

[122] Maes LD, Herbin M, Hackert R, et al. Steady locomotion in dogs: temporal and associated spatial coordination patterns and the effect of speed. J Exp Biol 2008;211:138–49.

[123] Stigall AR, Farr BD, Ramos MT, et al. A formalized method to acclimate dogs to voluntary treadmill locomotion at various speeds and inclines. Animals (Basel) 2022;12.

[124] Mickelson MA, Vo T, Piazza AM, et al. Influence of trial repetition on lameness during force platform gait analysis in a heterogeneous population of clinically lame dogs each trotting at its preferred velocity. Am J Vet Res 2017;78:1284–92.

[125] Nordquist B, Fischer J, Kim SY, et al. Effects of trial repetition, limb side, intraday and inter-week variation on vertical and craniocaudal ground reaction forces in clinically normal Labrador Retrievers. Vet Comp Orthop Traumatol 2011;24:435–44.

[126] Rincon Alvarez J, Anesi S, Czopowicz M, et al. The effect of calibration method on repeatability and reproducibility of pressure mat data in a canine population. Vet Comp Orthop Traumatol 2020;33:428–33.

[127] Jevens DJ, Hauptman JG, DeCamp CE, et al. Contributions to variance in force-plate analysis of gait in dogs. Am J Vet Res 1993;54:612–5.

[128] Lafuente MP, Provis L, Schmalz EA. Effects of restrictive and non-restrictive harnesses on shoulder extension in dogs at walk and trot. Vet Rec 2019;184:64.

[129] Weissenbacher A, Tichy A, Weissenbacher K, et al. Influence of two types of guide harnesses on ground reaction forces and step length of guide dogs for the blind. Animals (Basel) 2022;12:2453.

[130] Kapatkin AS, Arbittier G, Kass PH, et al. Kinetic gait analysis of healthy dogs on two different surfaces. Vet Surg 2007;36:605–8.

[131] Kieves NR, Hart JL, Evans RB, et al. Comparison of three walkway cover types for use during objective canine gait analysis with a pressure-sensitive walkway. Am J Vet Res 2019;80:265–9.

[132] Colborne GR, Innes JF, Comerford EJ, et al. Distribution of power across the hind limb joints in Labrador Retrievers and Greyhounds. Am J Vet Res 2005;66:1563–71.

[133] Besancon MF, Conzemius MG, Evans RB, et al. Distribution of vertical forces in the pads of Greyhounds and Labrador Retrievers during walking. Am J Vet Res 2004;65:1497–501.

[134] Mölsä SH, Hielm-Björkman AK, Laitinen-Vapaavuori OM. Force platform analysis in clinically healthy Rottweilers: comparison with Labrador Retrievers. Vet Surg 2010;39:701–7.

[135] Humphries A, Shaheen AF, Gomez Alvarez CB. Biomechanical comparison of standing posture and during trot between German shepherd and Labrador retriever dogs. PLoS One 2020;15:e0239832.

[136] Bertram JE, Lee DV, Case HN, et al. Comparison of the trotting gaits of Labrador Retrievers and Greyhounds. Am J Vet Res 2000;61:832–8.

[137] Brady RB, Sidiropoulos AN, Bennett HJ, et al. Evaluation of gait-related variables in lean and obese dogs at a trot. Am J Vet Res 2013;74:757–62.

Advances in Small Animal Care 4 (2023) 21–35

ADVANCES IN SMALL ANIMAL CARE

Patient-Centered Physical Rehabilitation in Companion Animals

Arielle Pechette Markley, DVM, cVMA, CVPP, CCRT, DAIPM, DACVSMR[a],*,
Nina R. Kieves, DVM, DACVS, DACVSMR[a], David Levine, PT, PhD, DPT, MPH, CCRP[b],
Denis J. Marcellin-Little, DEDV, DACVS, DACVSMR[c]

[a]Department of Clinical Sciences, The Ohio State University College of Veterinary Medicine, 601 Vernon L Tharp Street, Columbus, OH 43210, USA; [b]Department of Physical Therapy, University of Tennessee at Chattanooga, 615 McCallie Avenue, Chattanooga, TN 37403, USA; [c]Veterinary Orthopedic Research Laboratory, School of Veterinary Medicine, University of California, Davis, 1285 Veterinary Medicine Drive, VM3A Room 4206, Davis, CA 95616, USA

KEYWORDS

- Physical rehabilitation • Companion animals • Patient-centered care • Client education
- Collaborative goal setting • Client-specific outcome measures • Shared decision-making

KEY POINTS

- Patient-centered physical therapy is a recently introduced process in human medicine that places the patient at the center of their care and leads to improved outcomes.
- Patient-centered therapy is based on communication, collaborative goal setting, shared decision-making, individualized treatment planning, biopsychosocial perspective, respect and empowerment, and education.
- Patient-centered physical rehabilitation follows principles similar to patient-centered physical therapy in human medicine but presents challenges because both the animal and the owner must be considered.

INTRODUCTION

Patient-centered care is increasingly advocated in human health care to improve quality care and patient outcomes. Although the definition of patient-centered care is not standardized, its general concept involves a shift in focus from care services offered to treat specific diseases to an individualized holistic approach to care of the whole person taking into account biological, psychosocial, personal preference, past experiences, and autonomy [1–5]. With this approach, the patient is seen as a partner in their care, not just a receiver of care, and their input and participation are essential. In human health care, a patient-centered approach has been shown to be positively associated with improved health outcomes, including functional mobility, quality of life, and overall well-being [1,6–8].

Physical rehabilitation is an essential aspect of veterinary care, particularly for pets recovering from injury and/or surgery or when managing chronic conditions. Although the concept of patient-centered rehabilitation in veterinary medicine is not new, past recommendations have primarily been focused on the physical aspects of rehabilitation [9–13]. This historic approach included individualized treatment plans incorporating various modalities based on the particular disease or surgery, the phase of tissue healing, degree of physical disability, and targeted interventions such as exercise programs for the patient. However, veterinary rehabilitation therapy is inherently multidimensional. The historical focus on the physical aspects of the rehabilitation plan leaves out a number of components critical to the success of physical rehabilitation therapy, including

*Corresponding author, E-mail address: markley.125@osu.edu

https://doi.org/10.1016/j.yasa.2023.05.002

the owner or handler of the patient, psychological and behavioral status of the patient, and anticipated future work or activities. All of these other components need to be considered to create genuine patient-centered care plans, which are needed to improve quality of care and patient outcomes. As physical rehabilitation plans are often based on functional improvement, with less emphasis on disease management, patient-centered therapy is especially important in this field. This article outlines a framework for veterinary patient-centered care focused on physical rehabilitation.

PATIENT-CENTERED CARE MODELS IN HUMAN HEALTH CARE

As part of the growing focus on patient-centered care in human health care, much work has focused on developing defined models and frameworks to help providers deliver consistent patient-centered care in a variety of settings and populations. An increasing number of studies on patient-centered care in musculoskeletal rehabilitation and physiotherapy have been published. These studies identified significant gaps in current interventions and the implementation thereof [4,14–18]. Most investigators note that many of the patient care frameworks are lacking critical components, particularly the components "developing a coping plan" and "follow-up," and the lack of inclusion of some of these components may result in suboptimal patient outcomes. Coping plans include the identification of potential barriers to the implementation of therapeutic recommendations and problem-solving around these barriers. These studies voice the need for more research on model development and how framework components impact patient outcomes.

CHALLENGES TO FRAMEWORK DEVELOPMENT IN VETERINARY MEDICINE

Most of the patient-centered models and frameworks in human medicine, particularly in rehabilitation, are based on the clinician–patient dyad where the patient is able to communicate with the clinician to participate in their care decisions. The challenge to developing patient-centered care frameworks for any setting or population in veterinary medicine is the addition of the third-party proxy which, in most situations, is the pet owner. This creates a care triad between the clinician, pet owner, and patient. The clinician must consider not only the needs and best course of care for their patient but also the needs, expectations, and circumstances of the pet

owner. In addition, we as clinicians make inferences on what the patient is experiencing as well as their needs, as they cannot directly communicate with us. This makes many of the components of patient care frameworks more challenging to create and implement because all members of the care triad must be considered. This becomes particularly challenging when the expectations of the client are unrealistic, or the client is unwilling or unable to manage the pet adequately.

Other challenges for patient-centered care framework development and implementation in veterinary medicine mirror the obstacles noted in human medicine: the lack of knowledge about patient-centered care, lack of training for professionals on communication and patient-centered care strategies, limited consultation time, and lack of skills to implement the framework components [17,19–21]. Currently, very limited research on patient-centered care in veterinary medicine is available. Most studies focus on "relationship-centered care" and the client communication component of the care paradigm [22–24]. Studies evaluating the use of patient-centered care in the veterinary rehabilitation setting are not available.

RECOMMENDED FRAMEWORK

Based on the review of the various frameworks in human medicine, the following key components are recommended for a proposed framework in veterinary physical rehabilitation (Fig. 1).
1. Communication
2. Collaborative goal setting
3. Shared decision-making
4. Individualized treatment planning
5. Biopsychosocial perspective
6. Respect and empowerment
7. Education

Although several of these categories overlap, it is important to consider each individually when planning patient care to ensure that all components are thoroughly met.

COMMUNICATION

Communication is the foundation of patient-centered care. Communication between the rehabilitation provider and pet owner is essential throughout the rehabilitation process. It is critical for the provider to develop a partnership with the pet owner and maintain ongoing dialogue. The following are recommendations for developing comprehensive, patient-based communication strategies in the veterinary rehabilitation setting,

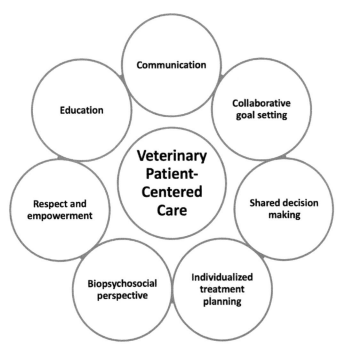

FIG. 1 The components of veterinary patient-centered care involve the patient, owner, and clinicians providing and overseeing care.

adapting guidelines from the Gothenburg person-centered care and the Canadian Occupational Performance Measure [25,26].

Initial development of partnership between therapist and owner

Establishing a partnership with the client: A meaningful partnership is one in which both the patient and clinician feel seen, heard, and appreciated. Establishing meaningful connections is a foundational component of the therapeutic relationship, also known as the therapeutic alliance. Therapeutic alliance is a term used in human rehabilitation to describe the development of a bond and subsequent positive feelings between the client and therapist [27].

There is strong evidence that an enhanced therapeutic alliance can improve outcomes in human physical rehabilitation [28]. The therapeutic alliance in small animal rehabilitation extends to the relationship between the practitioner and the owner. A strong therapeutic alliance has been proposed to be central to patient-centered care, with better quality relationships associated with improved outcomes, satisfaction, and compliance [29–33]. Veterinary rehabilitation therapists and their team members should be intentional

in establishing a meaningful connection with the pet owner during the course of rehabilitation therapy.

Obtain a narrative about the patient covering everyday life: A patient narrative is created through the dialogue between the pet owner and the rehabilitation professionals (therapists, technicians, assistants, and others involved). Understanding the goals for the pet and owner is imperative in decision-making throughout the process of physical rehabilitation to achieve the best outcome. It is the therapist's responsibility to initiate this conversation, which will allow for gathering the narrative. It is important to gather as much information as possible about the pet's normal daily life, as these details will be used to formulate the goals and individualized treatment plan.

Explore client needs, preferences, expectations, motivations, resources, and circumstances: Because veterinary medicine involves a care triad, the pet owner's narrative is just as critical to obtain as that of the pet itself. The needs, preferences, and expectations of the pet owner will influence the goals and treatment planning. Their resources, motivations, and circumstances can act as facilitators or barriers to rehabilitation care. These factors need to be considered when creating the treatment plan so that the plan can be successful.

Tailoring Communication Styles

Patient-centered care requires a collaborative communication style and tailoring the communication to the individual pet owner. In human patient-centered care,
this particular communication style is referred to as
"person-focused communication," as it takes the patient narrative and puts it in the context of the patient's
entire life, rather than just in the context of their health
care [34]. This approach to communication facilitates
the development of the therapeutic relationship and
improved outcomes [35,36]. Effective communication
relies on verbal and nonverbal communication and
the process and content communication. Patient-
centered communication strategies can be intimidating
for the clinician to implement due to potential lack of
training and the time-intensive nature of collaborative
communication. In human health care, developed
frameworks help improve clinician–patient communication, including the Calgary–Cambridge guide, yet
no similar frameworks exist in veterinary medicine
[37]. Similar frameworks may need to be considered
in veterinary medicine to improve patient-centered
care, particularly in the rehabilitation setting where patients often have complex chronic conditions that
require long-term therapy and an effective therapeutic
collaboration between owners and clinicians.

Collaborative goal setting and shared decision-making

Collaborative goal setting and shared decision-making
are discussed in more detail below, but it is important
to note that communication, the development of a partnership between the therapist and owner, obtaining a
narrative, and exploring the psychosocial factors are all
critical to the collaborative goal setting and shared
decision-making process. These goals should be revisited
frequently, whereas care is being provided to meet the
needs of the owner and the patient as they evolve.

Ongoing dialogue

The veterinarian should provide regular updates on the
pet's progress and adjust the rehabilitation plan as
needed based on the pet's response. The communication and reevaluation rates should be adapted to the
speed of progression of medical conditions, problems
that evolve rapidly may require daily communications,
and chronic problems may be effectively managed with
monthly communications. Selecting a communication
coordinator and establishing communication standard
protocols decreases the burden and increases the effectiveness of the process.

Rehabilitation team communication

It is important to setup robust, efficient, and consistent
internal communication protocols for all those
involved in a patient's care. This is particularly relevant
when multiple clinicians are involved in a case. Communications should be summarized and documented
in the medical record in a timely fashion, including
objective data and plan of care [38]. Effective medical
communication is open, clear, respectful, and nonpuni-
tive and includes regular and routine communication
and information sharing. There should be clear, designated roles and tasks for team members as well as
defined decision-making procedures. Effective communication in a team environment requires access to
needed resources, appropriate balance of member
participation, acknowledgment and processing of conflict, shared responsibility for team success, and a mechanism to evaluate outcomes and adapt care based on
those outcomes.

Communication with other providers

Because rehabilitation patients may be referred, a
communication plan with referring veterinarians
should be implemented. The communication rate
should be consistent, generally after the initial evaluation and at predetermined milestones, for example, during the transition from acute care to subacute care and
from subacute care to chronic care. Communication
methods should be adapted to match the methods
preferred by referral practices (ie, verbal vs electronic
communication).

COLLABORATIVE GOAL SETTING

Goal setting has been shown to be one of the most
important components of rehabilitation based on
studies in human physical therapy [14,16,39–41].
Goal setting is defined as the iterative process of setting
goals, determining how to achieve the goals with a specific rehabilitation plan and evaluating and redefining
the goals based on outcome measures [41]. Setting
meaningful goals seems to improve the rehabilitation
process and outcomes for people [16]. Traditional
goal setting, both in human and veterinary medicine,
has been clinician-based. Clinician-based goal setting
relies on impairment-based assessments, such as range
of motion, strength, lameness, muscle girth, and others,
to develop an interventional plan. The transition toward patient-centered goal setting should consider the
individual's experiences, situations, expectations, and
levels of disability, and in the case of veterinary

rehabilitation, this should include consideration of both the individual patient and the individual owner(s) of the patient. Collaborative goal setting, therefore, merges the patient-centered goals and the clinician-defined rehabilitation goals.

Although a substantial number of studies on goal setting are available in human rehabilitation practice and specifically in association with patient-centered care [14–16,39,41], there are no similar studies in veterinary medicine. Therefore, the following recommendations are extrapolated from human studies.

Clinician-centered goal development

A comprehensive patient assessment is critical for developing rehabilitation goals, individualized treatment plans, and outcome measures. Detailed discussion on performance of a comprehensive rehabilitation assessment is beyond the scope of this review and is available in other resources [42–44]. In brief, patient assessment should include stance and gait analysis during a walk, trot, or other activities such as stairs, a full physical examination, orthopedic and neurologic examinations, evaluation of joint motion and stability, range of motion using goniometry, limb girth measurements, functional mobility, and strength assessments. Assessment should include detailed documentation of subjective and objective measures so that progress can be objectively evaluated. The therapist's rehabilitation goals based on impairments should then be considered in context with the following patient-centered approach to goal setting.

Identify personally meaningful daily activities that the patient is having a hard time performing

As part of the initial owner interview, it is important to identify meaningful daily activities that the patient is having a hard time performing [45]. The key to making this patient-centered is identifying activities that are "personally meaningful," which, in this case, would be those that are meaningful to the owner of the patient. This allows for development of goals that are relevant in the patient's environment, rather than what the rehabilitation therapist assumes is important for the patient. These activities can include a very wide range of activities depending on the patient and the owner, ranging from basic elimination activities and mobility around the house to pleasure and human–animal bonding activities. The importance and prioritization of these activities will be unique to each human-animal pair.

It is also vital to gather detailed and specific data regarding daily activities. The more specific the details are, the more easily the goals can be defined and measured. This requires a conscious effort on the part of all the team members who are collecting the initial history and client–patient narrative. Although this is time-consuming initially, performing this work up-front will be beneficial over the course of the patient's care. Several communication strategies, including the use of active listening skills, asking open-ended questions, and following up to narrow down specifics, are helpful to support data gathering. For example, if the client says that their dog is "slowing down," it is imperative to clarify that further. Is the dog slower to rise from a down to a sit or slower to rise from a sit to a stand? Did the dog used to walk 1 mile twice a day, but can now only walk half of a mile? Has the speed of the walk decreased? Identifying specific challenges allows for creation of measurable goals and gives the owner a way to objectively track progress. The specific information collected during follow-up questions also provides valuable information about the likely source of a problem, for example, the general loss of fitness, a pain response to propulsion in the forelimbs or hind limbs, or a pain response to specific joint movements. All of these will require a different management approach; therefore, delineating the problem initially is imperative. These potential problems can be confirmed during focused reexaminations.

It is important to note that multiple client-specific outcome measurement (CSOM) tools are available in veterinary medicine. These are often used to increase the objectivity of the evaluation of client-reported feedback in research settings. However, they can be used practically and successfully in clinical rehabilitation practice. A variety of instruments ranging from acute pain and chronic pain scoring, mobility evaluation, and quality of life scoring are available at no charge to users [46–55]. Targeted patients and the degree and level of validation vary widely between CSOMs. Although these CSOMs do have benefit in veterinary rehabilitation practice as a way to provide more objective data tracking, they are not recommended as a sole tool in patient-centered goal setting and outcome assessment, as they are not personalized to the patient or owner and may not accurately reflect the needs and desires of the owner–patient dyad.

Set goals for activities the patient needs to perform

2The initial goal setting requires identification of the activities that the patient needs to perform. These become the nonnegotiable and top prioritization goals when it comes to creating an individualized rehabilitation treatment plan. These activity needs are going to be dependent on the needs and circumstances of the owner, which is why establishing the initial narrative is essential. Therapeutic plans must consider ingress and egress from home and motor vehicles. For example, if the owner lives in a split-level house with multiple sets of stairs, has a set of four stairs that the dog must be able to navigate to get into the yard, or lives on the third floor of an apartment complex with no elevator, then comfort, range of motion, proprioception, and the strength needed to perform stairs will be prioritized and the utilization of supplies and equipment such as a sling/harness or a ramp will be considered. Once again, these goals need to be quantitatively and qualitatively as specific as possible to create an optimally individualized treatment plan and to assess outcomes. Because stairs vary widely in height and texture, setting a goal of "be able to do stairs" does not provide enough information to tailor the rehabilitation approach or evaluate success of the rehabilitation plan. Although the rehabilitation strategies for improving joint mobility, range of motion, proprioception, and strength are going to be similar for all patients with the need to do stairs, the exact therapeutic plan, timeline, and determining successful outcome are going to vary significantly between the patient that needs to navigate four stairs and the patient that needs to navigate three flights of stairs. These goals can be short-term goals (eg, ability to climb four stairs in 2 weeks) or longer term goals (eg, navigating three flights of stairs in 2 months). Knowledge of these specifics also enables the clinician to give the owner a reasonable timeline to achieve their goal.

Set goals for activities owner wants the patient to perform

The next set of goals are based on the activities that the owner wants the patient to perform. For working dogs, goal setting includes the standard activities needed to recertify or perform the work. For sporting dogs, goal setting requires a discussion with the owner regarding their perspective on return to performance or potential retirement. The list of wants will vary based on the owner's preferences, highlighting again the importance of the initial client narrative. The same activity, such as the ability to navigate stairs or jump up, may be on the wish list of one owner but may be a critical need for another owner. Differentiating between the two is important for creating meaningful goals and therapeutic plans and for setting realistic owner expectations.

Collaboration to merge client and therapist goals

Collaborative goal setting has been shown to improve psychosocial outcomes in the rehabilitation setting [56]. Some clients may prefer more therapist direction, whereas others may prefer to take the lead in setting goals. In an optimal situation, realistic and achievable goals are discussed and set collaboratively. This collaborative process ensures that the client understands the risks, benefits, and possible outcomes of different treatment options and feels empowered to make decisions about the care that is right for both their pet and themselves. This directly leads to, and is integrated into, the concept of the shared decision-making, which is discussed in more detail below.

Developing outcome measures that assess goals

Practical outcome measures commensurate with collaborative goals are selected at the onset of therapy. The optimal outcome measures are specific, valid (accurate and repeatable), convenient, and affordable. Disease-specific outcome measures may include pain scoring, muscle girth measurements, goniometry, and weight bearing [48,50,57–64]. Functional outcome measures are often more challenging to assess in veterinary patients due to the requirement for specialized equipment for validated, objective kinetic and kinematic gait analysis, and the lack of validation for many of the more convenient outcome measures, such as strength testing or task-specific challenges that are commonly used in human physical therapy [65–70]. A recent study recommended specific development of functional tests for canine geriatric patients to evaluate strength, endurance, mobility, and proprioception [43]. Some of these tests include timed up and go, Cavaletti rails, figure 8 turns, and down to stand [43]. These can also be simple patient-specific outcome measures, mutually agreed on, such as the ability to ambulate for a 10-minute walk with the owner, or at a higher level, performing agility-specific obstacles (such as weave poles) with no lameness after training. Developing outcome measures that match the goals set during the collaborative goal setting process is critical for monitoring progress, managing expectations, improving client satisfaction, and can improve overall outcomes.

Plan strategies by identifying barriers and facilitators of participation in rehabilitation activities

Assessing barriers to rehabilitation helps to prevent the formulation of unattainable goals. Unattainable goals are discouraging for the pet owner and result in reduced compliance, decreased satisfaction, and may result in the owner choosing to not start or to discontinue their pet's involvement in rehabilitation therapy [71].

Identifying barriers and facilitators can help the owner and rehabilitation therapy team recognize potential challenges and plan mitigation strategies in advance. Examples of barriers include resources (money, time), logistics (travel, ability to get pet in a motor vehicle), owners' physical abilities, patient behavior (fear, anxiety, and aggression), patient obesity, and so forth. Examples of facilitators include a motivated owner, households with multiple individuals who share the burden of care, continuity of care by the same providers, hospitalizing the patient for rehabilitation if the caregiver burden is too great, goal setting and frequent communication to review of these goals, and so forth. Collaboration between the owner and clinician can help minimize the impact of barriers related to resources and logistics.

Formulation of coping plan

Setting up a coping plan is important when managing chronic conditions that often lead to permanent or progressive problems, including impaired mobility, chronic pain, and urinary or fecal incontinence. Formulation of a coping plan has been noted to be an underused but important component of rehabilitation goal setting in human medicine [16]. In human studies, this coping plan primarily focuses on identifying barriers to the rehabilitation plan and patient goals and creating preemptive strategies to overcome these barriers [16]. However, because the veterinary physical rehabilitation relationship is a triad, there must be consideration of creating coping plans to help the client manage the pet's condition but also taking into account the caregiver burden.

The caregiver care burden has been thoroughly documented in human medicine but has only recently garnered attention in veterinary medicine [72]. Studies in veterinary medicine have shown that the owners of sick pets have greater symptoms of depression, anxiety, and stress [73,74]. The caregiver burden is also associated with poorer psychosocial function in veterinary clients. Higher levels of caregiver burden are associated with more serious illness of the pet, though the severity of the disease alone does not fully account for burden [73,74]. Other studies have explored the relationship between caregiver burden, anticipatory grief, quality of life, and euthanasia, and greater burden significantly predicts an owner's consideration of euthanasia [74]. It is important to note that studies have shown that enhancing owner satisfaction may mitigate factors contributing to burden, in turn reducing the decision of premature euthanasia, and that the use of a collaborative approach to treatment planning is the key to enhancing owner satisfaction [75]. Therefore, creation of a coping plan to help the owner identify and address the barriers to their goals, as well creating a plan to reduce specific factors implicated in increasing the caregiver burden is likely to improve overall treatment outcomes [76,77].

On the opposite end of the spectrum of dealing with severe illness and quality of life is the challenge of managing a high-intensity active dog during physical rehabilitation therapy. Exercise restriction can be incredibly challenging, a source of significant owner frustration, and a primary source of compliance issues during the postoperative or post-injury period. Generally, restrictions to exercise are recommended for an allotted amount of time, without any further recommendations to help an owner successfully navigate this period of time. Working with the owner to develop a coping plan to ensure the dog is mentally and physically stimulated, whereas staying within the confines of the exercise restriction can be beneficial for compliance and owner satisfaction. Options for mental management include adding in puzzles, frozen food toys, low impact training techniques such as scent work, tracking, and so forth. [78–86] Combined physical and mental stimulation may include training the low movement components of sports such as rally and obedience and an increased number of targeted home exercises as dictated by the therapist [87,88]. Pharmaceutical management may also be needed as part of the coping plan for some patients or for some duration of the exercise restriction period. Providing the owner with a plan and tools for management of the exercise restriction period may help increase compliance with exercise restrictions, resulting in better outcomes and a lower likelihood of complications and injury recurrence and increasing ongoing owner satisfaction.

Follow-up and ongoing monitoring

Over the course of rehabilitation therapy, patient functioning and health change, but also the owner's desires and expectations can change. Goals and therapeutic plans should be monitored for appropriateness and adjusted as needed throughout the rehabilitation process. Continuously reevaluating goals also provide the opportunity to evaluate goal progress and to observe goal achievement. This can improve owner satisfaction and active engagement in their pet's rehabilitation therapy and can increase commitment. It is therefore recommended that goal evaluation and modification should be scheduled as part of regular rehabilitation therapy reevaluations or at any time when owners have concerns.

Development of goal setting models

Models have been created to provide guidance for clinicians in the collaborative goal setting process within the larger context of patient-centered care. For example, a three-goal model has been introduced in human medicine to manage patients with multiple medical problems (Table 1). The three goals are disease goals, functional goals, and fundamental goals [89]. Fundamental goals relate to life priorities; these can be discussed explicitly or implicitly when setting collaborative goals. This concept could be readily adapted to the rehabilitation therapy of companion animals.

These goals can be compromised if owners are noncompliant, do not fully understand the goals and/or plan, or have health issues themselves preventing implementation of the plan. Goals should be mutually agreed on, and communication and owner education are critical for buy-in. Goals should be revisited frequently and adjusted as needed with the owner. Suitable outcome measures must be used to evaluate the progress (or lack of progress) for goals to assure meaningful interventions are used.

SHARED DECISION-MAKING

Shared decision-making is an important component of patient-centered care and can increase satisfaction, engagement, and compliance [17,19,35,89–93]. Shared decision-making takes into account the owner's context, knowledge, needs, values, and goals [35,89–92]. Communication is the key to shared decision-making. Once goals are developed, human shared decision-making models suggest using a three-talk model. This model involves (1) "Goal-Team talk," which is the work needed to form a partnership and support decision-making; (2) "Goal-Option talk," which includes discussion of the risks, benefits, and alternatives;

TABLE 1
The Goals of Rehabilitation Therapy in Human and Companion Animals

Types of Goals	Examples
Fundamental goals	Independent function within the house
Functional goals	Ambulate independently for 5 min; climbing up/down one flight of the owners' stairs without assist
Disease-related goals	Decrease joint pain; weight loss

and (3) "Goal-Decision talk," which involves helping patients explore their preferences and reach a specific decision [94]. A similar approach could be implemented into the shared decision-making in veterinary physical rehabilitation and may also improve client satisfaction, engagement, and compliance.

Shared decision-making is often underused in human medicine due to time constraints and lack of training in the skills needed to be effective in the process [95]. As a consequence, various models and guidelines to help with implementation of the shared decision-making process have been designed for practice [96]. Patient decision aids intended to help patients participate in decisions that involve weighing the benefits and risks of various treatment options have also been developed and recommendations for their use are available. Decision aids can be pamphlets, videos, or Web-based tools. They describe the options available and make the decision explicit. Studies in human medicine have shown that decision aids reduce decisional conflict related to feeling uninformed, reduce the feeling that the patient's personal values are unheard, decrease the proportion of people who are passive in decision-making, and reduce the proportion of people who remain undecided post-intervention [96,97]. Similar development of shared decision-making models and decision aids for the veterinary physical rehabilitation setting may be beneficial in improving efficiency and utilization of this approach in busy clinical practice settings.

INDIVIDUALIZED TREATMENT PLANNING

Treatment planning should be individualized, coordinated, holistic, and integrated among caregivers. There also needs to be an awareness of changing needs of patients over time. Individualized treatment planning considers factors such as age, activity level, premorbid, and comorbid conditions and is centered on treating each patient's unique condition. These plans are individually tailored for the patient instead of "one size fits all" protocols. For example, after tibial plateau leveling osteotomy (TPLO) surgery, protocols are commonly implemented that may not take into consideration the individual factors of the case such as chronicity, owner needs and abilities, and overall fitness of the patient. Consideration of all factors is what makes patient-centered care advantageous to achieving optimal outcomes.

BIOPSYCHOSOCIAL PERSPECTIVE

In human medicine, the biopsychosocial model describes the interconnectedness between the biological factors of the disease, the psychological implications (emotions, distress, fear, and coping strategies), and the social (socioeconomic, cultural, and family circumstances) factors and how these complex relationships affect patient disease, treatment, and outcomes. When that model is applied to companion animal therapy, the psychological and emotional impacts of rehabilitation care need to be considered for both the patient and the owner in the context of their experiences, beliefs, expectations, and perceptions. If stress, anxiety, and fear are minimized for the patient as well as the client, there can be more effective execution of the treatment plan, better communication, improved outcomes, and overall enhanced quality of care. The owner's social factors also need to be considered when devising the treatment program and anticipated outcomes.

Client

The development of a biopsychosocial perspective for the client is based on the initial narrative where the client needs, preferences, expectations, motivations, resources, and circumstances are established. This also involves establishing the biopsychosocial consequences of their pet's condition, which includes the support that the owner may need to overcome challenges and barriers to managing their pet as well as addressing the factors related to the caregiver burden. Components of the biopsychosocial perspective may include what the owner can do physically, the living environment, the owner's support system at home, what the owner's capacity for patient exercise is, time and financial restraints, and ability to carry out tasks such as bladder expression, wound care, mobility management, among others. This biopsychosocial perspective must be taken into account with communication strategies, during the collaborative goal setting and shared decision-making processes, when planning strategies to address barriers and when providing owner education.

Patient

Developing a biopsychosocial perspective of the patient is more challenging due to both the nonverbal nature of the patient and the inability to explain the rehabilitation therapies and processes to the patient. The responsibility of managing fear, anxiety, and stress in the patient falls directly on the rehabilitation team. This requires a thorough understanding of animal behavior, as well as training principles, both of which are often overlooked in veterinary and rehabilitation training programs.

Assessment of the patient's needs, preferences, motivations, and circumstances relies on detailed information gathering from the owner. Asking the owner to describe

what types of situations and activities increase/decrease fear and anxiety in their pet, what motivates their pet, and what training techniques they use at home can all help the rehabilitation team tailor their physical rehabilitation approach to the patient. In practice, some patients may be very comfortable with manual therapy but may not be willing to exercise, whereas other patients may prefer a hands-off approach and may be very willing to exercise but may not tolerate manual therapy.

One of the most important behavior and training principles that should be considered in the rehabilitation setting is "the learner determines what is reinforcing" and, on the flip side, "the learner determines what is aversive." [98] Reinforcement strategies will not be equal between patients, and communication with the owner and monitoring the behavior of the patient will help determine the most effective reinforcement during physical rehabilitation therapy, whether that is food (and what kind), toys, praise, petting, and so forth. Although physical rehabilitation is generally intended to be low stress, some seemingly non-harmful rehabilitation techniques can be very aversive to some patients and their preferences and needs must be taken into consideration. For example, the recommendation to bump patients during walks to cause perturbations and weight shifting may not bother some dogs, but pressure-sensitive or touch-sensitive dogs, or patients with allodynia, may experience it as quite aversive.

Although some rehabilitation techniques may only be aversive to certain patients due to their personalities and individual behavior needs, some common recommendations are likely aversive to most patients, such as taping a syringe cap to the bottom of a paw to compel weight shifting through discomfort. It is important for the rehabilitation team to carefully monitor the patient's reaction and behavior throughout their therapy visits to minimize the accidental use of aversive events, as aversive training has been shown to increase stress-related behaviors and cortisol levels in dogs and can negatively impact the human–dog relationship and the overall welfare of the patient [99–101].

Veterinary visits, by their nature, are socially invasive for companion animal patients. Recognition of this, as well as increased awareness of the negative effects of fear, stress, and anxiety, has resulted in the development of the "Fear Free" initiative [102]. The Fear Free platform provides education for veterinary professionals and pet owners with the goal of improving emotional well-being of the pet. The Fear Free certification course for veterinary professionals includes training on concepts of touch and handling, stress-response, basic learning theory, body language, behavioral modification, providing low stress transportation and hospital environments, and pharmaceutical regimens [102]. These learning concepts and techniques may be beneficial resources for the rehabilitation team when developing patient-centered physical rehabilitation plans that are tailored to support the emotional well-being of the patient. The veterinary rehabilitation team also needs to have an awareness of, and be proactive regarding, the need for pharmaceutical intervention to reduce anxiety and stress during therapy visits. This is particularly important as veterinary physical rehabilitation patients are usually making frequent visits, often multiple times a week, for therapy. Collaboration with a board-certified behaviorist may be indicated in some instances. In other, albeit rare cases, the patient may simply not be amenable to a formal physical rehabilitation setting and at-home care provided by the owner may be more achievable.

In the broader context of the patient-centered care framework, the biopsychosocial perspective for both the owner and the patient needs to be considered during the collaborative goal setting and shared decision-making process, during individualized treatment planning and in regard to coordination and communication with the rehabilitation care team. Taking the owner and patient's needs, preferences, expectations, motivations, and circumstances into account may improve owner satisfaction, patient outcome, and the emotional well-being of both the owner and the patient.

RESPECT AND EMPOWERMENT

Respect between the owner and the clinician can improve outcomes and facilitate owner education. Respect also builds the partnership and feelings of trust between those involved. Listening to understand is a core principle as is attention to detail, encouragement, and empathy. Empowerment is a process through which people gain greater control over decisions and actions affecting the health of their pet. By empowering owners to take responsibility for the management of the pet, it may enhance medical outcomes. Empowerment is primarily achieved by education but is also enhanced through collaborative goal setting and reassessment. Education on exercise and diet are commonly used in rehabilitation, and owners who can directly see improvements will be more empowered to continue the care.

EDUCATION

Owner education is a critical component in managing expectations, empowering and engaging owners in the care of their pet, and ensuring compliance. Qualitative information is available about methods clinicians should use to educate pet owners [103,104]. Little information is available about the quantity of information that should be shared with owners and the timing of that education. However, human studies indicate that written education is often not perceived as individualized or patient-centered by the patients themselves and that the education should be tailored to the patients' needs and goals [105,106]. The lack of owner compliance with veterinary recommendations can be challenging and a barrier to treatment success [107–109]. This can potentially be improved through the use of videos for home exercise programs that are common in canine rehabilitation as this approach has been shown to improve compliance in human medicine [110,111]. In addition to video-based instruction, follow-up calls or reminders via email of phone applications can also help improve compliance [112].

Support

Studies of human rehabilitation participants indicate that many people struggle with the transition from the hospital environment to the home environment [15,113–116]. Participants report having a hard time with integration of daily life tasks, difficulty implementing home rehabilitation and exercise plans, and experiencing social challenges. They believe that there is a need for more support after discharge. Although there are no studies detailing these challenges in the veterinary physical rehabilitation setting, it can be assumed that owners experience similar hardships when bringing a pet home after surgery or injury. The studies in human rehabilitation suggest using patient follow-up phone calls as a method of providing additional postdischarge support, but they note that what constitutes an optimal design for follow-up support is not clear [15,113–116]. Leveraging the veterinary care team to assist in predetermined follow-up protocols, such as phone calls and emails to check in with the owner regarding the care and status of their pet, may help to improve owner satisfaction and compliance.

SUMMARY

Although physical rehabilitation in human medicine has been, and often remains, disease- and function-based, efforts to incorporate the patient and their family/caregivers into the plan of care and treatment objectives have led to improved outcomes and patient satisfaction. In companion animal rehabilitation, physical rehabilitation should be centered over the patient's response and the owner's objectives. Patient-centered physical rehabilitation will likely enhance the experience and outcome for both the patient and its owner.

CLINICS CARE POINTS

- When taking a patient-centered approach to physical rehabilitation planning in companion animals, the process must incorporate the clinician, the owner, and the patient with collaboration and communication at the forefront. The clinician assesses the patient's medical problems and provides the potential management approaches. The owner expresses their needs, preferences, expectations, motivations, and resources. The patient's profile, prior training, and behavior must be considered and influence therapy choices.
- The goals of therapy should be based on meaningful daily activities that the patient needs to be able to perform and should be developed collaboratively with the pet owner. The outcome measures of therapy assess these specific goals.
- Challenges to implementation of therapy are explored at the onset of therapy and a coping plan is made. Therapy is adapted to address both the facilitators and barriers to care.
- Treatments are individualized to minimize the burden of care on the owner and patient.
- Clinic protocols should be developed to ensure that owner education, ongoing communication, and follow-up are consistent.

DISCLOSURE

The authors have nothing to disclose.

REFERENCES

[1] Morgan S, Yoder LH. A concept analysis of person-centered care. J Holist Nurs 2012;30(1):6–15.
[2] McCormack B. A conceptual framework for person-centred practice with older people. Int J Nurs Pract 2003;9(3):202–9.
[3] Yun D, Choi J. Person-centered rehabilitation care and outcomes: A systematic literature review. Int J Nurs Stud 2019;93:74–83.
[4] Wijma AJ, Bletterman AN, Clark JR, et al. Patient-centeredness in physiotherapy: What does it entail? A systematic review of qualitative studies. Physiother Theory Pract 2017;33(11):825–40.
[5] Hansen LS, Præstegaard J, Lehn-Christiansen S. Patient-centeredness in Physiotherapy - A literature mapping review. Physiother Theory Pract 2022;38(12):1843–56.
[6] Olsson L-E, Jakobsson Ung E, Swedberg K, et al. Efficacy of person-centred care as an intervention in controlled trials - a systematic review. J Clin Nurs 2013;22(3–4):456–65.
[7] Larsson I, Fridlund B, Arvidsson B, et al. OP0204-HPR Biological therapy can be monitored more cost effectively by a nurse-led rheumatology clinic. Ann Rheum Dis 2014;73(Suppl 2):139–40.
[8] Moore CL, Kaplan SL. A framework and resources for shared decision making: opportunities for improved physical therapy outcomes. Phys Ther 2018;98(12):1022–36.
[9] Baltzer WI. Rehabilitation of companion animals following orthopaedic surgery. N Z Vet J 2020;68(3):157–67.
[10] Marcellin-Little DJ, Levine D, Millis DL. Multifactorial rehabilitation planning in companion animals. Advances in Small Animal Care 2021;2:1–10.
[11] Mosley C, Edwards T, Romano L, et al. Proposed Canadian consensus guidelines on osteoarthritis treatment based on OA-COAST stages 1-4. Front Vet Sci 2022;9:830098.
[12] Frank LR, Roynard PFP. Veterinary neurologic rehabilitation: the rationale for a comprehensive approach. Top Companion Anim Med 2018;33(2):49–57.
[13] Kirkby Shaw K, Alvarez L, Foster SA, et al. Fundamental principles of rehabilitation and musculoskeletal tissue healing. Vet Surg 2020;49(1):22–32.
[14] Melin J, Nordin Å, Feldthusen C, et al. Goal-setting in physiotherapy: exploring a person-centered perspective. Physiother Theory Pract 2021;37(8):863–80.
[15] Eggen L, Thuesen J. Goals and action plans across time and place - A qualitative study exploring the importance of "context" in person-centered rehabilitation. Front Rehabil Sci 2022;3:788080.
[16] Kang E, Kim MY, Lipsey KL, et al. Person-centered goal setting: A systematic review of intervention components and level of active engagement in rehabilitation goal-setting interventions. Arch Phys Med Rehabil 2022;103(1):121–30.e3.
[17] Hutting N, Caneiro JP, Ong'wen OM, et al. Patient-centered care in musculoskeletal practice: Key elements to support clinicians to focus on the person. Musculoskelet Sci Pract 2022;57:102434.
[18] Daluiso-King G, Hebron C. Is the biopsychosocial model in musculoskeletal physiotherapy adequate? An evolutionary concept analysis. Physiother Theory Pract 2022;38(3):373–89.
[19] Hutting N, Caneiro JP, Ong'wen OM, et al. Person-centered care for musculoskeletal pain: Putting principles into practice. Musculoskelet Sci Pract 2022;62:102663.
[20] van den Heuvel C, van der Horst J, Winkelhorst E, et al. Experiences, barriers and needs of physiotherapists with regard to providing self-management support to people with low back pain: A qualitative study. Musculoskelet Sci Pract 2021;56:102462.

[21] Unsgaard-Tøndel M, Søderstrøm S. Building therapeutic alliances with patients in treatment for low back pain: A focus group study. Physiother Res Int 2022; 27(1):e1932.

[22] Küper AM, Merle R. Being nice Is not enough - Exploring relationship-centered veterinary care with structural equation modeling. A quantitative study on German pet owners' perception. Front Vet Sci 2019;6: 56.

[23] Merle R, Küper AM. Attitude of veterinarians toward self-Informed animal owners affects shared decision making. Front Vet Sci 2021;8:692452.

[24] Küeper AM, Merle R. Partners in sickness and in health? Relationship-centered veterinary care and self-educated pet owners in Germany: A structural equation model. Front Vet Sci 2020;7:605631.

[25] Ekman I, Swedberg K, Taft C, et al. Person-centered care – Ready for prime time. Eur J Cardiovasc Nurs 2011; 10(4):248–51.

[26] McColl MA, Denis CB, Douglas K-L, et al. A clinically significant difference on the COPM: A review. Can J Occup Ther 2023;90(1):92–102.

[27] Bordin ES. The generalizability of the psychoanalytic concept of the working alliance. Psychother Theory Res Pract 1979;16(3):252–60.

[28] Kinney M, Seider J, Beaty AF, et al. The impact of therapeutic alliance in physical therapy for chronic musculoskeletal pain: A systematic review of the literature. Physiother Theory Pract 2020;36(8):886–98.

[29] Bright FAS, Boland P, Rutherford SJ, et al. Implementing a client-centred approach in rehabilitation: an autoethnography. Disabil Rehabil 2012;34(12): 997–1004.

[30] McCabe E, Miciak M, Roduta Roberts M, et al. Development of the physiotherapy therapeutic relationship measure. Eur J Physiother 2022;24(5):287–96.

[31] Miciak M, Mayan M, Brown C, et al. The necessary conditions of engagement for the therapeutic relationship in physiotherapy: an interpretive description study. Arch Physiother 2018;8:3.

[32] Ferreira PH, Ferreira ML, Maher CG, et al. The therapeutic alliance between clinicians and patients predicts outcome in chronic low back pain. Phys Ther 2013; 93(4):470–8.

[33] Adams CL, Frankel RM. It may be a dog's life but the relationship with her owners is also key to her health and well being: communication in veterinary medicine. Vet Clin North Am Small Anim Pract 2007;37(1):1–17 [abstract: vii].

[34] Bellows J, Young S, Chase A. Person-focused care at Kaiser Permanente. Perm J 2014;90–1. https://doi.org/10.7812/TPP/13-165.

[35] Lin I, Wiles L, Waller R, et al. What does best practice care for musculoskeletal pain look like? Eleven consistent recommendations from high-quality clinical practice guidelines: systematic review. Br J Sports Med 2020; 54(2):79–86.

[36] Pinto RZ, Ferreira ML, Oliveira VC, et al. Patient-centred communication is associated with positive therapeutic alliance: a systematic review. J Physiother 2012;58(2): 77–87.

[37] Silverman J, Kurtz S, Draper J. Skills for Communicating with Patients. 3rd ed. CRC Press; 2013. https://doi.org/10.1201/9781910227268.

[38] O'Daniel M, Rosenstein AH. Professional communication and team collaboration. In: Hughes RG, editor. Patient Safety and quality: an evidence-based Handbook for Nurses. Advances in patient safety. Rockville, MD: Agency for Healthcare Research and Quality (US); 2008. p. 271–81.

[39] Rosewilliam S, Roskell CA, Pandyan AD. A systematic review and synthesis of the quantitative and qualitative evidence behind patient-centred goal setting in stroke rehabilitation. Clin Rehabil 2011;25(6):501–14.

[40] Leach E, Cornwell P, Fleming J, et al. Patient centered goal-setting in a subacute rehabilitation setting. Disabil Rehabil 2010;32(2):159–72.

[41] Smit EB, Bouwstra H, Hertogh CM, et al. Goal-setting in geriatric rehabilitation: a systematic review and meta-analysis. Clin Rehabil 2019;33(3):395–407.

[42] Millis DL, Ciuperca IA. Evidence for canine rehabilitation and physical therapy. Vet Clin North Am Small Anim Pract 2015;45(1):1–27.

[43] Frye C, Carr BJ, Lenfest M, et al. Canine geriatric rehabilitation: considerations and strategies for assessment, functional scoring, and follow up. Front Vet Sci 2022; 9:842458.

[44] Montalbano C. Canine comprehensive mobility assessment. Vet Clin North Am Small Anim Pract 2022;52(4): 841–56.

[45] Gingerich DA, Strobel JD. Use of client-specific outcome measures to assess treatment effects in geriatric, arthritic dogs: controlled clinical evaluation of a nutraceutical. Vet Ther 2003;4(4):376–86.

[46] Hercock CA, Pinchbeck G, Giejda A, et al. Validation of a client-based clinical metrology instrument for the evaluation of canine elbow osteoarthritis. J Small Anim Pract 2009;50(6):266–71.

[47] Hielm-Björkman AK, Rita H, Tulamo R-M. Psychometric testing of the Helsinki chronic pain index by completion of a questionnaire in Finnish by owners of dogs with chronic signs of pain caused by osteoarthritis. Am J Vet Res 2009;70(6):727–34.

[48] Innes JF, Morton MA, Lascelles BDX. Minimal clinically-important differences for the "Liverpool Osteoarthritis in Dogs" (LOAD) and the "Canine Orthopedic Index" (COI) client-reported outcomes measures. PLoS One 2023;18(2):e0280912.

[49] Brown DC. The Canine Orthopedic Index. Step 1: Devising the items. Vet Surg 2014;43(3):232–40.

[50] Brown DC, Boston RC, Coyne JC, et al. Development and psychometric testing of an instrument designed to measure chronic pain in dogs with osteoarthritis. Am J Vet Res 2007;68(6):631–7.

[51] Reid J, Nolan AM, Scott EM. Measuring pain in dogs and cats using structured behavioural observation. Vet J 2018;236:72–9.

[52] Reid J, Wiseman-Orr L, Scott M. Shortening of an existing generic online health-related quality of life instrument for dogs. J Small Anim Pract 2018;59(6):334–42.

[53] Hall SS, Brown BJ, Mills DS. Developing and assessing the validity of a scale to assess pet dog quality of life: Lincoln P-QoL. Front Vet Sci 2019;6:326.

[54] Roberts C, Armson B, Bartram D, et al. Construction of a conceptual framework for assessment of health-related quality of life in dogs with osteoarthritis. Front Vet Sci 2021;8:741864.

[55] Chen FL, Ullal TV, Graves JL, et al. Evaluating instruments for assessing healthspan: a multi-center cross-sectional study on health-related quality of life (HRQL) and frailty in the companion dog. Geroscience 2023. https://doi.org/10.1007/s11357-023-00744-2.

[56] Levack WMM, Weatherall M, Hay-Smith EJC, et al. Goal setting and strategies to enhance goal pursuit for adults with acquired disability participating in rehabilitation. Cochrane Database Syst Rev 2015;2015(7):CD009727.

[57] Giuffrida MA, Brown DC, Ellenberg SS, et al. Development and psychometric testing of the Canine Owner-Reported Quality of Life questionnaire, an instrument designed to measure quality of life in dogs with cancer. J Am Vet Med Assoc 2018;252(9):1073–83.

[58] Hielm-Björkman AK, Kuusela E, Liman A, et al. Evaluation of methods for assessment of pain associated with chronic osteoarthritis in dogs. J Am Vet Med Assoc 2003;222(11):1552–8.

[59] Jaeger G, Marcellin-Little DJ, Levine D. Reliability of goniometry in Labrador Retrievers. Am J Vet Res 2002;63(7):979–86.

[60] Clarke E, Aulakh KS, Hudson C, et al. Effect of sedation or general anesthesia on elbow goniometry and thoracic limb circumference measurements in dogs with naturally occurring elbow osteoarthritis. Vet Surg 2020;49(7):1428–36.

[61] Sabanci SS, Ocal MK. Comparison of goniometric measurements of the stifle joint in seven breeds of normal dogs. Vet Comp Orthop Traumatol 2016;29(3):214–9.

[62] Kim AY, Elam LH, Lambrechts NE, et al. Appendicular skeletal muscle mass assessment in dogs: a scoping literature review. BMC Vet Res 2022;18(1):280.

[63] McCarthy DA, Millis DL, Levine D, et al. Variables affecting thigh girth measurement and observer reliability in dogs. Front Vet Sci 2018;5:203.

[64] Freund KA, Kieves NR, Hart JL, et al. Assessment of novel digital and smartphone goniometers for measurement of canine stifle joint angles. Am J Vet Res 2016;77(7):749–55.

[65] Horak FB, Wrisley DM, Frank J. The Balance Evaluation Systems Test (BESTest) to differentiate balance deficits. Phys Ther 2009;89(5):484–98.

[66] Bohannon RW, Tudini F. Unipedal balance test for older adults: a systematic review and meta-analysis of studies providing normative data. Physiotherapy 2018;104(4):376–82.

[67] Podsiadlo D, Richardson S. The timed "Up & Go": A test of basic functional mobility for frail elderly persons. J Am Geriatr Soc 1991;39(2):142–8.

[68] Perry J, Weiss WB, Burnfield JM, et al. The supine hip extensor manual muscle test: a reliability and validity study. Arch Phys Med Rehabil 2004;85(8):1345–50.

[69] Millor N, Lecumberri P, Gómez M, et al. An evaluation of the 30-s chair stand test in older adults: frailty detection based on kinematic parameters from a single inertial unit. J NeuroEng Rehabil 2013;10:86.

[70] Bohannon RW. Sit-to-stand test for measuring performance of lower extremity muscles. Percept Mot Skills 1995;80(1):163–6.

[71] Riediger M, Freund AM. Interference and facilitation among personal goals: differential associations with subjective well-being and persistent goal pursuit. Pers Soc Psychol Bull 2004;30(12):1511–23.

[72] Adelman RD, Tmanova LL, Delgado D, et al. Caregiver burden: a clinical review. JAMA 2014;311(10):1052–60.

[73] Spitznagel MB, Cox MD, Jacobson DM, et al. Assessment of caregiver burden and associations with psychosocial function, veterinary service use, and factors related to treatment plan adherence among owners of dogs and cats. J Am Vet Med Assoc 2019;254(1):124–32.

[74] Spitznagel MB, Anderson JR, Marchitelli B, et al. Owner quality of life, caregiver burden and anticipatory grief: How they differ, why it matters. Vet Rec 2021;188(9):e74.

[75] Spitznagel MB, Patrick K, Gober MW, et al. Relationships among owner consideration of euthanasia, caregiver burden, and treatment satisfaction in canine osteoarthritis. Vet J 2022;286:105868.

[76] Spitznagel MB, Mueller MK, Fraychak T, et al. Validation of an abbreviated instrument to assess veterinary client caregiver burden. J Vet Intern Med 2019;33(3):1251–9.

[77] Spitznagel MB, Jacobson DM, Cox MD, et al. Caregiver burden in owners of a sick companion animal: a cross-sectional observational study. Vet Rec 2017;181(12):321.

[78] Flint HE, Atkinson M, Lush J, et al. Long-lasting chews elicit positive emotional states in dogs during short periods of social isolation. Animals (Basel) 2023;13(4). https://doi.org/10.3390/ani13040552.

[79] Rooney N, Gaines S, Hiby E. A practitioner's guide to working dog welfare. J Vet Behav 2009;4(3):127–34.

[80] Rooney NJ, Clark CCA, Casey RA. Minimizing fear and anxiety in working dogs: A review. J Vet Behav 2016;16:53–64.

[81] Wells DL. A review of environmental enrichment for kennelled dogs, Canis familiaris. Appl Anim Behav Sci 2004;85(3–4):307–17.

[82] Schipper LL, Vinke CM, Schilder MBH, et al. The effect of feeding enrichment toys on the behaviour of

kennelled dogs (Canis familiaris). Appl Anim Behav Sci 2008;114(1–2):182–95.

[83] Wallis L.J., Range F., Kubinyi E., et al., Utilising dog-computer interactions to provide mental stimulation in dogs especially during ageing. In: Proceedings of the Fourth International Conference on Animal-Computer Interaction - ACI2017. November 21 - 23, 2017; Milton Keynes, United Kingdom, ACM Press; 2017:1-12. https://doi.org/10.1145/3152130.3152146.

[84] Murtagh K, Farnworth MJ, Brilot BO. The scent of enrichment: Exploring the effect of odour and biological salience on behaviour during enrichment of kennelled dogs. Appl Anim Behav Sci 2020;223:104917.

[85] Amaya V, Paterson MBA, Phillips CJC. Effects of olfactory and auditory enrichment on the behaviour of shelter dogs. Animals (Basel) 2020;10(4). https://doi.org/10.3390/ani10040581.

[86] Hunt RL, Whiteside H, Prankel S. Effects of environmental enrichment on dog behaviour: pilot study. Animals (Basel) 2022;12(2). https://doi.org/10.3390/ani12020141.

[87] Flaherty MJ. Therapy exercises following cranial cruciate ligament repair in dogs. Vet Clin North Am Small Anim Pract 2023. https://doi.org/10.1016/j.cvsm.2023.02.013.

[88] Drum MG, Marcellin-Little DJ, Davis MS. Principles and applications of therapeutic exercises for small animals. Vet Clin North Am Small Anim Pract 2015;45(1):73–90.

[89] Vermunt NP, Harmsen M, Elwyn G, et al. A three-goal model for patients with multimorbidity: A qualitative approach. Health Expect 2018;21(2):528–38.

[90] Elwyn G, Edwards A, Wensing M, et al. Shared decision making: developing the OPTION scale for measuring patient involvement. Qual Saf Health Care 2003; 12(2):93–9.

[91] Spatz ES, Krumholz HM, Moulton BW. Prime time for shared decision making. JAMA 2017;317(13):1309–10.

[92] Bomhof-Roordink H, Gärtner FR, Stiggelbout AM, et al. Key components of shared decision making models: a systematic review. BMJ Open 2019;9(12): e031763.

[93] Syed H, Zubaria K, Tanoli AQ, et al. Conceptual approach of shared decision making in physical therapy: An approach for betterment of patients? Int J Endorsing Health Sci Res (IJEHSR) 2019;7(3):131.

[94] Elwyn G, Vermunt NPCA. Goal-based shared decision-making: Developing an integrated model. J Patient Exp 2020;7(5):688–96.

[95] Stevens A, Köke A, van der Weijden T, et al. The development of a patient-specific method for physiotherapy goal setting: a user-centered design. Disabil Rehabil 2018;40(17):2048–55.

[96] Overview | Shared decision making | Guidance | NICE. Available at: https://www.nice.org.uk/guidance/ng197. Accessed April 13, 2023.

[97] Stacey D, Légaré F, Col NF, et al. Decision aids for people facing health treatment or screening decisions. Cochrane Database Syst Rev 2014;1:CD001431.

[98] Skinner BF. Contingencies of reinforcement: a Theoretical analysis (B. F. Skinner Reprint Series; Edited by Julie S. Vargas Book 3). Acton MA: Copley Publishing Group; 2014. p. 325.

[99] Vieira de Castro AC, Fuchs D, Morello GM, et al. Does training method matter? Evidence for the negative impact of aversive-based methods on companion dog welfare. PLoS One 2020;15(12):e0225023.

[100] Casey RA, Naj-Oleari M, Campbell S, et al. Dogs are more pessimistic if their owners use two or more aversive training methods. Sci Rep 2021;11(1):19023.

[101] Deldalle S, Gaunet F. Effects of 2 training methods on stress-related behaviors of the dog (Canis familiaris) and on the dog–owner relationship. J Vet Behav 2014; 9(2):58–65.

[102] Fear Free Pets - Taking the "Pet" Out of "Petrified" for All Animals. Available at: https://fearfreepets.com. Accessed April 13, 2023.

[103] Schollen M. Research report: The relationship between education and age on pet ownership in the Netherlands. December 2014. Available at: https://edepot.wur.nl/328813. Accessed April 13, 2023.

[104] Providing Education to Pet Owner. Available at: https://www.aaha.org/aaha-guidelines/2021-aaha-nutrition-and-weight-management-guidelines/practice-opportunities/opportunities-and-resources-to-leverage-the-value-of-proper-nutrition-in-your-practice/. Accessed April 13, 2023.

[105] Cooper K, Smith BH, Hancock E. Patient-centredness in physiotherapy from the perspective of the chronic low back pain patient. Physiotherapy 2008;94(3): 244–52.

[106] Kidd MO, Bond CH, Bell ML. Patients' perspectives of patient-centredness as important in musculoskeletal physiotherapy interactions: a qualitative study. Physiotherapy 2011;97(2):154–62.

[107] Kamleh M, Khosa DK, Verbrugghe A, et al. A cross-sectional study of pet owners' attitudes and intentions towards nutritional guidance received from veterinarians. Vet Rec 2020;187(12):e123.

[108] Eschle S, Hartmann K, Rieger A, et al. Canine vaccination in Germany: A survey of owner attitudes and compliance. PLoS One 2020;15(8):e0238371.

[109] Porsani MYH, Teixeira FA, Amaral AR, et al. Factors associated with failure of dog's weight loss programmes. Vet Med Sci 2020;6(3):299–305.

[110] Toci GR, Green A, Mubin N, et al. Patient adherence with at-home hand and wrist exercises: A randomized controlled trial of video versus handout format. Hand (N Y) 2021. https://doi.org/10.1177/15589447211052750 15589447211052750.

[111] Katt BM, Tawfik AM, Imbergamo C, et al. Patient comprehension of operative instructions with a paper handout versus a video: A prospective randomized control trial. J Hand Surg Am 2023;48(3):311.e1–8.

[112] Yaşarer Ö, Yilmaz HG, Doğan H. Comparison of two different delivery methods of home-based exercise on

neck pain. Somatosens Mot Res 2023;1–8. https://doi.org/10.1080/08990220.2023.2194389.

[113] Dager TN, Kjeken I, Berdal G, et al. Rehabilitation for patients with rheumatic diseases: Patient experiences of a structured goal planning and tailored follow-up programme. SAGE Open Med 2017;5:2050312117739786.

[114] Hamnes B, Berdal G, Bø I, et al. Patients' experiences with goal pursuit after discharge from rheumatology rehabilitation: A qualitative study. Muscoskel Care 2021;19(3):249–58.

[115] Wade D. Rehabilitation - a new approach. Part four: a new paradigm, and its implications. Clin Rehabil 2016;30(2):109–18.

[116] Stauner M, Primdahl J. A sanctuary from everyday life: rheumatology patients' experiences of in-patient multidisciplinary rehabilitation - a qualitative study. Disabil Rehabil 2022;44(10):1872–9.

Advances in Small Animal Care 4 (2023) 37–52

ADVANCES IN SMALL ANIMAL CARE

Clinical Instruments for the Evaluation of Orthopedic Problems in Dogs and Human Patients, a Review

Heli K. Hyytiäinen, PT, MSc, PhD[a],*, David Levine, PT, PhD, MPH, DPT, CCRP[b], Denis J. Marcellin-Little, DEDV, DACVS, DACVSMR[c]

[a]Department of Equine and Small Animal Medicine, Faculty of Veterinary Medicine, University of Helsinki, PO Box 57 (Viikintie 49), 00014 Helsinki, Finland; [b]Department of Physical Therapy, University of Tennessee at Chattanooga, 615 McCallie Avenue, Chattanooga, TN 37403, USA; [c]Veterinary Orthopedic Research Laboratory, School of Veterinary Medicine, University of California, 1285 Veterinary Medicine DR, VM3A Room 4206, Davis, CA 95616, USA

KEYWORDS

• Assessment methods   • Outcome measurement tools   • Quantification   • Physiotherapy   • One health

KEY POINTS

- When investigating orthopedic problems in dogs, questions for owners can be combined to form specific questionnaires. Several physical tests can also be combined to form specific testing instruments.
- These questionnaires and instruments can be validated to make sure that have acceptable accuracy and consistency.
- In human patients, outcomes assessing most orthopedic diagnoses and treatment procedures include the use of one validated instrument or more.
- In dogs, the use of validated instruments to evaluate the severity of a problem and the response to therapy is increasing.

The collection of measurements of musculoskeletal function in dogs is critically important to diagnose problems, to evaluate the severity of these problems, and to assess their progression and response to therapy. Measurements are often grouped to form standardized sets of questions or tests that can be validated for accuracy and consistency within and among observers. These sets of questions or tests are referred to as instruments or batteries to be completed by owners (questionnaires) and clinicians (instruments). Some components of instruments are objective in nature, and others are subjective. These components quantify patient impairments, for example, the pain response to palpation or joint motion, lack of joint motion, or loss of muscle mass. These measurements ensure that the initial assessment is complete and inform future

evaluations. The difference between the findings of the same instruments over time represents disease progression or response to therapy.

PSYCHOMETRIC PROPERTIES OF INSTRUMENTS

Clinicians select instruments with attention to their relevance to the problem being treated, their validity, reliability, responsiveness, and their convenience. Instrument validity (*are the results true?*) and reliability (*are the results similar when the instrument is used by several observers or by one observer over time?*) should be evaluated to fully validate an instrument. These characteristics of instruments are named psychometric characteristics.

*Corresponding author, *E-mail address:* heli.hyytiainen@helsinki.fi

---

https://doi.org/10.1016/j.yasa.2023.05.007

The validity of an instrument is critically important [1]. Validity includes face validity (*does the instrument make sense for what is being evaluated?*) and content validity (*does the instrument include all aspects of what is being evaluated and nothing more?*). The sensitivity of a test describes the test's ability to detect a problem when it is present. Its specificity describes the test's ability to rule out the problem when it is absent [2]. Validity, sensitivity, and specificity are tested by comparing the results of the measurement tool with the results of other, already validated, gold standard measurement method(s). The purpose of the test dictates the appropriate level and proportions between sensitivity and specificity: a sensitivity of 90% means that 10% of problems will go undetected, and a specificity of 90% means that 10% of detected problems are actually not a problem. Clinicians should take test sensitivity and specificity into account when interpreting the results of measurements.

The intra-rater repeatability, also named intraobserver repeatability, is the comparison of repeated evaluations of the same patient collected by one rater over a relatively short period of time, a process also named *test-retest*. Repeatability provides information about the sensitivity of an instrument [3]. When testing repeatability, differences among measurements are due to the instrument itself and to the procedure used to collect information. The interobserver reproducibility, also named consistency or inter-rater reliability, is the comparison of evaluations of the same patient collected by several raters. Reproducibility provides information about differences in interpretation among raters. Because observers vary in their personality and experience level and because the evaluation of reproducibility includes repeated measurements with their own repeatability, the repeatability of an instrument should be higher than its reproducibility. Repeatability and reproducibility are calculated as intraclass correlation coefficient (ICC) values, ranging from 0 (worst reliability) to 1 (perfect reliability). In human medicine, ICC values < 0.50 are considered to represent poor reliability, values $\geq$ 0.50 and less than 0.75 are considered to represent moderate reliability, values $\geq$ 0.75 and less than 0.90 are considered to represent good reliability, and values $\geq$ 0.90 are considered to represent excellent reliability [4]. The capacity of an instrument to detect change over time is named responsiveness [5]. Responsiveness is an important aspect of an instrument when it is intended to evaluated the outcome of an intervention.

Instrument validation also includes a comparison to another testing method, for example, a comparison to another instrument or other objective test. For example, in orthopedics, an instrument can be compared with an objective measure of limb use, such as the forces generated on force plates at a trot [6]. This type of validation is named cross-validation or parallel testing, because the results of 2 tests are collected in parallel. Validity and reliability are related to each other, but are not dependent on each other. Test that have a low reliability are not valid. To be reliable, tests should be consistent (precise) and accurate (free from bias). Tests can have a ceiling effect, where most test results are clustered at the upper end of scale, or a floor effect, where results are clustered at the lower end of the scale. Floor and ceiling effect indicate a lack of criterion validity, where the parameters measured are either too stringent or too lenient to detect changes over time. The minimum clinically important difference (MCID) is the smallest change in instrument results that represent a perceived positive or negative patient impact [7]. The measurement of MCID is dogs is made more challenging than in people by their nonverbal nature. However, information regarding the MCID of instruments used to evaluate dogs is emerging [8].

GENERAL EVALUATION OF DOG HEALTH AND MOBILITY

Several instruments are used to measure dogs' health and mobility. These are observational, often based on subjective assessments of the dog's behavior and function or locomotion, commonly in questionnaire format, directed to the owner or the clinician. These instruments have been systematically reviewed [9–11].

The Canine Brief Pain Inventory (CBPI) was introduced in 2007 to assess pain in patients with osteoarthritis (OA) [12]. The CBPI has 10 questions regarding the severity of the dog's pain and their effects function, each graded on scale from 0 to 10 and 1 question regarding the dog's overall quality of life, graded from 1 to 5. The CBPI has good validity, reliability, and responsiveness [12–14]. The Swedish version of the CBPI has been validated [15]. Criterion and construct validity of the CBPI has been further assessed against other equivalent instruments (visual analog scale [VAS], Liverpool Osteoarthritis in Dogs [LOAD] questionnaire, and Canine Orthopedic Index [COI]), and shown to be acceptable [16]. The CBPI has also been validated in French, Italian, and Portuguese [17–19], and a generic linguistic validation of the instrument has been done for Australia, China, Germany, Hungary, Ireland, Japan, Netherlands, and Portugal [20].

The Helsinki Chronic Pain Index (HCPI) was developed to measure chronic OA pain in dogs with OA, and introduced in 2009 based on preliminary work reported in 2003 [21,22]. The owner-directed HCPI consists of 11 questions regarding the dog's behavior and locomotion. The questions are answered on a 5-point scale (0–4), with a total score ranging from 0 to 44. The instrument has high predictive validity, internal consistency, and test-retest reliability (ICC 0.92), as well as high sensitivity [14,21]. This instrument is valid, reliable, and responsive, when tested on dogs with hip or elbow OA.

The owner-directed COI was developed and tested in 3 stages, reported in 2014 [23–25]. The instrument assesses stiffness, gait, function, and quality of life in dogs with OA with an acceptable level of validity and reliability [25]. Scoring is done through 16 questions, each scored on a qualitative 5-point scale. Unlike other test sections, the quality of life section of the test may not be responsive to nonsteroidal anti-inflammatory therapy [24]. The minimal clinically important difference (MCID) for COI has been suggested to be 14 [8]. Criterion and construct validity of the COI has been further assessed against other equivalent instruments (VAS, CBPI, and LOAD), and shown to be acceptable [16]. The COI has also been modified and translated to Swedish and validated as such [26]. That version had sufficient validity and reliability to be used in clinical practice in Swedish for dogs with chronic elbow OA. The criterion and construct validation of the Portuguese version of the COI have also been reported [27].

The LOAD is a questionnaire for owners of dogs with OA introduced in 2009 [28]. It had good reliability and was responsive, but its criterion validity was poor when tested in a cohort of dogs with OA of the elbow [28]. In another study in dogs with OA affecting various joints, its construct and criterion validity were deemed acceptable for clinical use [14]. Criterion and construct validity of the LOAD were further assessed against other equivalent instruments (VAS, CBPI, and COI) and were shown to be acceptable [16].

The LOAD assesses dog's mobility through 13 questions with 5-point scale descriptive answers, resulting in total score ranging from 0 to 52. The MCID for LOAD has been suggested to be 4 [8]. The LOAD has also been tested for its criterion and construct validity in Portuguese [29].

A VAS was reported to be a reliable and responsive method for assessing outcome after a surgical treatment of cranial cruciate ligament (CCL) deficiency in 1998 [30]. The VAS was deemed valid and with good repeatability when tested against the HCPI in 2011 [31]. The

authors concluded that a VAS is a reliable instrument to assessing chronic OA-related pain in dogs. However, at baseline, it may have poor face validity with untrained users (ie, with owners). In 2004, the VAS was applied to a 19-question questionnaire directed to owners regarding the function of their dog with a lameness [32]. The questionnaire was found to be valid and repeatable when assessing mild or moderate lameness. Criterion and construct validity of the Hudson's VAS has also been assessed against other equivalent instruments (CBPI, LOAD, and COI) and shown to be acceptable [16].

The Glasgow University Health-related Dog Behavior Questionnaire (GUVQuest), a quality of life-related questionnaire, was introduced in 2004 and validated in 2006 [33,34]. The questionnaire assesses dog's activity, pain, sociability, aggression, anxiety, enthusiasm, happiness, and mobility. It consists of 109 questions, each with 7-point answers. Another, generic quality of life questionnaire focused on wellbeing was introduced in 2022 [35]. It has 32 questions, related to day-time and feeding-time behaviors, querying whether the dog is energetic, mobile, happy, sociable, relaxed, interested, and satisfied. Scoring is done through 7-point scales. The questionnaire appears to have acceptable validity but needs to be further validated.

Several methods are used to evaluate the general physical performance of dogs. A Canine Timed Up and Go (CTUG) test, adapted from the human Time Up and Go test used to evaluate mobility, has been independently proposed by several authors [36,37]. In one validation study where dogs rose from a recumbent position and walked 7 m (23 feet), the test had acceptable intra- and inter-tester repeatability [36]. However, the responsiveness and floor and ceiling effects of the CTUG have not evaluated. Similarly, a CTUG test was proposed where dogs were timed as they rose and walked 10 body lengths, but that test has not been validated [37].

Activity monitors have been used to evaluate mobility in dogs, for example, to estimate a response to the medical management of OA. In one study, activity counts increased by 20% when dogs with OA received a nonsteroidal anti-inflammatory drug but did not increase when they received a placebo [38]. Activity monitors are influenced by several factors, including where and how tightly they are worn; however, they lack precision and their validation remains limited [39].

Algometers have been used to evaluate pressure-pain (mechanical nociceptive) thresholds in dog limbs. In one study, a modified algometer was validated during an intervention (morphine and saline in a cross-over study). Pressure-pain thresholds were tested on metacarpal and metatarsal pads, the tibia, the femur, and the abdomen [40]. The tests were described as repeatable but information about validity was limited.

The distribution of weight among dog limbs (ie, location of the center of mass) while standing can be measured using scales. The accuracy of a pressure sensitive platform was confirmed in one study [41]. In a study describing weight distribution measurements collected from 20 normal dogs using a weight distribution platform, measurements had acceptable repeatability when methods were consistent [42]. In another study evaluating 46 dogs with naturally occurring pelvic limb lameness that used a different weight distribution platform, pelvic limb symmetry index measurements had acceptable repeatability, but forelimb stance measurements were not repeatable [43].

Kinetics of dog gait is also evaluated using force plates and pressure sensitive walkways. Primary outcome variables include peak vertical force, vertical impulse, and acceleration/deceleration. Symmetry indices can be calculated from primary variables. The accuracy of force plate measurements of dogs at a walk and trot has been well documented [44–46]. Measurements acquired using 1 or 2 force plates do not appear to differ [46,47]. Trial measurements are influenced by several factors, including but not limited to speed, speed changes, changes in head posture during trials, handler position, and constraint method [48]. For these reasons, trials are generally limited to dogs within a relatively limited body mass range (eg, 20–40 kg) and are conducted within a narrow range of speed (eg, 1.7–2.1 m/s) and speed change (± 0.5 m/s^2). Bilateral limb problems greatly complicate the analysis of the outcome measures of force plates measurements because symmetry indices may not change over time. In one review, the authors stated that "force plate data may be difficult to interpret in the presence of multiple arthritic joints" [49]. Pressure-sensitive walkways have also been validated, including through comparisons with force plates [50–53]. Their use to evaluate dog gait is increasing. Measurements are influenced by the speed, changes in posture during the trial, handler position and control, and type of force walkway cover [54].

JOINT-SPECIFIC INSTRUMENTS
Outcome measure scales for joint function, limb function, and quality of life are widely used in human medicine as functional baseline and to compare the effects of different treatments such as surgery, rehabilitation, medications, and other interventions. Outcome scales have been adapted for all joints. Some scales are filled by clinicians, requiring physical measurements, and others, without physical measurements, can be filled by patients (patient-reported outcome measures [PROM]). The scales with widest clinical use are described below.

Hip Joint
In human medicine, objective measures specific to the hip including passive range of motion (ROM) are commonly used to gather data on pain, function, motion, gait, and health-related quality of life (HRQOL). Some hip outcome measures are better suited to specific conditions such as OA, hip arthroscopy, postsurgical total hip arthroplasty or certain situations such as return to work, geriatric function, or athletic performance. The Harris hip score (HHS), first published in 1969 [55], was developed to assess the results of hip surgery and to evaluate hip disabilities in the adult population. Pain and impaired physical function are the 2 primary domains measured in the HHS. The HHS has been used in over 7500 human studies worldwide and is available open access [56,57]. The modified HHS was introduced in 2000. The clinician measurement domains such as ROM were removed to allow it to be used as a PROM [58]. In a systematic review of 59 studies, an unacceptable ceiling effect ($\geq 15\%$ of patients) was present in 31 studies (53% of studies), suggesting that the HHS is suboptimal to evaluate long-term outcomes [59].

The Oxford hip score (OHS), introduced in 1996 [60], was designed to assess outcomes after total hip arthroplasty (THA). The OHS measures patients' perceptions regarding pain and function. It was updated in 2007, introducing a new scoring system applicable across clinical settings. It is available open access [61,62]. The OHS is commonly used to evaluate hip OA [63]. Its ceiling effect appears lower than the HHS. It was responsive 1 year after THA surgery [64]. The Hip Disability and Osteoarthritis Outcome Score (HOOS) was published in 2003 as an extension of the Western Ontario and McMaster Universities Osteoarthritis Index (WOMAC) instrument to assess patient opinions on their hip conditions [65]. The HOOS can be used in adults with or without hip disability or OA. It freely available and validated in 2 versions (LK 1.1 and LK 2.0) [66,67]. The HOOS is valuable for active individuals, since it contains a *sports and recreational activities* subscale, in addition to 4 other subscales *(symptoms/stiffness, pain, function/daily living, function, and quality of life)* [68]. In a systematic review, the HOOS was recommended when following patients with hip OA over time [69]. The HOOS-PS, derived from the HOOS, was created as the result of an initiative between the Osteoarthritis Research Society International (OARSI) and Outcome Measures in Rheumatology (OMERACT) organizations to create a short and fast outcome measure using only 5 items from the 21-item HOOS [70]. These items included consist entirely of functional activities such as descending stairs and running, and are rated solely on the difficulty of performing them, with no rating of pain.

The International Hip Outcome Tool 33 (iHOT-33) [71] and a shortened version (iHOT-12) measure health-related quality of life following treatment of hip disorders in more active patients are commonly used after arthroscopic hip surgery [68]. Both the HOOS and iHOT-12 have good validity and responsiveness in patients undergoing arthroscopic hip surgery [68].

Pain and difficulty in functional activities impacting HRQOL are the common denominators in contemporary hip outcome measures to allow them to be completed quickly and independently by the patient without the need for objective measurements such as ROM or gait parameters. The activities of function and daily living included in the scales have been well validated in humans. Which activities might be included in canine scales, their reliability and validity, responsiveness, and floor and ceiling effects have not been investigated; however, these human scales give us insight into building useful canine hip scales in the future.

In dogs, no functional testing batteries are available specifically for hip joint-related dysfunction. Laxity of the hip joint can be evaluated with palpable or audible reduction of a subluxated femoral head during dorsal force being applied to the femur (Barlow sign), with added abduction (Ortolani sign) or through the lateral displacement of greater trochanter by more than 2 mm during manual limb translation or adduction (Barden's sign) [56]. However, these are diagnostic tests, and thus should not be used by other veterinary medicine professionals than veterinarians. A technique of measuring the ROM of the hip with a plastic universal goniometer was described, and its validity and intra-rater and inter-rater reliability were tested [72]. Reliability was tested against radiographs. The mean intra-rater variability in measurements was 3° (range, 1°–6°). Sedation did not influence the goniometric measurements [72]. Normal passive ROM has been reported for Labrador retrievers (50°–162°), German shepherd dogs (44°–155°), and

greyhounds (72°–128°) [72–74]. The decreased motion reported in the greyhound hip was most likely due to the fact that, in that study, the authors elected to keep the stifle joint in extension while the hip was being manipulated [73].

Knee (Stifle) Joint

In human medicine, the Lysholm Knee Scoring Scale (LKSS) was published in 1982 [75]. It was designed to evaluate knee stability after ligamentous surgical repair. An update was published in 1985 [76]. The LKSS can be freely accessed online [77]. The scale includes 8 items, varying from limping, locking, instability, inflammation/pain, and functional activities. The scores are interpreted from 0 (lowest) to 100 (best). A systematic review of 73 articles comparing 41 knee measures found that the LKSS had good validation and was best suited for generalized knee disorders [78]. Also, the scale has minimal administrative and respondent burden, and floor and ceiling effects are not problematic.

The Cincinnati Knee Rating System (CKRS) was originally published in 1999 [79]. It can be freely accessed online [80]. A modified version of the CKRS was created in 1990 The CKRS was designed for evaluation of patients after anterior cruciate ligament surgery [81]. The modified CKRS has 8 questions pertaining to symptoms, function, and activities of daily living. The Cincinnati Knee Rating System was found to demonstrate high test-retest reliability, validity, and did not possess any floor effects, and a ceiling effect in a small percentage of patients. The CKRS is an adequate choice for evaluating anterior cruciate ligament conditions.

The Lower Extremity Functional Scale (LEFS) was developed in 1999 with the purpose of determining an individual's lower extremity functionality [82]. The LEFS includes 20 items, each with a maximum score of 4, denoting a full score of 80 that represents high function. A systematic review of 27 articles found good test-retest reliability, high internal consistency, and no floor or ceiling effects in various populations [83]. Of this systematic review, the most common populations studied have been hip OA, knee OA, total knee replacement, and THA. The LEFS is a versatile tool that can be applied to generalize to numerous lower extremity conditions. The LEFS can be freely accessed online [84].

The Knee Injury and Osteoarthritis Outcome Score (KOOS) was published in 1998 and includes 42 items divided among pain, symptoms, activities of daily living, sport, and quality of life. Items are scored from none (0) to extreme (4) [85]. The KOOS has been found to have adequate validity, reliability, psychometric qualities, and responsiveness. Further, it is a useful patient-reported tool to gauge knee function in individuals with knee OA, and combinations of ACL, meniscus, and cartilage injury. The KOOS can be freely accessed online [86]. Versions of KOOS have been tailored to children, joint replacement, patellofemoral pain, and physical function. These have also been found to be responsive.

In dogs, measurements of the ROM of the stifle joint with universal goniometer were found to be reliable [72]. Landmarks for the measurement were defined, and the ROM was measured with the dog in lateral recumbency. Passive ROM of the stifle has been reported to vary between breeds (Table 1) [72,74,87–89]. Limb circumference has been measured using a tape measure to indirectly evaluate hind limb muscle mass in dogs. Validity has been examined in several studies. The reliability of that method is questionable overall, because several factors affect it: the type of tape measure, the presence or absence of haircoat, limb position, and the site of measurement [90,91]. Some studies reported high intra- and inter-rater reliability when confounding factors are controlled [90]. Other studies found otherwise [91–93]. In one study, limb circumference was considered less sensitive than ultrasound measurements of thigh muscle thickness on the proximal and lateral aspect of the thigh [94]. Sedation does not seem to affect thigh circumference measurements [90]. Inter-rater reliability was poor in one study: variations

in measurements were 3.6 times higher than intra-rater variation [92]. This high variability could be controlled by having measurements collected by a single rater and, since tape measures vary, by using a single type of tape measure. In 2012, bathroom scales were found to be a reliable method for assessing distribution of static weight bearing between hind limbs in dogs with stifle OA [95]. The intra-rater repeatability of measurements was high (81%) in limbs with OA and was substantial (70%) in healthy limbs. The method had high specificity (85%) but low sensitivity (40%).

In addition to measurement of passive ROM with universal goniometer and the static weight bearing, in 2013, the validity and sensitivity of 9 other commonly used clinical individual assessment methods was also studied in relation to stifle pathologies [96]. The ability of the methods to recognize stifle joints with surgically treated CCL injury and with stifle OA from healthy stifle joint was tested. The assessment of muscle atrophy, evaluation of asymmetry in a sitting and lying position and symmetry of thrust up from these positions, manual and measured static weight bearing, and measurement of stifle PROM were best. The validity of the methods was tested by comparing the results of them with the results of 6 gold standards (orthopedic examination, imaging assessment, and force platform analysis). Despite differences in agreement between the testing methods and the gold standard results, these methods ranked overall in the best half of the tested methods. Highest sensitivities (means above 65%) were seen in palpatory assessment of thigh muscle mass symmetry, assessment of symmetry of sitting position and symmetry of thrust up from sitting, and manual evaluation of static weight bearing. Lowest ranking methods with least sensitivity included visual lameness assessment, diagonal position on straight line locomotion, and walking up and down stairs [96].

Three functional testing batteries for stifle patients have been published. The first was the Finnish Canine Stifle Index (FCSI) published in 2018 [97]. The FCSI was developed based on the above-mentioned examination and testing of individual evaluation methods, and their validity, sensitivity, and ranking [96]. The FCSI applies to patients with any type of stifle dysfunction, regardless of the pathology. It consists of 8 tasks: visual evaluation of functional active ROM: sitting and lying positions, and symmetry of thrust up from these positions, manual evaluation of symmetry of thigh muscle mass, measurement of symmetry of static weight bearing between hind limbs, and measurement of stifle flexion and extension passive ROM with a universal goniometer. Each task has specific scoring system provided: some

TABLE 1
Mean Stifle Joint Flexion and Extension Across Breeds of Dogs

Breed	Stifle Flexion	Stifle Extension
Belgian Shepherd (Malinois)	29°	156°
Boxer	39°	159°
Doberman Pinscher	30°	164°
French Bulldog	59°	173°
German Shepherd dog	33°	153°
	34°	151°
Golden retriever	34°	156°
Labrador retriever	42°	162°
	38°	157°
Rottweiler	34°	154°
	45°	161°

tasks result in comparative 0 or 2 scores, some had scores 0 to 3, with a multiplier applied at the end to allow dogs to skip some tasks. The final total score varies from 0 to 263, where 0 is the best possible score and 263 the worst. There are 2 cut-off lines for the total score: scores from 0 to 60 are considered to represent adequate level of function, 60 to 120 compromised function, and 120 to 263 severely compromised function—the latter with high sensitivity (83%) and specificity (89%) [97,98]. The testing battery gives a score to both hind limbs, but as some of the tasks are comparative, the worst of the 2 limbs at the day of testing represents the actual result. Thus, it is directed to unilateral assessment, but can be used to evaluate patients with bilateral problems. The FCSI does not discriminate any sizes of breeds of dogs, and allows dogs to skip some of the tasks without it influencing the score and clinical interpretation. The FCSI has been tested for its validity, reliability, and responsiveness. Gold standards, against which the FCSI was tested, were orthopedic examination, radiological and force platform analysis, and a conclusive assessment (combination of previous). This was done in attempts to capture the functionality aspect to the gold standards, as directly functional gold standards did not otherwise exist in veterinary medicine yet. The sensitivity (90%) and specificity (90.5%) of the FCSI were both excellent. Cronbach's alpha for internal reliability of the FCSI score was adequate (0.727). The FCSI is responsive to change, and has also good inter-tester reliability, as well as moderate to good intraclass correlation (0.780). It has not been tested for floor or ceiling effects [97,98]. The testing battery is designed to be used by veterinarians and physical therapists, as it is noninvasive, not diagnostic and does not contain diagnostic tasks, but is purely a tool for assessing the level of stifle dysfunction. It is also an outcome measurement tool.

Another test for stifle patients, the Bologna Healing Stifle Injury Index (BHSII) was developed in 2019 [99]. This is a questionnaire format outcome measurement tool, designed for owners and clinicians of dogs who have gone through a surgical treatment of CCL injury. The questionnaire consists of 34 multiple choice questions, out of which 24 are for the owner of the dog, and 10 for the clinician treating the dog. Each question is answered with a score from 0 to 4, where 0 would indicate no problems, and 4 severe problems. The instrument was reported to be valid and reliable (ICC ≥ 0.9, Cronbach's alpha = 0.84 for the owner questionnaire section), have high accuracy, and show responsiveness based on assumed healing over time [99].

A third outcome measurement tool for stifle patients combining functional elements, the Stifle Function Score, was published in 2022 [100]. This testing battery is developed for unilateral CCL patients and consists of 14 assessments: limb use at a walk, limb use at a trot, lameness at a walk, lameness at a trot, stair climbing, sit-to-stand, dancing, pain response, stifle effusion, thigh circumference/muscle atrophy, stifle extension, stifle flexion, and cranial drawer/tibial thrust. Each assessment is scored either from 0 to 10 or 0 to 5, with final score of 0 to 100, where 100 is the best possible score. The Stifle Function Score was tested against ground reaction force-based symmetry index to confirm its validity [100]. This measurement tool has not been tested for reliability nor responsiveness. Interestingly, this testing battery contains several maneuvers (cranial drawer test, tibial thrust) that are generally considered diagnostic in veterinary medicine. Also, the reliability of these tests in nonsedated dogs appears suboptimal [101]. Dogs should be sedated to perform these reliably, which makes the test invasive and may decrease its applicability for use by nonveterinarians in clinical practice.

Ankle (Hock) Joint

The Foot and Ankle Ability Measure (FAAM) was published in 2005 to establish an accepted self-reported instrument for individuals with lower extremity disorders [102]. FAAM consists of a 21-item activities of daily living (ADL) and 8-item sports subscale. Each item is rated 4 to 0, ranging from no difficulty to inability to complete, with total collective scores ranging from 0 to 84. In a systematic review of 39 articles, FAAM received the most positive ratings for clinimetric evaluation in populations with a variety of foot and ankle problems [103]. Although more research is required, it appears FAAM may be useful for individuals with chronic ankle instability [103] and for patients undergoing ligament reconstruction [104]. There does not appear to be any floor or ceiling effect to the FAAM. A free pdf document of FAAM can be accessed online [105].

The Foot and Ankle Disability Index (FADI) was originally described in 1999 [106]. It consists of 22 functional items and 4 pain-related questions. The scoring is graded from 4 (done with no difficulty) to 0 (unable to do). The maximum score is 106, meaning full functionality. A systematic review of 669 articles found that FADI has been found to be sensitive and reliable with measuring outcomes in athletic populations with chronic ankle instability [107]. The FADI can be freely accessed online [108]. An alternative version, the FADI Sport, has also been published to identify deficits more specific to sport. The FADI Sport contains the same functional activities combined with more vigorous physical activities with the same scoring mechanism. The FADI Sport can be freely accessed online [109]. Both FADI and FADI sport appear sensitive and reliable.

The Bristol Foot Score (BFS) was published in 2005 in an attempt to produce a patient-centered assessment tool [110]. The BFS has 3 subscales composed of questions relating to pain, footwear, foot health, and mobility. There is a total of 15 items scored 1 (best) to 3 to 6 (worse) with a range of 15 (best) to 73 (worst). The BFS has limited psychometric properties and has unknown values for minimal detectable change. More research is required to properly validate BFS and, currently, its clinical utility may be limited [111].

The Foot and Ankle Module (FAM) was developed by the American Academy of Orthopedic Surgeons (AAOS). It was designed to evaluate patient perception of foot health and measure surgical outcomes [47] It consists of questions about pain, function, inflammation, and shoe comfort. The FAM includes 25 questions scored from 1 to 5 or 1 to 6, with 1 being best and 5 or 6 being worst [111]. The AAOS-FAM has been shown to have acceptable internal and a retest reliability comparable with other accepted outcome measures [112]. However, the tool does not account for psychological, efficacy, or quality of life components [111]. It is recommended that the FAM be used in conjunction with other outcome measures such as the Short Form 36 (SF-36) to ensure accurate measurements of the foot health effects on quality of life [111]. A free version for AAOS-FAM could not be readily found online.

In dogs, no specific tarsal evaluation method has been reported, beyond measurements of ROM in Labrador retrievers (39°–164°) and German Shepherd dogs (30°–149°) [72,74].

Shoulder Joint

The Disabilities of the Arm, Shoulder, and Hand (DASH) outcome measure was created in 1996 by the AAOS Outcomes Research Committee and the Institute for Work and Health [113]. DASH was created due to other outcome measures having too narrow or having too generalized patient perspective. DASH is designed to provide information on physical function and be applicable to a wide range of conditions of the upper extremity. The DASH includes 30 questions scored from 1 to 5. And the results are interpreted as 0 to 100, 0 representing no disability and 100 representing the maximal disability [114]. In a systematic review of 28 articles comparing 16 shoulder disability outcome measures, DASH received the highest clinimetric properties

[115]. These properties included a checklist analyzing validity, responsiveness, practical burden, and interpretability. In addition, DASH had no floor or ceiling effect. This suggests that the versatility of DASH allows for the use of a variety of shoulder conditions. The QuickDASH alternative outcome tool was produced in 2005 with 11 questions designed to be more efficient while maintaining measurement properties [116,117]. The QuickDASH is effective in monitoring shoulder function.

The Western Ontario Rotator Cuff (WORC) Index was introduced in 2003 [118]. The WORC Index was designed to identify HRQoL factors in individuals with disorders of the rotator cuff; it has 21 questions covering different domains: physical symptoms, work, lifestyle, recreation, and emotion [119]. The WORC is one of the most responsive questionnaires for rotator cuff disorders [120]. An abbreviated version named short-WORC was published in 2012. short-WORC has only 7 questions and has comparable results of the standard questionnaire [121]. A systematic review of 1881 articles evaluating 39 outcome instruments for patients with rotator cuff disease found that WORC had the highest psychometric properties, suggesting that WORC is the most effective tool for these patients [122]. No floor effects were observed for the WORC at baseline or at 6 months and for the short-WORC at 6 months. However, floor effects were observed at baseline for 19% of patients for the short-WORC [123].

The Shoulder Pain and Disability Index (SPADI) was published in 1991 to measure pain and disability correlated with shoulder pathologies. SPADI has 13 questions used to quantify pain and disability [124,125]. In the SPADI, each question is graded from 0 (absence of pain or disability) to 10 (extreme pain and maximum difficulty). A systematic review of 85 studies, 32 tools, and 111 validations found the SPADI had the highest methodological quality for measuring shoulder pain [126]. The SPADI has proven to be consistent since its publication in 1991 and responsive in individuals following shoulder arthroplasty and is recommended for this group. No floor or ceiling effects have been observed for the SPADI [127].

The Western Ontario Shoulder Instability (WOSI) index was published in 1998 [128,129]. The WOSI was designed to accurately measure instability of the shoulder, analyzing 4 components: direction, frequency, cause, and degree. The WOSI has 21 items with the domains of physical symptoms, sports, recreation, work, lifestyle, and emotions. The optimal score (0) signifies no impact of shoulder-related issues compared to the maximum score (2100). A meta-analysis of 91 studies analyzing outcome measures for shoulder instability found that the WOSI had the highest rating, reinforcing its reliability, validity, and responsiveness [130]. For individuals with shoulder instability, the use of the WOSI is recommended in conjunction with additional outcome measures to ensure that all domains are addressed [130].

In the dog shoulder, passive ROM measurements with a universal goniometer are reliable (57°–165° in Labrador retrievers, 47°–159° in German shepherd dogs) [72,74] but no other shoulder joint-specific functional tests or testing batteries have been proposed or validated.

Elbow Joint

The Upper Extremity Functional Index (UEFI-20), originally published in 2001, has 20 functional items scored from 0 (worst) to 4 (best), with a maximum score of 80 [131,132]. The UEFI-20 has excellent retest reliability with upper extremity conditions and has strong clinimetric properties [133]. A reduced version of the UEFI contains 15 items (UEFI-15) [134]. In a Rasch analysis [135], the UEFI-15 was valid, whereas the UEFI-20 was not [136]. A prospective longitudinal study of general upper extremity dysfunction found that the UEFI and UEFI-15 had comparable reliability and validity [137]. However, the UEFI-15 is recommended due to its one-dimensionality and its shorter length, in conjunction with an outcome measure focused on pain. There is limited evidence discussing the use of the UEFI-20 or UEFI-15 for specific elbow conditions, However, given its versatility, it can be utilized for general upper extremity conditions.

The Liverpool Elbow Score (LES) was originally published in 2004 due to the lack of validated elbow-specific questionnaires and to incorporate patient perception (9 subjective questions about pain and function) and clinician assessment (6 assessments of elbow ROM or strength) [138]. Each of the 15 items is scored from 0 (worst) to 4 (best), with a total score of 60. The LES has been found to be responsive, without floor or ceiling effects in individuals with a total elbow replacement [139]. The LES also is an appropriate outcome measure for patients with elbow stiffness and for patients undergoing arthrolysis [140].

The American Shoulder and Elbow Surgeons elbow scoring system (ASES-e) consists of 18 total patient reported questions: 5 pain items, 12 function items, and 1 satisfaction item. The pain questions are rated as 0 (painless) to 10 (worst pain), function items are rated as 0 (inability) to 3 (not difficult), and satisfaction is rated as 1 (not satisfied) to 10 (very satisfied). The ASES-e also has a physician component that assesses motion, stability, strength, and physical findings [141,142]. In a systematic review of 9 articles, the ASES-e had high test-retest reliability and responsiveness [143]. The satisfaction portion of the ASES-e has a moderate ceiling effect at approximately 43%; it is therefore advised that this portion of the tool not be integrated into the total score [143]. ASES-e is an adequate tool for assessing elbow pathologies.

As above, passive ROM measurements with a goniometer are a reliable method for measuring range of elbow motion (36°–165° in Labrador retrievers, 25°–155° in German Shepherd dogs) [72,74]. A craniocaudal sliding caliper measurement has been shown to be a valid tool for measuring elbow joint swelling, with high intra-tester reliability (ICC = 0.95) and low inter-rater reliability (ICC = 0.59) [144]. A tape measure has been shown to be a valid tool for measuring elbow joint swelling [144]. Tape measurements also reliably measure the circumference of antebrachium distal to the elbow, but not brachium proximal to the elbow [93].

Carpal Joint

The Patient-Rated Wrist Evaluation (PRWE) was developed in 2008 to measure wrist pain and disability in ADL [145]. Wrist pain and disability is rated with a pain subscale with 5 items and a function subscale with specific activities (6 items) and usual activities (4 items). All items are rated from 1 (best) to 10 (worst), for a total score ranging from 0 to 150. The PRWE is freely available online [146]. The Patient-Rated Wrist/Hand Evaluation (PRWHE) is a modified version of the PRWE that differs only in the fact that the term "wrist" is replaced with "wrist/hand" and that is includes an optional question about hand cosmesis.

In dogs, the assessment of passive carpal ROM in the sagittal plane using a goniometer has been validated (32°–196° in Labrador retrievers, 34°–198° in German Shepherd dogs) [72,74]. Passive motion of the carpus in the frontal plane has also been validated in Labrador Retrievers (7° of varus, 12° of valgus) [72]. However, limb conformation varies widely in dogs, particularly as a result of chondrodystrophy and chondrodysplasia. Several studies reported carpal motion in chondrodystrophic dogs and have highlighted differences between chondrodystrophic and non-chondrodystrophic dogs [147,148]. Weight-bearing goniometric methods to measure valgus of the distal portion of the radius and external rotation of the forelimb have been described [148]. Measurements of valgus of the distal portion of the radius were collected using a modified 7.5 cm diameter goniometer centered over the carpus with short arms aligned with the lateral epicondyle and the third digit, respectively. Mean ± SD angulation was 9 + 4° in non-chondrodystrophic dogs and 23 ± 11° in chondrodystrophic dogs. The method was highly repeatable intra-tester in non-chondrodystrophic (ICC = 0.819) and chondrodystrophic dogs (ICC = 0.937). Inter-tester repeatability (reliability) was moderate in chondrodystrophic (ICC = 0.740) dogs but low in non-chondrodystrophic dogs (ICC = 0.292). Measurements of external rotation were collected when dogs stepped on a goniometer whose arms are parallel to the spine and the third digit, respectively. Mean ± SD external rotation was 14 ± 5° in non-chondrodystrophic dogs and 30 ± 13° in chondrodystrophic dogs. That method was highly repeatable intra-tester in chondrodystrophic dogs (ICC = 0.942) but had a low repeatability in non-chondrodystrophic dogs (ICC = 0.505). Inter-tester repeatability (reliability) was moderate in chondrodystrophic (ICC = 0.646) dogs and was low in non-chondrodystrophic dogs (ICC = 0.390) [148]. Instruments for assessments of carpal function in dogs have not been reported.

DISCUSSION

Testing batteries and functional measurement tools for dogs are emerging and are becoming more commonplace; however, the gap between human and veterinary medicine is substantial, both in number of tools and the rigor of their psychometric testing. Practitioners should be aware of key psychometric properties (validity, reliability, floor and ceiling effects) of the tests they choose to use, and the accompanied false positive and false negative rates as well as their responsiveness to the condition they are targeting. Sensitivity, specificity, likelihood ratios, and other statistical analyses are not commonly reported in small animal research but may be very helpful in examining which tests are best suited for individual patients.

In a study where 58 dogs with lameness due to OA were examined using force plate analysis and an owner-assessed and veterinarian-assessed lameness scales, lameness as rated by the owner or the veterinarians did not relate to the true status of the dogs measured using a force plate [149]. The unconscious desire to see improvement when none is present is named caregiver placebo. In that study, the caregiver placebo effect when evaluating lameness was present in 57% of owners and 40% to 45% of veterinarians. The caregiver placebo effect is also present in human medicine. Because objective outcome measures are not influenced by caregiver placebo, it is important to

rely on objective outcome measures rather than subjective impressions both when managing patients and conducting clinical research.

Also, patient-reported outcomes used in human medicine are collected directly from the patient and are therefore more precise than outcomes collected from owners and a clinician regarding outcomes in dogs. The outcome measures provided by owners about their pet's health, quality of life, and functional status are influenced on several factors. These factors alter the perceived response to therapy. Although they provide useful information, the results of owner-reported questionnaires need to be examined against validated objective measures as often as possible. Because little is known regarding the sources of discrepancy between owner-reported outcome measures and objective outcome measures [6], it is important to continue to study these discrepancies.

Unfortunately, replication of studies done on many of the functional scales and measures in veterinary medicine remains highly unusual. We commonly prioritize novelty over replication in research; however, the National Institutes of Health (NIH) considers reproducibility of research to be an integral part of research practice [150]. In the field of psychology, 100 experiments with varied designs were repeated by 270 investigators and, surprisingly, fewer than 50% reached the same results, showing the importance of replicating studies [151]. A seminal study examining validity and reliability of goniometry in Labrador retrievers [72] has been replicated many times using a similar technique in various breeds (see Table 1), which has helped to validate the results and has expanded our knowledge of joint motion across dog breeds. Individual studies are a window into the area being studied, but replication increases (or decreases) confidence in the results, makes results more generalizable, and provides information about potential sources of variability among dogs and medical conditions. Ceiling and floor effects while discussed extensively in human medicine are rarely studied or discussed in veterinary medicine.

It is also critically important to determine MCID for the functional measures and instruments currently use and for those that are already developed [152,153]. For current instruments used in dogs, a single study reported an MCID, for the LOAD in dogs 6 weeks after CCL stabilization surgery [8].

Although much has been accomplished in the past decade to address the needs for clinical instruments useful in dogs for quantifying pain, function, and joint mobility, large research gaps remain. Such gaps currently limit the development of evidence-based approaches for optimal interventions. Psychometric properties (reliability, validity, and responsiveness) of instruments including owner reported and clinical reported outcomes need to be examined and replicated in various breeds, ages, and conditions. The development of specific outcome measures for key diseases (eg, OA, CCL injury, intervertebral disc disease), joints (hip, stifle, elbow), and surgical interventions is warranted.

In conclusion, outcome measure instruments are a critical component of the management of chronic conditions such as OA in dogs. Tools are emerging and are partially validated. Their use when managing clinical cases and in clinical research provide extremely valuable information.

CLINICS CARE POINTS

- Several outcome measure questionnaires such as the Canine Brief Pain Inventory, the COI, the HCPI, and the LOAD questionnaires have sufficient validation for use in many clinical situations. With approximately 10 questions, these questionnaires are easy to use and convenient. The same questionnaire or questionnaires should be used over time.

- Outcome measure questionnaires are critically important when managing chronic musculoskeletal problems in dogs. The questionnaire is initially filled and used as a baseline. The questionnaire is filled again at a later date to evaluate response to therapy and disease progression.

- For each questionnaire, the MCID is the number of points change in score that reflects a positive response to therapy. For the Canine Brief Pain Inventory, the MCID is 4 points.

REFERENCES

[1] Mosier CI. A critical examination of the concepts of face validity. Educ Psychol Meas 1947;7(2):191–205.
[2] Altman DG, Bland JM. Diagnostic tests. 1: Sensitivity and specificity. BMJ 1994;308(6943):1552.
[3] Bartlett JW, Frost C. Reliability, repeatability and reproducibility: analysis of measurement errors in continuous variables. Ultrasound Obstet Gynecol 2008;31(4):466–75.
[4] Portney LG, Watkins MP. Foundations of clinical research: applications to practice. 3rd edition. Upper Saddle River, NJ: Prentice Hall; 2008.
[5] Stratford PW, Binkley JM, Riddle DL. Health status measures: strategies and analytic methods for assessing change scores. Phys Ther 1996;76(10):1109–23.
[6] Brown DC, Boston RC, Farrar JT. Comparison of force plate gait analysis and owner assessment of pain using the Canine Brief Pain Inventory in dogs with osteoarthritis. J Vet Intern Med 2013;27(1):22–30.
[7] Copay AG, Subach BR, Glassman SD, et al. Understanding the minimum clinically important difference: a review of concepts and methods. Spine J 2007;7(5):541–6.
[8] Innes JF, Morton MA, Lascelles BDX. Minimal clinically-important differences for the 'Liverpool Osteoarthritis in Dogs' (LOAD) and the 'Canine Orthopedic Index' (COI) client-reported outcomes measures. PLoS One 2023;18(2):e0280912.
[9] Radke H, Joeris A, Chen M. Evidence-based evaluation of owner-reported outcome measures for canine orthopedic care - a COSMIN evaluation of 6 instruments. Vet Surg 2022;51(2):244–53.
[10] Belshaw Z, Yeates J. Assessment of quality of life and chronic pain in dogs. Vet J 2018;239:59–64.
[11] Fulmer AE, Laven LJ, Hill KE. Quality of Life Measurement in Dogs and Cats: A Scoping Review of Generic Tools. Animals (Basel) 2022;12(3).
[12] Brown DC, Boston RC, Coyne JC, et al. Development and psychometric testing of an instrument designed to measure chronic pain in dogs with osteoarthritis. Am J Vet Res 2007;68(6):631–7.
[13] Brown DC, Boston RC, Coyne JC, et al. Ability of the canine brief pain inventory to detect response to treatment in dogs with osteoarthritis. J Am Vet Med Assoc 2008;233(8):1278–83.
[14] Walton MB, Cowderoy E, Lascelles D, et al. Evaluation of construct and criterion validity for the 'Liverpool Osteoarthritis in Dogs' (LOAD) clinical metrology instrument and comparison to two other instruments. PLoS One 2013;8(3):e58125.
[15] Essner A, Zetterberg L, Hellstrom K, et al. Psychometric evaluation of the canine brief pain inventory in a Swedish sample of dogs with pain related to osteoarthritis. Acta Vet Scand 2017;59(1):44.
[16] Alves JC, Santos A, Jorge P, et al. Evaluation of Four Clinical Metrology Instruments for the Assessment of Osteoarthritis in Dogs. Animals (Basel) 2022;12(20).
[17] Alves JC, Santos A, Jorge P. Initial psychometric evaluation of the Portuguese version of the Canine Brief Pain Inventory. Am J Vet Res 2022;84(1).
[18] Ragetly GR, Massey L, Brown DC. Initial psychometric testing and validation of the French version of the Canine Brief Pain Inventory. Vet Anaesth Analg 2019;46(5):667–72.
[19] Della Rocca G, Di Salvo A, Medori C, et al. Initial Psychometric Testing and Validation of the Italian Version of the Canine Brief Pain Inventory in Dogs With Pain Related to Osteoarthritis. Front Vet Sci 2021;8:736458.
[20] Wells JR, Young AL, Crane A, et al. Linguistic Validation of the Canine Brief Pain Inventory (CBPI) for Global Use. Front Vet Sci 2021;8:769112.

[21] Hielm-Bjorkman AK, Rita H, Tulamo RM. Psychometric testing of the Helsinki chronic pain index by completion of a questionnaire in Finnish by owners of dogs with chronic signs of pain caused by osteoarthritis. Am J Vet Res 2009;70(6):727–34.

[22] Hielm-Bjorkman AK, Kuusela E, Liman A, et al. Evaluation of methods for assessment of pain associated with chronic osteoarthritis in dogs. J Am Vet Med Assoc 2003;222(11):1552–8.

[23] Brown DC. The Canine Orthopedic Index. Step 1: Devising the items. Vet Surg 2014;43(3):232–40.

[24] Brown DC. The Canine Orthopedic Index. Step 3: Responsiveness testing. Vet Surg 2014;43(3):247–54.

[25] Brown DC. The Canine Orthopedic Index. Step 2: Psychometric testing. Vet Surg 2014;43(3):241–6.

[26] Andersson A, Bergstrom A. Adaptation of the Canine Orthopaedic Index to evaluate chronic elbow osteoarthritis in Swedish dogs. Acta Vet Scand 2019;61(1):29.

[27] Alves JC. Initial Psychometric Evaluation of the Portuguese Version of the Canine Orthopedic Index. Vet Comp Orthop Traumatol 2023. https://doi.org/10.1055/s-0043-1768231.

[28] Hercock CA, Pinchbeck G, Giejda A, et al. Validation of a client-based clinical metrology instrument for the evaluation of canine elbow osteoarthritis. J Small Anim Pract 2009;50(6):266–71.

[29] Alves JC, Jorge P, Santos A. Initial psychometric evaluation of the Portuguese version of the Liverpool Osteoarthritis in Dogs. BMC Vet Res 2022;18(1):367.

[30] Innes JF, Barr AR. Can owners assess outcome following treatment of canine cruciate ligament deficiency? J Small Anim Pract 1998;39(8):373–8.

[31] Hielm-Bjorkman AK, Kapatkin AS, Rita HJ. Reliability and validity of a visual analogue scale used by owners to measure chronic pain attributable to osteoarthritis in their dogs. Am J Vet Res 2011;72(5):601–7.

[32] Hudson JT, Slater MR, Taylor L, et al. Assessing repeatability and validity of a visual analogue scale questionnaire for use in assessing pain and lameness in dogs. Am J Vet Res 2004;65(12):1634–43.

[33] Wiseman-Orr ML, Nolan AM, Reid J, et al. Development of a questionnaire to measure the effects of chronic pain on health-related quality of life in dogs. Am J Vet Res 2004;65(8):1077–84.

[34] Wiseman-Orr ML, Scott EM, Reid J, et al. Validation of a structured questionnaire as an instrument to measure chronic pain in dogs on the basis of effects on health-related quality of life. Am J Vet Res 2006;67(11):1826–36.

[35] Schmutz A, Spofford N, Burghardt W, et al. Development and initial validation of a dog quality of life instrument. Sci Rep 2022;12(1):12225.

[36] Hesbach A. A proposed canine movement performance test: the canine timed up and go test (CTUG). Orthoped Phys Ther Pract 2003;15:26.

[37] Frye C, Carr BJ, Lenfest M, et al. Canine Geriatric Rehabilitation: Considerations and Strategies for Assessment, Functional Scoring, and Follow Up. Front Vet Sci 2022;9:842458.

[38] Brown DC, Boston RC, Farrar JT. Use of an activity monitor to detect response to treatment in dogs with osteoarthritis. J Am Vet Med Assoc 2010;237(1):66–70.

[39] Conzemius MG, Scott R, Lascelles BDX, et al. Measuring distance traveled with an activity monitor in normal dogs participating in a 5K race (Abstr). Vet Comp Orthop Traumatol 2018.

[40] Kaka U, Chen HC, Goh YM, et al. Validation of a modified algometer to measure mechanical nociceptive thresholds in awake dogs. BioMed Res Int 2015;2015:375421.

[41] Bosscher G, Tomas A, Roe SC, et al. Repeatability and accuracy testing of a weight distribution platform and comparison to a pressure sensitive walkway to assess static weight distribution. Vet Comp Orthop Traumatol 2017;30(2):160–4.

[42] Phelps HA, Ramos V, Shires PK, et al. The effect of measurement method on static weight distribution to all legs in dogs using the Quadruped Biofeedback System. Vet Comp Orthop Traumatol 2007;20(2):108–12.

[43] Wilson ML, Roush JK, Renberg WC. Single-day and multiday repeatability of stance analysis results for dogs with hind limb lameness. Am J Vet Res 2019;80(4):403–9.

[44] Jevens DJ, Hauptman JG, DeCamp CE, et al. Contributions to variance in force-plate analysis of gait in dogs. Am J Vet Res 1993;54(4):612–5.

[45] Volstad NJ, Sandberg G, Robb S, et al. The evaluation of limb symmetry indices using ground reaction forces collected with one or two force plates in healthy dogs. Vet Comp Orthop Traumatol 2017;30(1):54–8.

[46] Stejskal M, Torres BT, Sandberg GS, et al. Variability of vertical ground reaction forces collected with one and two force plates in healthy dogs. Vet Comp Orthop Traumatol 2015;28(5):318–22.

[47] Pettit EM, Sandberg GS, Volstad NJ, et al. Evaluation of Ground Reaction Forces and Limb Symmetry Indices Using Ground Reaction Forces Collected with One or Two Plates in Dogs Exhibiting a Stifle Lameness. Vet Comp Orthop Traumatol 2020;33(6):398–401.

[48] McLaughlin RM Jr, Roush JK. Effects of subject stance time and velocity on ground reaction forces in clinically normal greyhounds at the trot. Am J Vet Res 1994;55(12):1666–71.

[49] Sharkey M. The challenges of assessing osteoarthritis and postoperative pain in dogs. AAPS J 2013;15(2):598–607.

[50] Avendano JN, Langenbach A, Brunke MW, et al. Ground reaction forces, temporospatial parameters, range of motion, and limb characteristics were analyzed for small and medium size sound dogs with the use of pressure sensitive walkway. Am J Vet Res 2023;84(6):1–9.

[51] Seibert R, Marcellin-Little DJ, Roe SC, et al. Comparison of body weight distribution, peak vertical force, and vertical impulse as measures of hip joint pain and efficacy of total hip replacement. Vet Surg 2012;41(4):443–7.

[52] Rincon Alvarez J, Anesi S, Czopowicz M, et al. The Effect of Calibration Method on Repeatability and Reproducibility of Pressure Mat Data in a Canine Population. Vet Comp Orthop Traumatol 2020;33(6):428–33.

[53] Sandberg G, Torres B, Berjeski A, et al. Comparison of Simultaneously Collected Kinetic Data with Force Plates and a Pressure Walkway. Vet Comp Orthop Traumatol 2018;31(5):327–31.

[54] Kieves NR, Hart JL, Evans RB, et al. Comparison of three walkway cover types for use during objective canine gait analysis with a pressure-sensitive walkway. Am J Vet Res 2019;80(3):265–9.

[55] Harris WH. Traumatic arthritis of the hip after dislocation and acetabular fractures: treatment by mold arthroplasty. An end-result study using a new method of result evaluation. J Bone Joint Surg Am 1969;51(4):737–55.

[56] Harris Hip Score. https://www.orthopaedicscore.com/scorepages/harris_hip_score.html.

[57] Marchetti P, Binazzi R, Vaccari V, et al. Long-term results with cementless Fitek (or Fitmore) cups. J Arthroplasty 2005;20(6):730–7.

[58] Byrd JW, Jones KS. Prospective analysis of hip arthroscopy with 2-year follow-up. Arthroscopy 2000;16(6):578–87.

[59] Wamper KE, Sierevelt IN, Poolman RW, et al. The Harris hip score: Do ceiling effects limit its usefulness in orthopedics? Acta Orthop 2010;81(6):703–7.

[60] Dawson J, Fitzpatrick R, Carr A, et al. Questionnaire on the perceptions of patients about total hip replacement. J Bone Joint Surg Br 1996;78(2):185–90.

[61] Murray DW, Fitzpatrick R, Rogers K, et al. The use of the Oxford hip and knee scores. J Bone Joint Surg Br 2007;89(8):1010–4.

[62] Oxford Hip Score. http://www.orthopaedicscore.com/scorepages/oxford_hip_score.html.

[63] Martinelli N, Longo UG, Marinozzi A, et al. Cross-cultural adaptation and validation with reliability, validity, and responsiveness of the Italian version of the Oxford Hip Score in patients with hip osteoarthritis. Qual Life Res 2011;20(6):923–9.

[64] Weel H, Lindeboom R, Kuipers SE, et al. Comparison between the Harris- and Oxford Hip Score to evaluate outcomes one-year after total hip arthroplasty. Acta Orthop Belg 2017;83(1):98–109.

[65] Klässbo M, Larsson E, Mannevik E. Hip disability and osteoarthritis outcome score. An extension of the Western Ontario and McMaster Universities Osteoarthritis Index. Scand J Rheumatol 2003;32(1):46–51.

[66] Nilsdotter AK, Lohmander LS, Klassbo M, et al. Hip disability and osteoarthritis outcome score (HOOS)–validity and responsiveness in total hip replacement. BMC Musculoskelet Disord 2003;4:10.

[67] Questionnaires, user's guides and scoring files. http://www.koos.nu/.

[68] Kemp JL, Collins NJ, Roos EM, et al. Psychometric properties of patient-reported outcome measures for hip arthroscopic surgery. Am J Sports Med 2013;41(9):2065–73.

[69] Thorborg K, Roos EM, Bartels EM, et al. Validity, reliability and responsiveness of patient-reported outcome questionnaires when assessing hip and groin disability: a systematic review. Br J Sports Med 2010;44(16):1186–96.

[70] Davis AM, Perruccio AV, Canizares M, et al. The development of a short measure of physical function for hip OA HOOS-Physical Function Shortform (HOOS-PS): an OARSI/OMERACT initiative. Osteoarthritis Cartilage 2008;16(5):551–9.

[71] Mohtadi NG, Griffin DR, Pedersen ME, et al. Arthroscopy of the Hip Outcomes Research, The development and validation of a self-administered quality-of-life outcome measure for young, active patients with symptomatic hip disease: the International Hip Outcome Tool (iHOT-33). Arthroscopy 2012;28(5):595–605, quiz 606-10 e1.

[72] Jaegger G, Marcellin-Little DJ, Levine D. Reliability of goniometry in Labrador retrievers. Am J Vet Res 2002;63(7):979–86.

[73] Nicholson HL, Osmotherly PG, Smith BA, et al. Determinants of passive hip range of motion in adult Greyhounds. Aust Vet J 2007;85(6):217–21.

[74] Thomas TM, Marcellin-Little DJ, Roe SC, et al. Comparison of measurements obtained by use of an electrogoniometer and a universal plastic goniometer for the assessment of joint motion in dogs. Am J Vet Res 2006;67(12):1974–9.

[75] Lysholm J, Gillquist J. Evaluation of knee ligament surgery results with special emphasis on use of a scoring scale. Am J Sports Med 1982;10(3):150–4.

[76] Tegner Y, Lysholm J. Rating systems in the evaluation of knee ligament injuries. Clin Orthop Relat Res 1985;198:43–9.

[77] Lysholm Knee Scoring Scale. http://www.lakarhuset.com/docs/lysholmkneescoringscale.pdf.

[78] Chamorro-Moriana G, Perez-Cabezas V, Espuny-Ruiz F, et al. Assessing knee functionality: Systematic review of validated outcome measures. Ann Phys Rehabil Med 2022;65(6):101608.

[79] Barber-Westin SD, Noyes FR, McCloskey JW. Rigorous statistical reliability, validity, and responsiveness testing of the Cincinnati knee rating system in 350 subjects with uninjured, injured, or anterior cruciate ligament-reconstructed knees. Am J Sports Med 1999;27(4):402–16.

[80] Symptom Rating Form - Cincinnati Knee Rating System - F02. https://noyeskneeinstitute.com/wp-content/uploads/2019/07/SymptonRating.pdf.

[81] Free Online Modified Cincinnati Knee Rating System Calculator — OrthoToolKit. https://orthotoolkit.com/cincinnati/.

[82] Binkley JM, Stratford PW, Lott SA, et al. The Lower Extremity Functional Scale (LEFS): scale development, measurement properties, and clinical application. North American Orthopaedic Rehabilitation Research Network. Phys Ther 1999;79(4):371–83.

[83] Mehta SP, Fulton A, Quach C, et al. Measurement properties of the lower extremity functional scale: A systematic review. J Orthop Sports Phys Ther 2016;46(3):200–16.

[84] Lower Extremity Functional Scale (LEFS) https://www.emoryhealthcare.org/ui/pdfs/msk-pt-forms/hip-lefs.pdf.

[85] Collins NJ, Misra D, Felson DT, et al. Measures of knee function: International Knee Documentation Committee (IKDC) Subjective Knee Evaluation Form, Knee Injury and Osteoarthritis Outcome Score (KOOS), Knee Injury and Osteoarthritis Outcome Score Physical Function Short Form (KOOS-PS), Knee Outcome Survey Activities of Daily Living Scale (KOS-ADL), Lysholm Knee Scoring Scale, Oxford Knee Score (OKS), Western Ontario and McMaster Universities Osteoarthritis Index (WOMAC), Activity Rating Scale (ARS), and Tegner Activity Score (TAS). Arthritis Care Res 2011;63(0 11):S208–28.

[86] KOOS Knee Survey. http://www.koos.nu/koos-english.pdf.

[87] Formenton MR, de Lima LG, Vassalo FG, et al. Goniometric assessment in French bulldogs. Front Vet Sci 2019;6:424.

[88] Sabanci SS, Ocal MK. Comparison of goniometric measurements of the stifle joint in seven breeds of normal dogs. Vet Comp Orthop Traumatol 2016;29(3):214–9.

[89] Mendonça GBN. Goniometria em cães de raça Rottweiler [V. Titulo]. Goiânia, Goiás, Brasil: Universidade Federal de Goiás; 2009.

[90] McCarthy DA, Millis DL, Levine D, et al. Variables affecting thigh girth measurement and observer reliability in dogs. Front Vet Sci 2018;5:203.

[91] Bascuñán AL, Kieves N, Goh C, et al. Evaluation of factors influencing thigh circumference measurement in dogs. Vet Evidence 2016;1(2):1–12.

[92] Baker SG, Roush JK, Unis MD, et al. Comparison of four commercial devices to measure limb circumference in dogs. Vet Comp Orthop Traumatol 2010;23(6):406–10.

[93] Smith TJ, Baltzer WI, Jelinski SE, et al. Inter- and intra-tester reliability of anthropometric assessment of limb circumference in labrador retrievers. Vet Surg 2013;42(3):316–21.

[94] Frank I, Duerr F, Zanghi B, et al. Diagnostic Ultrasound Detection of Changes in Femoral Muscle Mass Recovery after Tibial Plateau Levelling Osteotomy in Dogs. Vet Comp Orthop Traumatol 2019;32(5):394–400.

[95] Hyytiäinen HK, Mölsä SH, Junnila JT, et al. Use of bathroom scales in measuring asymmetry of hindlimb static weight bearing in dogs with osteoarthritis. Vet Comp Orthop Traumatol 2012;25(5):390–6.

[96] Hyytiäinen HK, Mölsä SH, Junnila JT, et al. Ranking of physiotherapeutic evaluation methods as outcome measures of stifle functionality in dogs. Acta Vet Scand 2013;55(1):29.

[97] Hyytiäinen HK, Mölsä SH, Junnila JJT, et al. Developing a testing battery for measuring dogs' stifle functionality: the Finnish Canine Stifle Index (FCSI). Vet Rec 2018;183(10):324.

[98] Hyytiäinen HK, Morelius M, Lappalainen AK, et al. The Finnish Canine Stifle Index: responsiveness to change and intertester reliability. Vet Rec 2020;186(18):604.

[99] Pinna S, Lambertini C, Grassato L, et al. Evidence-based veterinary medicine: A tool for evaluating the healing process after surgical treatment for cranial cruciate ligament rupture in dogs. Front Vet Sci 2019;6:65.

[100] Gundersen K, Millis D, Zhu X. Development and testing of a stifle function score in dogs. Front Vet Sci 2022;9:895567.

[101] Carobbi B, Ness MG. Preliminary study evaluating tests used to diagnose canine cranial cruciate ligament failure. J Small Anim Pract 2009;50(5):224–6.

[102] Martin RL, Irrgang JJ, Burdett RG, et al. Evidence of validity for the Foot and Ankle Ability Measure (FAAM). Foot Ankle Int 2005;26(11):968–83.

[103] Eechaute C, Vaes P, Van Aerschot L, et al. The clinimetric qualities of patient-assessed instruments for measuring chronic ankle instability: a systematic review. BMC Musculoskelet Disord 2007;8:6.

[104] Roos EM, Brandsson S, Karlsson J. Validation of the foot and ankle outcome score for ankle ligament reconstruction. Foot Ankle Int 2001;22(10):788–94.

[105] Foot and Ankle Ability Measure (FAAM). https://www.princetonhcs.org/-/media/files/forms/princeton-rehabilitation/foot-and-ankle-ability-measure.pdf.

[106] Martin RL, Burdett RG, Irrgang JJ. Development of the Foot and Ankle Disability Index (FADI) [abstr]. J Orthop Sports Phys Ther 1999;29:A32–3.

[107] Hale SA, Hertel J. Reliability and sensitivity of the Foot and Ankle Disability Index in subjects with chronic ankle instability. J Athl Train 2005;40(1):35–40.

[108] The Foot & Ankle Disability Index (FADI) Score. http://www.blairpt.com/forms/FADI.pdf.

[109] The Foot and Ankle Disability Index (FADI) Score and Sports Module. https://www.reboundoregon.com/wp-content/uploads/Foot_and_Ankle_Disability_Index_and_Sports_Module_FADI.pdf.

[110] Barnett S, Campbell R, Harvey I. The Bristol Foot Score: developing a patient-based foot-health measure. J Am Podiatr Med Assoc 2005;95(3):264–72.

[111] Riskowski JL, Hagedorn TJ, Hannan MT. Measures of foot function, foot health, and foot pain: American Academy of Orthopedic Surgeons Lower Limb Outcomes Assessment: Foot and Ankle Module (AAOS-FAM), Bristol Foot Score (BFS), Revised Foot Function Index (FFI-R), Foot Health Status Questionnaire (FHSQ), Manchester Foot Pain and Disability Index (MFPDI), Podiatric Health Questionnaire (PHQ), and Rowan Foot Pain Assessment (ROFPAQ). Arthritis Care Res 2011;63(0 11):S229–39.

[112] Johanson NA, Liang MH, Daltroy L, et al. American Academy of Orthopaedic Surgeons lower limb outcomes assessment instruments. Reliability, validity, and sensitivity to change. J Bone Joint Surg Am 2004;86(5):902–9.

[113] Hudak PL, Amadio PC, Bombardier C. Development of an upper extremity outcome measure: the DASH (disabilities of the arm, shoulder and hand). The Upper Extremity Collaborative Group (UECG). Am J Ind Med 1996;29(6):602–8.

[114] The Disabilities of the Arm, Shoulder and Hand (DASH) Score. http://www.orthopaedicscore.com/scorepages/disabilities_of_arm_shoulder_hand_score_dash.html.

[115] Bot SD, Terwee CB, van der Windt DA, et al. Vet, Clinimetric evaluation of shoulder disability questionnaires: a systematic review of the literature. Ann Rheum Dis 2004;63(4):335–41.

[116] Beaton DE, Wright JG, Katz JN, et al. Development of the QuickDASH: comparison of three item-reduction approaches. J Bone Joint Surg Am 2005;87(5):1038–46.

[117] The Disabilities of the Arm, Shoulder and Hand Score (QuickDash). http://www.orthopaedicscore.com/scorepages/disabilities_of_arm_shoulder_hand_score_quick-dash.html.

[118] Kirkley A, Alvarez C, Griffin S. The development and evaluation of a disease-specific quality-of-life questionnaire for disorders of the rotator cuff: The Western Ontario Rotator Cuff Index. Clin J Sport Med 2003;13(2):84–92.

[119] The Western Ontario Rotator Cuff Index (WORC). https://orthop.washington.edu/sites/default/files/files/POOS-21_WORC.pdf.

[120] St-Pierre C, Desmeules F, Dionne CE, et al. Psychometric properties of self-reported questionnaires for the evaluation of symptoms and functional limitations in individuals with rotator cuff disorders: a systematic review. Disabil Rehabil 2016;38(2):103–22.

[121] Razmjou H, Stratford P, Holtby R. A shortened version of the Western ontario rotator cuff disability index: Development and measurement properties. Physiother Can 2012;64(2):135–44.

[122] Huang H, Grant JA, Miller BS, et al. A systematic review of the psychometric properties of patient-reported outcome instruments for use in patients with rotator cuff disease. Am J Sports Med 2015;43(10):2572–82.

[123] Dewan N, MacDermid JC, MacIntyre N. Validity and Responsiveness of the Short Version of the Western Ontario Rotator Cuff Index (Short-WORC) in Patients With Rotator Cuff Repair. J Orthop Sports Phys Ther 2018;48(5):409–18.

[124] Roach KE, Budiman-Mak E, Songsiridej N, et al. Development of a shoulder pain and disability index. Arthritis Care Res 1991;4(4):143–9.

[125] Shoulder Pain and Disability Index (SPADI). https://denalipt.com/wp-content/uploads/Shoulder-Pain-and-Disability-Index.pdf.

[126] Aldon-Villegas R, Ridao-Fernandez C, Torres-Enamorado D, et al. How to assess shoulder functionality: A systematic review of existing validated outcome measures. Diagnostics 2021;11(5):845.

[127] Roy JS, MacDermid JC, Woodhouse LJ. Measuring shoulder function: a systematic review of four questionnaires. Arthritis Rheum 2009;61(5):623–32.

[128] Kirkley A, Griffin S, McLintock H, et al. The development and evaluation of a disease-specific quality of life measurement tool for shoulder instability. The Western Ontario Shoulder Instability Index (WOSI). Am J Sports Med 1998;26(6):764–72.

[129] The Western Ontario Shoulder Instability Index (WOSI). https://www.aaos.org/globalassets/quality-and-practice-resources/patient-reported-outcome-measures/upper-extremity/wosi.pdf.

[130] Whittle JH, Peters SE, Manzanero S, et al. A systematic review of patient-reported outcome measures used in shoulder instability research. J Shoulder Elbow Surg 2020;29(2):381–91.

[131] Stratford P, Binkley JM, Startford DM. Development and initial validation of the Upper Extremity Functional Index. Physiother Can 2001;52:259–67.

[132] The Upper Extremity Functional Index (UEFI). https://www.rwjbh.org/documents/cmc/rehab/ue-functional-index.pdf.

[133] Arumugam V, MacDermid JC. Clinimetrics: Upper Extremity Functional Index. J Physiother 2018;64(2):125.

[134] Upper Extremity Functional Index-15. https://www.tac.vic.gov.au/__data/assets/pdf_file/0003/71508/Upper-Extremity-Functional-Index-15-FORM.pdf.

[135] Boone WJ. Rasch Analysis for Instrument Development: Why, When, and How? CBE-Life Sci Educ 2016;15(4).

[136] Hamilton CB, Chesworth BM. A Rasch-validated version of the upper extremity functional index for interval-level measurement of upper extremity function. Phys Ther 2013;93(11):1507–19.

[137] Chesworth BM, Hamilton CB, Walton DM, et al. Reliability and validity of two versions of the upper extremity functional index. Physiother Can 2014;66(3):243–53.

[138] Sathyamoorthy P, Kemp GJ, Rawal A, et al. Development and validation of an elbow score. Rheumatology 2004;43(11):1434–40.

[139] Vishwanathan K, Alizadehkhaiyat O, Kemp GJ, et al. Responsiveness of the Liverpool Elbow Score in elbow arthroplasty. J Shoulder Elbow Surg 2013;22(3):312–7.

[140] Sun Z, Fan C. Validation of the Liverpool Elbow Score for evaluation of elbow stiffness. BMC Musculoskelet Disord 2018;19(1):302.

[141] Longo UG, Franceschi F, Loppini M, et al. Rating systems for evaluation of the elbow. Br Med Bull 2008;87:131–61.

[142] ASES-E Scoring System. http://hokkaidogaisho.kenkyuu-kai.jp/images/sys%5Cinformation%5C20130328215447-F7813964C71CAB8FCF568A27231CAB98A0FF9A1F3A7053E8BAA7AFFBD3BF21CE.pdf.

[143] Vincent JI, MacDermid JC, King GJW, et al. Establishing the psychometric properties of 2 self-reported outcome measures of elbow pain and function: A systematic review. J Hand Ther 2019;32(2):222–32.

[144] S. Bergfors, Evaluation of four methods for the assessment of joint swelling in dogs, Uppsala, Sweden, 2012, p. 30.

[145] MacDermid JC, Turgeon T, Richards RS, et al. Patient rating of wrist pain and disability: a reliable and valid measurement tool. J Orthop Trauma 1998;12(8):577–86.

[146] Patient Rated Wrist Evaluation. https://www.ace-pt.org/wp-content/uploads/2019/10/PF-PRWHE.pdf.

[147] Reusing M, Brocardo M, W S. Goniometric evaluation and passive range of joint motion in chondrodystrophic and non- chondrodystrophic dogs of different sizes. VCOT Open 2020;3:e66–71.

[148] Pulkkinen HSM, Lappalainen AK, Hyytiäinen HK. Thoracic limb angular deformity in chondrodystrophic dogs: Repeatability of goniometric measurement of external rotation and carpal valgus. VCOT Open 2022;5:e123–30.

[149] Conzemius MG, Evans RB. Caregiver placebo effect for dogs with lameness from osteoarthritis. J Am Vet Med Assoc 2012;241(10):1314–9.

[150] Enhancing reproducibility through rigor and transparency. https://grants.nih.gov/policy/reproducibility/index.htm.

[151] Open Science C. Psychology. Estimating the reproducibility of psychological science. Science 2015;349(6251):aac4716.

[152] Copay AG, Chung AS, Eyberg B, et al. Minimum Clinically Important Difference: Current Trends in the Orthopaedic Literature, Part I: Upper Extremity: A Systematic Review. JBJS Rev 2018;6(9):e1.

[153] Copay AG, Eyberg B, Chung AS, et al. Minimum Clinically Important Difference: Current Trends in the Orthopaedic Literature, Part II: Lower Extremity: A Systematic Review. JBJS Rev 2018;6(9):e2.

Advances in Small Animal Care 4 (2023) 53–60

ADVANCES IN SMALL ANIMAL CARE

Musculoskeletal Problems in Sporting Dogs

Matthew W. Brunke, DVM, DACVSMR[a,*], David Levine, PT, PhD, MPH, DPT, CCRP, FAPTA[b],
Denis J. Marcellin-Little, DEDV, DACVS, DACVSMR[c],
Kirsten E. Oliver, RVT, CCRP, VTS (Physical Rehabilitation)[a],
Jennifer A. Barnhard, BVetMed (Hons), MS, MRCVS[a], Ashley A. Tringali, BS[a]

[a]Veterinary Surgical Centers, 124 Park Street Southeast, Vienna, VA 22180, USA; [b]Department of Physical Therapy, #3253, University of Tenn Chattanooga, 615 McCallie Avenue, Chattanooga, TN 37403, USA; [c]Veterinary Orthopedic Research Laboratory, School of Veterinary Medicine, University of California, 1285 Veterinary Medicine Drive, VM3A Room 4206, Dacis, CA 95616, USA

KEYWORDS
• Sporting dogs • Canine sports medicine • Canine rehabilitation • Agility • Flyball • Dock diving

KEY POINTS

- Many dog sports have similarities in the type of activities involved and the muscles being used to perform these activities, a pattern of injury is present in sporting dogs.
- Common sites of injuries include the shoulder joint, the spine, the iliopsoas muscle, and the feet and digits.
- A prompt and accurate diagnosis is important in sporting dogs to limit the impact of the initial injury on musculoskeletal tissues to minimize chronic changes to tissues resulting from delayed therapy, avoid unnecessary care, and minimize the time being sidelined.
- Although evidence-based information is often lacking for the management of musculoskeletal problems in sporting dogs, general principles of injury prevention and management used in human athletes can be used to inform therapy in injured sporting dogs.
- Training and physical rehabilitation requires collaboration and sustained communication between the owner, trainer/ handler, and clinician.

TRAINING AND CONDITIONING

Training and conditioning are activities done in preparation for the physical and psychological components of each sport: building adequate strength and power, developing cardiovascular and pulmonary endurance, and training the dog to perform the specific activities of the sport. Training and conditioning for an individual sport help prepare the dog both physically and behaviorally to optimally perform while minimizing the risk of injury. In comparison to sports for humans, in most instances, little is known about what methods are optimal for training and conditioning of sporting dogs. The general approach used to train dogs is to break a sport down into its components and practice these components individually. For example, dogs participating in flyball must sprint as rapidly as possible and jump over several hurdles to a spring-loaded box that shoots a tennis ball out when the dog presses the box while turning around. The dog must catch and carry the ball back over the hurdles to the finish line before

*Corresponding author. Veterinary Referral Associates, 500 Perry Parkway, Gaithersburg, MD 20877. E-mail address: drmattbrunke@gmail.com

https://doi.org/10.1016/j.yasa.2023.05.008
2666-450X/23/ © 2023 Elsevier Inc. All rights reserved.

www.advancesinsmallanimalcare.com

53

the next team member is released. Components of the sport include sprinting as rapidly as possible, jumping over hurdles, hitting the box and catching the ball, turning rapidly, and pushing off the box. These components can be taught and practiced individually before combining them. Short anaerobic sprints mimicking the course length (33 m or 100 feet) can be practiced to build hind limb propulsion and increase speed. Exercises that promote shoulder strength and stability such as Cavaletti rails and dynamic disc exercises for the forelimb can be used to increase shoulder strength and stability (Table 1). An oblique ramp can be used to practice box turns, starting at submaximal speed to train the muscles involved without overloading them. Training often starts with proprioceptive awareness (hind limb and forelimb placement), static weight-bearing exercises with proper posture, and challenges to core strength and balance. Dogs should be skeletally mature (ie, without open growth plates in long bones) before strenuous conditioning. The age of growth plate closure varies: closure occurs several months later in larger dogs compared with younger dogs. Explosive activity and concussive training should be avoided before skeletal maturity.

COMMON DOG SPORTS
Agility

Agility is one of the most popular dog sports in North America and its popularity in growing. In the United States, agility is overseen by a handful of organizations: the American Kennel Club (AKC), United Kennel Club (UKC), Canine Performance Events, North American Dog Agility Council, US Dog Agility Association, Australian Shepherd Club of America (ASCA), and Dogs on Course in North America. Agility events overseen by the AKC have more than one million entries per year. In agility, the handler directs the dog through a designed course consisting of equipment that includes some of the following: A-frames, see-saws, tire jumps, double and triple jumps, tunnels, weave poles, pause boxes/tables, hoop jumps, swing planks, and bridges. Courses have varying designs and degrees of difficulty depending on the overseeing organization and competition level. Penalty time is assessed for failure to complete certain tasks or missing the designated path of the course. The rules and obstacles vary according to each governing body.

Agility is a demanding sport that requires muscle strength and coordination in all planes of motion.

TABLE 1
Muscle use during therapeutic exercises in dogs

Muscle or Muscles	Exercises
Biceps femoris/hamstrings	Dancing backwards, up and over, walking, jogging, incline walking, sit-to-stands, reversing up a ramp, lateral limb lift, balance board
Gluteus medius	Walking, trotting, dancing backwards, jogging, Cavaletti rails, serpentine walking/hills, balance board, side stepping, lateral limb lifts
Quadriceps femoris, sartorius	Dancing forwards, up and over, jogging, sit-to-stands, side stepping, lateral limb lifts
Biceps brachii	FL balance discs, wheelbarrowing, Cavaletti rails, limb lifts, side stepping, static paws down, balance board, crawling
Subscapularis	FL balance discs, wheelbarrowing, Cavaletti rails, balance board, side stepping, balance board, crawling
Supraspinatus	FL balance discs, wheelbarrowing, Cavaletti rails, leg lifts, crawling/tunnels, side stepping
Triceps brachii	FL balance discs, pushups, wheelbarrowing, dynamic stabilization, balance board, crawling/tunnels
Infraspinatus/teres minor	FL balance discs, wheelbarrowing, balance board, crawling/tunnels
Epaxial muscles	Swimming, sit-stand-down, standing on unstable surfaces, lifting one limb at a time on unstable surfaces, Cavaletti rails, diagonal leg stands
Abdominal muscles	Sit pretty/beg, swimming, sit-stand-down, lifting one limb at a time on unstable surfaces, Cavaletti rails, diagonal leg stands

Abbreviation: FL, forelimb.
Data from Refs [53–57].

Agility requires explosive hind limb power for jumping, shoulder stability for weave poles and for jump landing, balance for see-saws and the dog walk, and overall endurance.

Several retrospective studies evaluated the frequency and risk of injury in agility dogs. The overall injury rate ranged from 14% to 42% [1–5]. Shoulder injuries, injuries to the spine, and injuries to the iliopsoas or groin region seem most commonly [5,6]. Although reported risk factors for injury vary among studies, being a border collie and having an increased weight to height ratio have been most consistently associated with increased risk of injury [5,7]. Owing to the high injury rate and physical demands of the sport, a recent study evaluated health research priorities as ranked by agility competitors: competitors across organizations and experience levels ranked the identification of risk factors for specific types of injuries as their top research priority [6]. Other research priorities included the safety of equipment and course design and strength and conditioning programs for the prevention of injury.

Dock Diving

Dock diving, also called big air or distance jumping, is a sport where dogs run along a dock with a nonskid surface measuring 13 m (40 feet) and jump as far as possible into a pool to retrieve a toy thrown by the handler with a timing and trajectory that maximizes the length of the jump. The distance is measured by most organizations to the point at which the base of the dog's tail breaks the water's surface. The body of water typically has a minimum depth of 0.9 m (3 feet deep) and a minimum length of 13 m (40 feet). Elite dogs can jump greater than 10 m (>33 feet). Vertical jump, also called extreme vertical or air retrieve, is another water event. In that event, the dog jumps vertically off the dock to retrieve a bumper toy extended from the edge of the dock. To succeed, a dog must retrieve or knock the bumper down. This requires neck extension strength and grasping the bumper with its teeth. Elite dogs can jump greater than 2.5 m (>8 feet). Other sports that are classified within dock diving such as speed retrieve have similar physical demands.

Dock diving requires powerful sprinting and jumping, and potential injuries include muscle strains (such as iliopsoas strain) from repetitive jumping, injuries from slips on the dock, impact injuries from hitting the water, and cervical injuries from neck extension when hitting the water to land with the head above the surface. In addition, neck injuries can also happen during vertical jumping from extension and grabbing the bumper in cervical extension.

Core strength (abdominals and back musculature) is important to maintain good posture and body control while in the air and to land in a straight position without twisting to achieve longer jumps and to better withstand the forces of impact with the water. Dogs typically flex their limbs before hitting the water using their abdominal muscles. Core stabilization exercises include sit-to-stands, rotation, and other exercises with all four limbs on unstable variable surfaces, and swimming exercises. Interval training performing sprinting for short distances mimicking the event can be incorporated. Stretching and flexibility of the rear limbs to promote full hip extension can be promoted through exercises such as high dancing and manual therapy. Improving rear limb power and explosive strength can help achieve greater speed when running down the dock and improve the distance of the jump. Plyometric exercises in which muscles exert maximum force in short intervals are optimal to build power. Exercises can include short jumps such as jumping up onto a platform from the floor.

Flyball

Flyball is a relay race between teams of dogs (four dogs/team), in which dogs sprint from the starting line, jump over four hurdles, turn around while catching a ball, jump the same four hurdles, and sprint to the starting line before the next dog is released. The hurdles start 1.8 m (6 feet) from starting line and are 3 m (10 feet) apart. The flyball box is 4.6 m (15 feet) after the fourth hurdle, making the course 16 m (51 feet) long and the event 32 m (102 feet) long. Governing bodies include the North American Flyball Association and the United Flyball League International. The hurdle height is determined by the shoulder height or the ulnar length of the smallest dog on the team, depending on the governing association.

Two surveys describing flyball injuries in North America reported that border collies and border collie mixes were the most common breeds participating in flyball [8,9]. One study included 375 flyball dogs and reported an injury rate of 39%. The most common injuries affected the forelimb (31%), hind limb (26%), and back or neck (15%). Specific areas most commonly affected were the nails/pads/digits ($n = 33$), shoulder ($n = 26$), neck/back ($n = 23$), iliopsoas ($n = 17$), and carpus ($n = 6$). Dogs over the age of 6 years were less likely to sustain injuries (odds ratio [OR] = 0.78, 95% CI 0.67–0.93), those that used carpal wraps had an increased risk of injury (OR = 2.46, 95% CI 1.52–3.94) [9]. Another study included 589 dogs that participated in flyball [8]. Within the past year, 23% of those dogs were reported to have been injured and 15% twice. The anatomic regions most commonly injured were pads/digits (24%), back (15%), shoulder (13%), or iliopsoas/groin (8.8%). Risk factors for injury included having sustained previous injuries (OR = 3.1), having a fast time less than 4.0 seconds (OR = 1.95, 95% CI 1.09–3.48), and being 3 to 7 years of age (OR = 4.08, 95% CI 1.44–11.58) or 8 year old or older (OR = 4.51, 95% CI 1.48–13.79). Risk factors for training and injury in flyball were also examined in another study involving 75 dogs with injury and 581 control dogs [10]. Results were similar to the previous study: being older than 10 years was associated with a higher injury risk compared with 6- to 9-year-old dogs (OR = 0.81, 95% CI 0.43–1.56) and 2- to 5-year-old dogs (OR = 0.25, 95% CI 0.11–0.55). Carpal bandaging, used by a fifth of dogs in that survey, was associated with increased injury risk. Speed correlated significantly with injury risk: dogs taking $\geq$ 6 seconds to complete the flyball course had the lowest injury risk, and those completing the course in less than 4 seconds had the greatest risk injury (OR = 2.7, 95% CI 0.80–9.09). The flyball box angle of 45° to 55° (relative to a horizontal plane) was associated with highest injury risk, whereas higher angles (66°–75°) were associated with a reduced injury risk (OR = 0.33, 95% CI 0.14–0.74).

When training flyball dogs, exercises that promote shoulder strength and stability such as Cavaletti rails and dynamic disc forelimb exercises should be considered. An oblique ramp can be used to practice box turns, starting at submaximal speed and at a higher angle (60°–75° relative to vertical) to train the muscles involved without overloading them. Plyometric exercises can include short jumps such as jumping up onto a platform from the floor. Core strengthening can provide stability for the landing and push off from the box and during hurdles.

Disc Dog

Disc dog (sometimes called Frisbee dog) uses a specialized set of flying discs that are thrown by the owner/handler and are caught by the dog. Working as team, competitions include distance catching, freestyle routines, accuracy events (such as bullseye), and others. In distance catching, where the goal is to complete a catch with the longest possible distance, dog speed and catching ability are required. Freestyle involves choreographed routines to music scored with an emphasis on success, variety, innovation, and the athletic skills of the dog handler. Routines most often last 1 and 2 minutes. Bullseye involves concentric circles

measuring 3.2, 7.4, and 13.8 m (4, 8, and 15 yards) in diameter. The throw originates in the circle center. Competitors have 1 minute to score points. Discs caught further and discs caught with all four limbs off the ground score more points.

Core strength is a key to maintaining posture and body control while in the air and to land safely. Core stabilization exercises include sit-to-stands or rotation with all four limbs on unstable variable surfaces and swimming exercises. Interval training, such as performing sprinting for short distances mimicking the event, can be incorporated. Stretching and flexibility of shoulder stabilizers and hip and stifle flexors/extensors with passive and active range of motion exercises accompanied with plyometric exercise can strengthen tendons, ligaments, and joints. The sport of disc dogs also requires excellent communication between handler and the dog, with care taken by the handler to throw the disc well to prevent the dog from overly twisting during the jump, catch, and landing, thus reducing the potential of injury.

Racing

Racing events include sprints and endurance races. Sprints range from 100 yards (Fast CAT) to 600 m (lure coursing) and greater. Endurance races can be greater than 1500 km long (>900 miles) such as the Iditarod Trail Sled Dog Race. All dog breeds can compete in Fast CAT races, where CAT stands for Coursing Ability Test or Coursing Aptitude Test [11]. Race time is converted into miles per hour multiplied by a handicap based on height at the withers (scapula) to earn points. Titles are awarded based on the number of points accumulated over time. Races are overseen by several organizations including the AKC, UKC, and American Sighthound Field Association. Rules regarding eligibility differ slightly among organizations. Lure coursing requires dogs to chase an artificial lure across a field, stimulating the instinctual response of hunting prey.

Sighthounds (greyhounds, whippets, Irish wolfhounds, borzoi, Scottish deerhounds, and so forth) are well suited for lure coursing. Races are run in groups of $\leq$ 3 dogs. Dogs follow the lure for 200 to 300 m (600–1000 feet) over a course that includes turns, which should not be excessively sharp to prevent injuries during turns. The lure remains in front of the dogs (10–30 m/yards), but at sufficient speed ($\leq$18 m/s [$\leq$ 40 mph]) so that dogs cannot catch or overtake the lure. The lure is pulled by a fishing line connected to pulleys. The course is inspected to ensure dogs cannot be ensnared in the line. Power to sprint requires powerful hind limb and forelimb muscle mass, cardiovascular conditioning, and core strength. Racing dogs can sustain soft tissue injuries associated within the hip flexor complex muscles and other muscles, shoulder region injuries, carpal and tarsal injuries, and cranial cruciate ligament injury occur [12–14]. Proper warming up before the race is common to acclimate the body for the race both for flexibility and cardiovascular preparation.

Although the greyhound racing industry is on a clear downward trend worldwide, greyhound medicine was a well-developed field in the past. Greyhounds are the fastest dogs and their muscles generate large extensor moments about the tarsus and hip joint [15]. The scientific literature focused on racing greyhounds injuries is substantial. Racing greyhounds can sustain injuries to approximately 20 muscles, particularly the gracilis, long head of the triceps brachii, and tensor fascia lata muscles [16,17]. Racing greyhounds sustain specific fractures in the tarsus (eg, central tarsal, calcaneus, fourth tarsal), carpus (accessory carpal), and long bone (radial, metacarpal, metatarsal) fractures [18–20]. Several racing greyhound fractures have been described as the "coalescence of stress fractures" [21], affecting the central tarsal bone, metacarpal/metatarsal bones, and acetabulum [22,23]. Greyhounds can race often, sometimes twice a week; their bones may not have time to adapt to the exercise regimen and microfractures may not have time to heal between races [24]. Stress fractures in sporting dogs seems mostly limited to racing greyhounds [22,25–27].

Sled dogs evolved from hunter gatherer travels over long distances during extreme cold weather north of the Arctic Circle. The Iditarod Trail Sled Dog Race is a multiday endurance race over packed snow and ice. Sled dog training includes a specific diet, cardiovascular endurance, limb strengthening, core strength and balance, and acclimation to cold temperatures [28]. Northern dog breeds, including chinook, huskies, and Samoyeds are bred for sled work. Injuries with sled dogs include shoulder and carpal injuries and paw pad abrasions [29]. Injuries appear less common in dogs with higher speed and in older dogs.

Muscle fiber types differ among sprinter and endurance racer dogs. Sprinting dogs have more fast-twitch (type II) muscle fibers with higher amounts of glycolic enzymes for anaerobic metabolism and smaller amounts of oxidative enzymes. Fast-twitch fibers generate a higher level of tension, shortening velocity but are less resistant to fatigue. Endurance racers have more slow-twitch (type I) muscle fibers with higher levels of oxidative enzymes that are recruited during aerobic activity and are resistant to fatigue. Racing dogs should receive adequate training and conditioning targeting bone remodeling and limb and core strength. Training and exercises prepare muscles for the specific tasks required when racing.

Obedience and Rally

Obedience is a formal competition where dogs complete a series of exercises with accuracy and precision. It can serve as a foundation of other dog sports and activities. The dog and handler need to communicate well, whereas the handlers ask the dog to retrieve, return, heal, and sit. The main governing bodies for obedience are the AKC, UKC, Canine Work and Games (C-WAGS), Companion Dog Sports Program, and ASCA [11]. During obedience, the dog often looks up at the handler and either to the left or to the right. This can place stress on the cervical musculature and core balance [30]. Exercises that encourage forelimb and hind limb proprioception (level step overs, reverse walking, reverse walking over obstacles), core strengthening, and cervical range of motion are recommended.

Rally, also named Rally Obedience or Rally-O, is more relaxed and more playful than formal obedience. Rally is more handler intensive, whereas obedience is more dog-intensive. In rally, handlers talk to their dog and can even treat their dogs under certain conditions, depending on the governing body. Rally has 10 to 20 stations set up as an obstacle course with signs of obedience commands [11]. Rally has several governing bodies: the AKC, UKC, C-WAGS, ASCA, and World Cynosport.

Injuries sustained in rally and obedience are similar. The dog observes the handler, causing cervical side flexion and rotation. Soft tissue injuries may occur with sudden starts and stops, jumps, tight turns, and slips on turns. Exercises that focus on general proprioception (eg, level step overs, side stepping with and without obstacles), core strength, and cervical flexibility are recommended.

DISCUSSION

The distribution of musculoskeletal injuries observed in sporting dogs differs from the distribution of musculoskeletal injuries observed in pets. Injuries in sporting dogs are more common and more varied, as anticipated based on the intensity of their physical activities. Sporting dogs sustain injuries to tendons around the shoulder joint (supraspinatus, biceps, infraspinatus, serratus ventralis, subscapularis muscles), the hip joint (iliopsoas muscle), and the hock (superficial digital flexor, common calcaneal tendon) [31–37]. Subjectively, sporting dogs do not appear to be at an increased risk of fracture, with the exception of racing greyhounds. Dogs that perform at a higher level have been shown to have an increased injury risk in several sports [8,10,38]. Injury risk is higher in older dogs in some studies [8], but not others [29]. Increased injury risk over time may be linked to the fact that the previous injuries predispose dogs to future injury [8]. The relationship of training intensity and musculoskeletal injury may not be linear. Some studies found that high training intensity was associated with an increased injury risk [4]; others have reported a protective effect of greatly increased training or increased competition frequency [7,39] possibly as a result of reaching peak athletic fitness. In human athletes, training at high speed (ie, training at racing speed or training above lactate thresholds) has been shown to increase injury risks [40,41].

Injuries in sporting dogs should be diagnosed promptly and specifically because management and prognosis vary based on the nature and severity of injuries. Because conventional radiographs lack sensitivity, identifying specific sporting injuries may require advanced medical imaging, including musculoskeletal ultrasound and computed tomography [42]. The use of musculoskeletal ultrasound to diagnose muscle and tendon injuries is increasing [33,37,43,44]. Computed tomography is used to diagnose fractures and fissures in geometrically complex areas [42]. PET is an emerging modality used to diagnose inflammation in musculoskeletal soft tissues and bone [45,46].

Once identified, injuries can be managed conservatively or surgically. Few prospective trials have compared the outcome of conservative and surgical management of sporting dog injuries, in part because randomization may be perceived to be unethical when managing injuries that may be perceived to require surgery. For example, most clinicians treat common calcaneal tendon injuries with surgery, even if the conservative management of these injuries can be successful in dogs and in human athletes [47,48]. There may also be a perception among owners and caregivers that recovery may take longer when musculoskeletal injuries are managed conservatively than when there are managed with surgery. Comparative information about recovery speed and rate with conservative and surgical management in human athletes is available. For example, for tendon ruptures, "… tendons that have nearby agonists can often be managed conservatively, but rupture of isolated prime mover tendons, such as the Achilles and patellar tendons, should be managed

surgically" [49]. In elite human athletes, the time to return to play after lumbar disc herniation does not differ between conservative and surgical management [50]. Because owners and handlers of sporting dogs expect a prompt and optimized recovery whether management is surgical or conservative, it is critical to implement physical rehabilitation proactively, in the immediate postoperative period, before the onset of chronic pain or limb disuse and before the onset of any biological or mechanical complication [51]. Principles of musculoskeletal tissue healing should be followed during recovery: manage injured tissues based on their anticipated recovery rate, individualize management, set measurable objectives, and use evidence-based rehabilitation methods [52].

In conclusion, musculoskeletal injuries occur commonly in sporting dogs; they should be diagnosed and managed promptly. Physical rehabilitation should be implemented in the immediate postoperative period to maximize safety and speed during recovery.

CLINICS CARE POINTS

- Sporting dogs have a high injury rate of approximately 25%. Injuries to the shoulder region, back, hip region, and digits are common and injuries to muscles and tendons are more common in sporting dogs than in sedentary pets.
- The workup of a sporting dog with a lameness should be prompt and focused on identifying the cause of lameness to focus therapy on a specific injury and avoid the development of a chronic problem and minimize time spent away from training or competing.
- Advanced imaging such as musculoskeletal ultrasound or computed tomography may be required to confirm the presence of a specific problem.

REFERENCES

[1] Cullen KL, Dickey JP, Bent LR, et al. Survey-based analysis of risk factors for injury among dogs participating in agility training and competition events. J Am Vet Med Assoc 2013;243(7):1019–24.
[2] Levy M, Hall C, Trentacosta N, et al. A preliminary retrospective survey of injuries occurring in dogs participating in canine agility. Vet Comp Orthop Traumatol 2009;22(4):321–4.
[3] Pechette Markley A, Shoben AB, Kieves NR. Internet Survey of Risk Factors Associated With Training and Competition in Dogs Competing in Agility Competitions. Front Vet Sci 2021;8:791617.

[4] Inkila L, Hyytiainen HK, Hielm-Bjorkman A, et al. Part II of Finnish Agility Dog Survey: Agility-Related Injuries and Risk Factors for Injury in Competition-Level Agility Dogs. Animals (Basel) 2022;12(3):227.

[5] Evanow JA, VanDeventer G, Dinallo G, et al. Internet survey of participant demographics and risk factors for injury in competitive agility dogs. VCOT Open 2021;4: e92–8.

[6] Sellon DC, Marcellin-Little DJ, McFarlane D, et al. Adverse health events and recommended health research priorities in agility dogs as reported by dog owners. Front Vet Sci 2023;10:1127632.

[7] Sellon DC, Marcellin-Little DJ. Risk factors for cranial cruciate ligament rupture in dogs participating in canine agility. BMC Vet Res 2022;18(1):39.

[8] Pinto KR, Chicoine AL, Romano LS, et al. An Internet survey of risk factors for injury in North American dogs competing in flyball. Can Vet J 2021;62(3): 253–60.

[9] Montalbano C, Gamble LJ, Walden K, et al. Internet Survey of Participant Demographics and Risk Factors for Injury in Flyball Dogs. Front Vet Sci 2019;6:391.

[10] Blake SP, Melfi VA, Tabor GF, et al. Injury Risk Factors Associated with Training and Competition in Flyball Dogs. Top Companion Anim Med 2023;53-54:100774.

[11] K. Burns, Jumping into canine sports. Canine sports and rehabilitation medicine growing by leaps and bounds, 2018. Available at: https://www.avma.org/javma-news/ 2018-07-15/jumping-canine-sports. Accessed February 2, 2023.

[12] Franini A, Entani MG, Colosio E, et al. Case report: Flexor carpi ulnaris tendinopathy in a lure-coursing dog treated with three platelet-rich plasma and platelet lysate injections. Front Vet Sci 2023;10:1003993.

[13] Miazga K, Szaluś-Jordanow O, Czopowicz M, et al. Exercise-induced Haematological and Blood Lactate Changes in Whippets Training for Lure Coursing. J Vet Res 2023; 67(1):139–46.

[14] Palmer AL, Rogers CW, Stafford KJ, et al. A retrospective descriptive analysis of race-day injuries of greyhounds in New Zealand. Aust Vet J 2021;99(6):255–62.

[15] Williams SB, Wilson AM, Rhodes L, et al. Functional anatomy and muscle moment arms of the pelvic limb of an elite sprinting athlete: the racing greyhound (Canis familiaris). J Anat 2008;213(4):361–72.

[16] Davis PE. Toe and muscle injuries of the racing greyhound. N Z Vet J 1973;21(7):133–46.

[17] Vaughan LC. Gracilis muscle injury in greyhounds. J Small Anim Pract 1969;10(6):363–75.

[18] Boudrieau RJ, Dee JF, Dee LG. Central tarsal bone fractures in the racing Greyhound: a review of 114 cases. J Am Vet Med Assoc 1984;184(12):1486–91.

[19] Johnson KA. Accessory carpal bone fractures in the racing greyhound. Classification and pathology. Vet Surg 1987; 16(1):60–4.

[20] Ost PC, Dee JF, Dee LG, et al. Fractures of the calcaneus in racing greyhounds. Vet Surg 1987;16(1):53–9.

[21] Payne R. Greyhound sports injuries: racing careers fractured by anatomical imperfections? Vet J 2013;196(3): 280–1.

[22] Wendelburg K, Dee J, Kaderly R, et al. Stress fractures of the acetabulum in 26 racing Greyhounds. Vet Surg 1988; 17(3):128–34.

[23] Bergh MS, Piras A, Samii VF, et al. Fractures in regions of adaptive modeling and remodeling of central tarsal bones in racing Greyhounds. Am J Vet Res 2012;73(3): 375–80.

[24] Goodship AE, Smith RKW. Skeletal physiology: Responses to exercise and training, equine exercise physiology: the science of exercise in the athletic horse. Philadelphia, PA, USA: Saunders Elsevier; 2008. p. 81–105.

[25] Johnson KA, Muir P, Nicoll RG, et al. Asymmetric adaptive modeling of central tarsal bones in racing greyhounds. Bone 2000;27(2):257–63.

[26] Lipscomb VJ, Lawes TJ, Goodship AE, et al. Asymmetric densitometric and mechanical adaptation of the left fifth metacarpal bone in racing greyhounds. Vet Rec 2001; 148(10):308–11.

[27] Muir P, Johnson KA, Ruaux-Mason CP. In vivo matrix microdamage in a naturally occurring canine fatigue fracture. Bone 1999;25(5):571–6.

[28] Calogiuri G, Weydahl A. Health challenges in long-distance dog sled racing: A systematic review of literature. Int J Circumpolar Health 2017;76(1):1396147.

[29] von Pfeil DJ, Liska WD, Nelson S Jr, et al. A survey on orthopedic injuries during a marathon sled dog race. Vet Med (Auckl) 2015;6:329–39.

[30] Harris H, Birch E, Boyd J. An examination of neck angle in obedience dogs whilst completing competition heelwork. Comp Exerc Physiol 2017; 13(1):31–6.

[31] Cullen KL, Dickey JP, Bent LR, et al. Internet-based survey of the nature and perceived causes of injury to dogs participating in agility training and competition events. J Am Vet Med Assoc 2013;243(7):1010–8.

[32] Jopp I, Reese S. Morphological and biomechanical studies on the common calcaneal tendon in dogs. Vet Comp Orthop Traumatol 2009;22(2):119–24.

[33] Mestieri MLA, Dos Santos BG, da Silva MNG, et al. Ultrasonographic diagnosis of bilateral partial rupture of the infraspinatus muscle in a racing greyhound. Braz J Vet Med 2021;43:e003120.

[34] Adrega Da Silva C, Bernard F, Bardet JF, et al. Fibrotic myopathy of the iliopsoas muscle in a dog. Vet Comp Orthop Traumatol 2009;22(3):238–42.

[35] Morey-Matamalas A, Corbetta D, Waine K, et al. Exercise-induced Acute Abdominal Haemorrhage due to Iliopsoas Trauma in Racing Greyhounds. J Comp Pathol 2020;177: 42–6.

[36] Frye CW, Hansen CM, Gendron K, et al. Successful medical management and rehabilitation of exercise-induced dorsal scapular luxation in an ultramarathon endurance sled dog with magnetic resonance imaging diagnosis of

grade II serratus ventralis strain. Can Vet J 2018;59(12):1329–32.

[37] von Pfeil DJF, Davis MS, Liska WD, et al. Orthopedic and ultrasonographic examination findings in 128 shoulders of 64 ultra-endurance Alaskan sled dogs. Vet Surg 2021;50(4):794–806.

[38] Sicard GK, Short K, Manley PA. A survey of injuries at five greyhound racing tracks. J Small Anim Pract 1999;40(9):428–32.

[39] A. Pechette Markley, A. Shoben, N. Kieves, Training load and relationship to injury risk in dogs competing in agility competitions (abstr), 2023 American College of Veterinary Sports Medicine and Rehabilitation Symposium, Charleston, SC, 2023.

[40] Meeuwisse WH, Fowler AR, Christie DJ. A prospective study of injury incidence among elite distance runners. Am J Sports Med 1989;17(5):669–76.

[41] van Gent RN, Siem D, van Middelkoop M, et al. Incidence and determinants of lower extremity running injuries in long distance runners: a systematic review. Br J Sports Med 2007;41(8):469–80 [discussion: 480].

[42] Butler D, Nemanic S, Warnock JJ. Comparison of radiography and computed tomography to evaluate fractures of the canine tarsus. Vet Radiol Ultrasound 2018;59(1):43–53.

[43] Mistieri ML, Wigger A, Canola JC, et al. Ultrasonographic evaluation of canine supraspinatus calcifying tendinosis. J Am Anim Hosp Assoc 2012;48(6):405–10.

[44] Abako J, Holak P, Glodek J, et al. Usefulness of Imaging Techniques in the Diagnosis of Selected Injuries and Lesions of the Canine Tarsus. A Review, Animals (Basel) 2021;11(6):1834.

[45] Frank I, Mann K, Duerr F. Fluorine-18-fluoro-2-deoxy-d-glucose PET-CT aids in detection of soft-tissue injuries for dogs with thoracic or pelvic limb lameness. Vet Radiol Ultrasound 2019;60(5):575–85.

[46] Spriet M. Positron emission tomography: a horse in the musculoskeletal imaging race. Am J Vet Res 2022;83(7):ajvr.22.03.0051.

[47] Mueller MC, Gradner G, Hittmair KM, et al. Conservative treatment of partial gastrocnemius muscle avulsions in dogs using therapeutic ultrasound – A force plate study. Vet Comp Orthop Traumatol 2009;22(3):243–8.

[48] Egger AC, Berkowitz MJ. Achilles tendon injuries. Curr Rev Musculoskelet Med 2017;10(1):72–80.

[49] Orchard J. Management of muscle and tendon injuries in footballers. Aust Fam Physician 2003;32(7):489–93.

[50] Sedrak P, Shahbaz M, Gohal C, et al. Return to Play After Symptomatic Lumbar Disc Herniation in Elite Athletes: A Systematic Review and Meta-analysis of Operative Versus Nonoperative Treatment. Sports Health 2021;13(5):446–53.

[51] Marcellin-Little DJ, Levine D, Millis DL. Multifactorial rehabilitation planning in companion animals. Adv Sm Anim Care 2021;2:1–10.

[52] Kirkby Shaw K, Alvarez L, Foster SA, et al. Fundamental principles of rehabilitation and musculoskeletal tissue healing. Vet Surg 2020;49(1):22–32.

[53] Bockstahler BB, Gesky R, Mueller M, et al. Correlation of surface electromyography of the vastus lateralis muscle in dogs at a walk with joint kinematics and ground reaction forces. Vet Surg 2009;38(6):754–61.

[54] Breitfuss K, Franz M, Peham C, et al. Surface Electromyography of the Vastus Lateralis, Biceps Femoris, and Gluteus Medius Muscle in Sound Dogs During Walking and Specific Physiotherapeutic Exercises. Vet Surg 2015;44(5):588–95.

[55] Lauer SK, Hillman RB, Li L, et al. Effects of treadmill inclination on electromyographic activity and hind limb kinematics in healthy hounds at a walk. Am J Vet Res 2009;70(5):658–64.

[56] McLean H, Millis D, Levine D. Surface Electromyography of the Vastus Lateralis, Biceps Femoris, and Gluteus Medius in Dogs During Stance, Walking, Trotting, and Selected Therapeutic Exercises. Front Vet Sci 2019;6:211.

[57] Miro F, Galisteo AM, Garrido-Castro JL, et al. Surface Electromyography of the Longissimus and Gluteus Medius Muscles in Greyhounds Walking and Trotting on Ground Flat. Up, and Downhill, Animals (Basel) 2020;10(6):968.

SECTION II: EMERGENCY AND CRITICAL CARE

Advances in Small Animal Care 4 (2023) 61–70

ADVANCES IN SMALL ANIMAL CARE

Extracorporeal Therapies in the Emergency Room and Intensive Care Unit

Leonel Londoño, DVM, DACVECC

Capital Veterinary Specialists, 3001 Hartely Road, Jacksonville, FL 32257, USA

KEYWORDS

• Hemodialysis • Therapeutic plasma exchange • Hemoperfusion • Extracorporeal blood purification
• Acute intoxication • Immune-mediated disease

KEY POINTS

- Extracorporeal blood purification therapies include conventional hemodialysis, hemoperfusion, and therapeutic plasma exchange.
- Extracorporeal therapies are applied based on the pharmacokinetic and pharmacodynamic properties of the toxin or endogenous compound targeted to be removed.
- In the emergency room, extracorporeal therapies are used to the remove toxins from systemic circulation, before it leads to severe systemic consequences, organ failure, and death.
- Therapeutic plasma exchange is an adjunct treatment of patients with severe immune-mediated disease not responding to conventional management with immunosuppression alone.
- In critically ill patients, extracorporeal blood purification can be used to treat fluid overload and potentially remove inflammatory cytokines to modulate their systemic inflammation.

INTRODUCTION

The demand for advanced level of care in veterinary patients, along with the versatility of extracorporeal blood purification (EBP) techniques, has led to a fairly rapid expansion of veterinary renal replacement programs for its applications in both renal and nonrenal diseases. The traditional use of EBP from a nephrology standpoint is targeted at the treatment of acute kidney injury and chronic kidney disease. The application of renal replacement therapies in this setting mainly focuses on urea and creatinine reduction as well as fluid and electrolyte homeostasis. Blood purification can also be applied to veterinary patients that require removal of a toxin or endogenous compound to prevent the systemic consequences of the toxin or help modulate their immune

response. The three main modalities of EBP in veterinary medicine include hemodialysis, hemoperfusion, and therapeutic plasma exchange (TPE) [1]. The application of these EBP modalities is based on the physicochemical profile of the substance aimed to be removed, which means that how the toxin or endogenous compound behaves in circulation. Standard intermittent hemodialysis (IHD) machines, continuous renal replacement therapy (CRRT) with membrane-based TPE cartridges, and centrifugal apheresis platforms have the potential to facilitate rapid clearance of a variety of toxins. The most common group of drugs cleared with EBP is nonsteroidal anti-inflammatories using membrane-based TPE or hemoperfusion [2]. TPE for management of immune-mediated conditions in dogs has shown promising results in

E-mail address: leolondonodvm@gmail.com

https://doi.org/10.1016/j.yasa.2023.05.004

decreasing the severity of clinical signs and speeding up recovery by removing immunoglobulins that directly target the tissues/cells in question [3–6]. It is vital to understand the physicochemical properties of the toxin or endogenous compound aimed to be removed to use the appropriate EBP technique that would provide the maximum clearance. In addition, patient characteristics such as body weight and hemodynamic status may prevent the use of EBP in the acute setting. Peritoneal dialysis is not considered an extracorporeal therapy and due to its slow clearance of toxins is not reviewed in this article.

TOXIN REMOVAL IN THE EMERGENCY ROOM

In dogs and cats presenting to the emergency room after an acute ingestion or iatrogenic exposure to a toxin or drug, extracorporeal therapies are indicated if one or more of the following apply.

- The patient fails to respond, or is not a candidate, to standard decontamination techniques (eg, injectable drugs or emesis cannot be induced due to neurologic signs).
- The dose of toxin exposure/ingestion suggests that severe morbidity or mortality is likely (eg, ethylene glycol).
- The normal route of elimination is impaired (eg, patient with chronic kidney disease exposed to a renally cleared drug/toxin).
- An antidote is not available (eg, nonsteroidal anti-inflammatory drugs).

TOXIN PHYSICOCHEMICAL PROPERTIES

The clinician should carefully consider the molecular weight (MW), solubility, protein binding, volume of distribution (V_d), charge, and rate of endogenous clearance when deciding if a toxin is amenable for extracorporeal purification. The ideal substance is a small molecule, with a low volume of distribution, low protein binding (<80%), and one that rapidly distributes from tissue to plasma. Most drugs and toxic compounds weigh less than 500 Da, and most conventional dialyzer membranes used in hemodialysis platforms can filter toxins of this size as long as they are water soluble and minimally bound to protein. Some membranes used in CRRT platforms are able to remove heavier toxins of up to 50,000 Da via convection [7,8]. The MW is not important when considering TPE or carbon hemoperfusion, as the toxins or drugs are either adsorbed by purified carbon particles or removed with other plasma components. When using conventional hemodialysis

for toxin removal, toxins diffuse against their concentration gradient by passive diffusion, decreasing the plasma concentration of the toxin. Most toxins then move from tissue to plasma relatively quickly allowing for rapid removal of the toxin from the entire system. Some toxins have a slower transit from tissues to plasma leading to a phenomenon called toxin-rebound, in which plasma concentrations increase several hours after hemodialysis [8].

Solubility refers to whether a substance dissolves more readily in water or lipid. Hydrophilic toxins have the potential to be effectively cleared with hemodialysis, as they cross into the water-based dialysate. Lipophilic solutes are not readily dialyzed and require other techniques for clearance such as hemoperfusion or TPE. A new technique called single pass lipid dialysis has been reported for the management of two dogs with ivermectin toxicity and ABCB1-1 gene mutation [9]. To remove a toxin or drug via EBP, the toxin should be present in significant quantities within the circulatory system; therefore, the volume of distribution (V_d) of the drug is the major determinant of clearance of the toxin. The volume of distribution refers to the estimated volume into which the drug is distributed in plasma compared with other body tissues. Toxins amenable to extracorporeal purification techniques have a small V_d (<1 L/kg) [8,10]. The closer the V_d of the toxin is to blood volume (0.06–0.09 L/kg), the more removable it becomes as most of the toxin remains within the intravascular space. Highly lipophilic drugs tend to have higher V_d and readily distribute into fat, rendering them relatively inaccessible to removal from the circulation. High V_d toxins (>1.5–2 L/kg) are generally less amenable to removal via EBP; however, extended duration during CRRT sessions, or repeated hemodialysis sessions, may be partially effective.

When drugs or toxins are highly bound to protein (>80%), they cannot be effectively removed via hemodialysis as plasma proteins have a large MW (eg, albumin 69,000 Da) and do not cross most dialyzer membranes [10,11]. Drugs or toxins that are highly protein bound such as non-steroidal ani-inflamtory drugs (NSAIDs) require removal via hemoperfusion or TPE. The algorithm in Fig. 1 shows a suggested approach to the use of EBP in acute intoxications.

HEMODIALYSIS

When considering hemodialysis for extracorporeal purification of selected toxins, IHD is preferred over CRRTs due to higher dialysate and blood flows achieved in IHD platforms compared with CRRT. In human

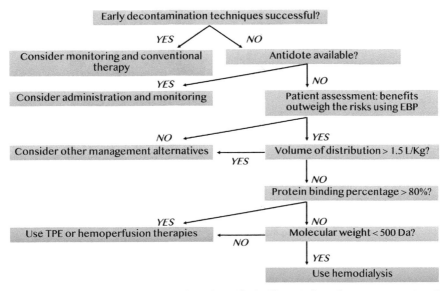

FIG. 1 Algorithm with suggested approach to the patient with acute ingestion or exposure to a toxin.

medicine, it is considered that CRRT for toxin removal has the potential benefits in patients with hemodynamic instability or when removing toxins with rebound characteristics due to slow movement from tissues to plasma, but most studies show that toxin clearance is higher when using IHD [12]. The toxins removed with hemodialysis must be hydrophilic with low MW (<500 Da), low protein binding percentage (<80%), and low volume of distribution (<1 L/kg). Certain deviations from these characteristics may be circumvented by using high-flux dialyzers and prolonged intermittent renal replacement therapies. The veterinary literature is scarce, and a very few case reports are published describing the use of hemodialysis for management of acute intoxications. The following toxins have been removed in acutely intoxicated dogs and cats using hemodialysis.

- Baclofen: dogs [13,14] and cat [15].
- Ethylene glycol: dogs [16,17].
- Ethanol: dog [18].
- Metaldehyde: dogs [19].

Hemoperfusion

Hemoperfusion is a method of EBP wherein a sorbent, most commonly activated charcoal, is used to selectively or non-selectively, and often reversibly, adsorb a circulating toxin. This modality is beneficial in cases of toxins that are not readily dialyzable with conventional IHD due to factors such as a high degree of protein-binding (>80%) or large MW (>500 Da). Hemoperfusion is often combined with other RRT

modalities to minimize complications associated with the nonselective adsorptive properties of activated charcoal. The use of hemoperfusion has fallen out of favor in human medicine accounting only for 1% of hemodialysis applications in United States [20]. Many reasons account for the decreased use of hemoperfusion filters both veterinary and human medicine. In veterinary medicine, the large priming volume required for the use of previous hemoperfusion devices (Fig. 2A) renders them not amenable for use in very small patients. New hemoperfusion devices with low priming volume (Fig. 2B) are currently being used successfully for removal of toxins with or without hemodialysis filters in series [21]. Hypocalcemia, hypoglycemia, and thrombocytopenia are possible sequelae to hemoperfusion performed in isolation [22]. When hemoperfusion and HD are performed in series, blood passes first through the HP cartridge, followed by the HD cartridge, allowing for normalization of electrolyte abnormalities (see Fig. 2A).

The rate of removal for toxins that are large or highly protein bound using HP will generally exceed that of HD alone. However, the HP sorbent column may become saturated at variable rates, resulting in a progressive decline in extraction ratios throughout the treatment. Saturation of HP columns can occur after 2 to 6 hours of continuous use. It results from deposition of cellular debris and plasma proteins from the HP column, with accumulation of adsorbed toxin contributing a relatively small degree to this saturation. To

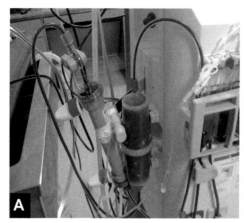 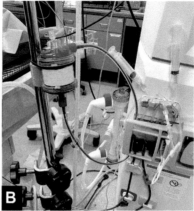

FIG. 2 (A) Charcoal hemoperfusion using the Adsorba 150 C cartridge in-series with an F-160 high-flux dialyzer in IHD platform. (B) Charcoal hemoperfusion using the Atlas V-100 AimaLojic column in an IHD platform bypassing the dialyzer.

minimize the effects of progressive HP column saturation, replacement of the cartridge every 3 to 4 hours may be necessary. In the majority of intoxications, a short treatment of 2 to 4 hours usually suffices to reverse toxic signs and reduce serum concentrations to a safer range. The following toxins or drugs have been successfully removed in companion animals with hemoperfusion in series with hemodialysis.

- Ethchlorvynol (Placidyl): dogs [23].
- Methotrexate: dog [24].
- Phenobarbital: dogs [25].
- Ibuprofen: dog [26].
- Carprofen: dogs [27].
- Cyclosporine: dog [28].

Therapeutic plasma exchange

TPE is a form of apheresis therapy in which plasma is separated from the cellular components of blood. The toxins removed via TPE are usually toxins with large MW ($\geq 15,000$ Da) or are highly protein bound (>80%) to make other, less expensive purification techniques unacceptably inefficient (eg, hemofiltration or high-flux dialysis), and the toxin has a small V_d (<1 L/kg) [29]. Three different ways of performing TPE are available in veterinary medicine including manual removal of small volumes of whole blood via a central line and manual centrifugation (manual TPE); extracorporeal centrifugation or extracorporeal membrane-based TPE [30,31]. In TPE via extracorporeal centrifugation, whole blood is pumped into a fast-rotating separation chamber. The blood components separate into layers based on their density, with the least dense portion, plasma, separating into a layer closest to the axis of rotation and extracted from the patient. In membrane-based TPE, whole blood flows through a bundle of parallel, single, hollow fibers confined in a plastic cylinder (TPE cartridge). Plasma is filtered through the pores of the membrane and a portion is collected, whereas other cellular components are returned to the patient.

A typical goal for each TPE treatment is the removal of one to one and a half plasma volumes and replacement with fluids such as albumin preparations, synthetic or natural colloids, and crystalloids. In humans, a combination of albumin and saline is used most commonly. However, due to complications associated with repeated administration of human albumin in dogs as well as limited availability of a species-specific product, combinations of balanced crystalloids (Lactated ringer's, Plasmalyte 148, Normosol-R) and fresh frozen plasma are typically used. Most of the literature evaluating the use of TPE for acute intoxication in companion animals has been focused on the removal of NSAIDs, the following drugs have been successfully removed with TPE in dogs.

- Ibuprofen: dogs [32–34].
- Meloxicam: dogs [33,35].
- Carprofen: dogs [34,36].
- Naproxen: dogs [33,34,37].
- Deracoxib: dogs [33].

Although the veterinary literature is limited to the management of NSAID intoxications, this platform represents an exciting opportunity for advancing the management of acutely poisoned patients. Further studies are indicated to determine efficacy of TPE in other specific intoxications.

Management of immune-mediated disease in the ICU

TPE is also capable of removing endogenous pathologic substances, including pathologic antibodies, immune complexes, endotoxins, cholesterol-containing lipoproteins, and cytokines [38]. Its use in people with immune-mediated disease is widely described [39]. Plasma exchange is considered a first-line therapy either as a primary, stand-alone treatment or in conjunction with other modes of treatment in people with conditions including Guillain–Barre Syndrome, Wegener granulomatosis, Goodpasture's syndrome, hyperviscosity in monoclonal gammopathies, paraproteinemic polyneuropathies, antibody-mediated transplant rejection, thrombotic thrombocytopenic purpura, and myasthenia gravis [38]. When treating immune-mediated diseases, TPE is generally prescribed every other day, allowing for redistribution of pathologic substances into the intravascular space and thus increasing efficiency of total body antibody removal. Clinical improvement is expected within three to five sessions. If no improvement is seen after this time, additional treatments are unlikely to be beneficial.

In veterinary patients, TPE has been used to treat patients with immune-mediated diseases that are severe in nature or refractory to conventional medical management. Successful use of TPE has been reported in the treatment of dogs immune-mediated hemolytic anemia [40,41]. In dogs with severe IMHA, the use of TPE has been shown to reduce blood transfusion requirements and improve survival (Fig. 3). The use of TPE has also been explored in dogs with immune-mediated thrombocytopenia and mixed hematological disorders (ie, Evan's syndrome) [42,43].

The use of TPE in the management of immune-mediated disease in dogs has also been explored for the management of severe refractory cases of myasthenia gravis, as an adjunct therapy or as a bridge to surgery [6]. The author of this article has also successfully used TPE for treatment of severe pemphigus foliaceus in dogs and a donkey. Specifically, three sessions of TPE in a mature female donkey with refractory pemphigus resulted in a 73% overall reduction in plasma immunoglobulin-G (IgG) levels and significant clinical improvement. The dogs treated also demonstrated marked improvement in clinical signs and therapeutic immunosuppressive de-escalation was possible following TPE (Fig. 4). However, as with most EBP treatments in veterinary patients, the literature on the use of TPE for immune-mediated diseases is limited to case reports and case series. Thus, randomized, controlled trials are indicated to definitively quantify the benefits of this treatment and to classify TPE as a first-line therapy in certain immune-mediated diseases.

Management of fluid overload in the ICU

Fluid overload due to overzealous fluid administration has been associated with increased morbidity and mortality in both human and veterinary ICUs [44,45]. The pathologic accumulation of body water that leads to interstitial and visceral edema worsens organ dysfunction. The cause of positive fluid balance in ICU patients is multifactorial.

- Liberal fluid therapy
- Inappropriate monitoring of fluid balance
- Renal dysfunction and development of oliguria/anuria
- Endothelial dysfunction and damage to the glycocalyx
- Hepatic dysfunction

The development of fluid overload also puts an increased demand on the kidneys which not only are responsible for clear excessive solutes and water delivered with intravenous fluids but also suffer the consequence of visceral edema, leading to increased intracapsular pressure, renal venous congestion, transtubular pressure, and reduced glomerular filtration rate [46]. Fluid overload can be treated with EBP, as water is considered a uremic toxin and hemodialysis can help reduce the water content by means of ultrafiltration. The early initiation of hemodialysis based on triggers such as development of oliguria regardless of creatinine levels has been shown to increase renal recovery rates and decreased mortality in people [47]. This is likely due to prevention of fluid overload associated with impaired renal function and overzealous fluid therapy. No current studies are available in small animals that describe the use of early hemodialysis to avoid the deleterious effects of fluid overload.

Slow continuous ultrafiltration

Slow continuous ultrafiltration (SCUF) is a form EBP that can be performed in a CRRT platform and intended to be performed in a true critical care setting for 24 hours per day. This modality of CRRT uses high-flux dialyzers and in people is mostly used for management of refractory heart failure and evidence of fluid overload that fails to respond to diuretic therapy [48]. This form of EBP uses low filtration rates and no substitution fluids; therefore, the clearance of other pathologic substances, besides water, is minimal compared with other forms of EBP. Its use is well-described in humans with non-

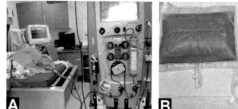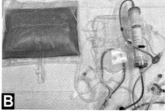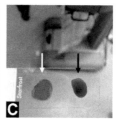

FIG. 3 (*A*) Therapeutic plasma exchange (TPE) in a 7-year-old mixed breed dog with severe immune-mediated hemolytic anemia. (*B*) The extracorporeal TPE-2000 circuit used and 2.4 L of plasma exchanged from the dog. (*C*) Degree of red blood cell microagglutination immediately before (*white arrow*) and after TPE (*black arrow*).

diuretic responsive congestive heart failure. In general, this extracorporeal therapy may represent a yet unexplored option for treating refractory heart failure in veterinary patients. More research is indicated to investigate its feasibility and efficacy in dogs and cats with diuretic-resistant fluid overload.

Management of liver failure and hyperbilirubinemia in the ICU

Many conditions associated with acute liver failure and secondary hepatic encephalopathy are commonly managed in the ICU, along with conditions leading to severe hyperbilirubinemia and secondary kernicterus. The use of TPE to reduce bilirubin levels has been previously evaluated in human patients and shown to significantly decrease total and direct bilirubin levels [49]. Two case reports have shown that TPE is an effective therapy that not only reduces plasma bilirubin

levels in dogs with hyperbilirubinemia secondary to immune-mediated hemolytic anemia but aids in resolving the neurologic signs associated with bilirubin encephalopathy, also known as kernicterus [50,51]. A single case report in a dog has also shown that TPE is an alternative method of rapidly reducing ammonia levels in dogs with hepatic encephalopathy [52]. Although no large-scale studies have been performed to evaluate the role of EBP in the management of severe hyperbilirubinemia and hyperammonemia in companion animals, these case studies show that TPE can be used for the management of these patients.

Patient considerations

Any extracorporeal treatment is defined by the prescription, which is developed based on the physical and clinical condition of the patient, as well as variations in body fluid volume and composition of the substance

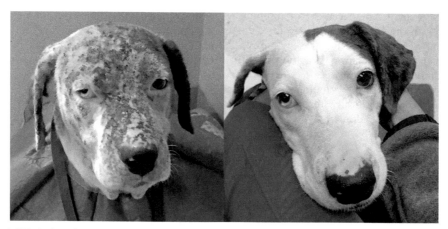

FIG. 4 Skin lesions in a 2-year-old intact female Catahoula Leopard Hog Dog with severe and refractory pemphigus foliaceus before treatment with TPE and 4 weeks after three TPE sessions 48 hours apart, using membrane-based-TPE.

being removed. The prescription should account for the physiologic, hematologic, and biochemical status of the patient before extracorporeal purification is initiated. Factors to consider in patient assessment include.

- Species
- Weight
- Hemodynamic stability (risk of hypovolemia and/or hypotension)
- Hematocrit and total plasma proteins
- Electrolyte and acid-base derangements
- Oxygenation capacity
- Coagulation status
- Current medications
- Recent surgery or healing wounds

It may be more challenging to perform EBP on patients that are small in size. In general, patients can tolerate loss of up to 20% of total blood volume before developing major clinical signs of hypovolemic shock, such as tachycardia, hypotension, and complete hemodynamic collapse. Thus, it is important to consider the volume of the extracorporeal circuit in relation to the patient's blood volume to decide whether the benefit of EBP outweighs risk to the patient. The species being treated is important as there are significant variations in blood volume according to each species; for example, in dogs, the blood volume is considered to be 80 to 90 mL/kg, whereas in cats, it is 50 to 60 mL/kg. Options to mitigate the risk of performing EBP in very small patients include using blood to prime the extracorporeal circuit. An alternate method is performing rapid transfusion directly to the patient as the extracorporeal circulation is started. Transfusion reactions are possible but are uncommon in clinical practice. Although these techniques may increase the cost of performing EBP, hemodynamic stability seems improved in small patients receiving a blood prime.

Coagulation status is also an important consideration when selecting patients for EBP. Various disease states may cause an increased risk of hypercoagulability during extracorporeal therapies, and in these patients, more aggressive anticoagulation protocols will be necessary. Severe systemic inflammation, immune-mediated disease, and neoplasia may affect the coagulation cascade in varying ways, so careful monitoring of clotting times during EBP is required to prevent clotting of the extracorporeal circuit and provide efficient EBP. Alternatively, patients in a preexisting hypocoagulable state also require special consideration. Clotting factor deficiencies, thrombocytopenia, thrombocytopathies, and hyperfibrinolysis may cause increased bleeding tendencies. In such patients, the risks of excessive hemorrhage from traditional unfractionated heparin

administration are too great despite the need to provide EBP, and the use of regional citrate may be preferred. Finally, patients with recent surgery or healing wounds may have delayed healing due to the removal of albumin and other immune components when performing TPE.

Complications of extracorporeal blood purification

Several retrospective studies have evaluated the rate of complications associated with EBP in companion animals. High rate of complications is reported, ranging between 33.8% and 54.5% [2,33,34]. Most complications were considered mild and self-resolving, and death was not reported as a complication associated with EBP in small animals. Some of the complications could not be directly attributed to EBP [2]. The most complications include.

- Mild hypotension
- Urticaria and facial swelling secondary to plasma transfusion during TPE
- Thrombocytopenia secondary to platelet activation during hemoperfusion
- External bleeding from the catheter insertion site due to systemic heparinization
- Excessive clotting of the TPE cartridge and discontinuation of therapy

Despite the high rate of complications associated with EBP, mortality rate was not significantly impacted by the high complication rates. In these studies, between 88.9% and 100% of patients who were treated with EBP survived to discharge from hospital [2,33,34]. Lower survival rates were associated with worse clinical signs of toxicity at presentation before the initiation of EBP in one study [2]. These findings suggest that the benefits of EBP outweigh the risks associated with the application of these therapies in small animals.

Present relevance and future avenues to consider or to investigate

As EBP advances and hemodialysis units become more available in veterinary ICUs, the role of EBP in the management of emergent and critically ill patients will become more evident. Controlled trials that evaluate the effect of EBP in patient outcomes and recovery are lacking. The biggest challenge is appropriate randomization of patients when considering that most dogs and cats presenting to the emergency room with an acute intoxication do not have a clear timeline or dose of toxin ingested, and the severity of immune-mediated conditions such as immune-mediated

hemolytic anemia, immune-mediated thrombocytopenia and others, is intrinsic to each patient. Despite
these challenges, research should be aimed at developing guidelines for the indications, prescription, and
adequate interventions when managing patients with
EBP in the critical care setting.

SUMMARY/DISCUSSION

The body of veterinary literature on EBP therapy in
small animals is exponentially growing with a fair number of case reports and multiple retrospective studies.
The use of EBP in acute intoxications not only has
been proven to be safe, but based on pharmacologic
monitoring of drugs levels in case reports, it has been
proven to be effective at removing circulating toxins
and preventing development of clinical signs associated
with acute intoxications and decreasing the likelihood
of organ damage and failure. Knowledge of the physicochemical properties of the toxin or drug in question is
essential when choosing the EBP technique and the
risk–benefit ratio associated with blood purification.
In the ICU, the role of EBP is expanding to the management of those refractory and severe cases of immune-
mediated disease not only as an adjunct therapy to
improve immunomodulation but also to reduce the
neurological effects of severe hyperbilirubinemia in
cases of hemolytic anemia and hyperammonemia in
cases of hepatic encephalopathy. Finally, EBP can be
used for the management of fluid overload due to renal
dysfunction and overzealous fluid therapy in small animals. EBP will likely play a role in the management of
critical illness, when enough evidence suggests that
cytokine removal can help modulate immune response
and endothelial dysfunction in severe sepsis and noninfectious causes of critical illness.

CLINICS CARE POINTS

- In dogs and cats with an acute intoxication and failure to respond to conventional decontamination techniques, blood purification techniques should be considered early in the course of treatment to decrease morbidity and mortality.
- Nonsteroidal anti-inflammatory drugs is the group of toxins most commonly treated with extracorporeal blood purification in veterinary patients, therapeutic plasma exchange should be considered as a therapeutic option to decrease the likelihood of organ damage, development of clinical signs and improve survival.

- In severe and refractory cases of immune-mediated disease (eg, immune-mediated hemolytic anemia, immune-mediated thrombocytopenia, myasthenia gravis or pemphigus), therapeutic plasma exchange should be considered as an adjunct therapy for control of clinical signs.
- In cases of severe hyperbilirubinemia and hyperammonemia leading to severe neurological signs, therapeutic plasma exchange can be considered to reduce the levels of these endogenous neurotoxicants.
- The high complication rates observed in veterinary patients with extracorporeal therapies should not be the reason to avoid referral, as these complications are for the most part self-limiting and not associated with mortality.

DISCLOSURE

The author mentioned the study Buckley GJ, Londoño L, Grabar RD, et al. Ex-vivo evaluation of ibuprofen removal by AimaLogic V100-Atlas hemoperfusion device from canine whole blood. J Vet Emerg Crit Care. 2020;30(S1):3. This study was financially supported by the company AimaLogic Animal Health. However, this support does not influence the data of this abstract article. In addition to this disclosure, the author has nothing to disclose.

REFERENCES

[1] Cowgill LD, Guillaumin J. Extracorporeal renal replacement therapy and blood purification in critical care. J Vet Emerg Crit Care 2013;23(2):194–204.
[2] Groover J, Londoño LA, Tapia-Ruano K, et al. Extracorporeal blood purification in acutely intoxicated veterinary patients: A multicenter retrospective study (2011–2018): 54 cases. J Vet Emerg Crit Care 2022;32:34–41.
[3] Francey T, Etter M, Schweighauser A. Evaluation of membrane-based therapeutic plasma exchange as adjunctive treatment for immune-mediated hematologic disorders in dogs. J Vet Intern Med 2021;35:925–35.
[4] Kopecny L, Palm CA, Naylor S, et al. Application of therapeutic plasma exchange in dogs with immune-mediated thrombocytopenia. J Vet Intern Med 2020;34:1576–81.
[5] Culler CA, Vigani A, Ripoll AZ, et al. Centrifugal therapeutic plasma exchange in dogs with immune-mediated hemolytic anemia (2016–2018): 7 cases. J Vet Emerg Crit Care 2022;32:645–52.
[6] Vitalo A, Buckley G, Londoño L. Therapeutic plasma exchange as adjunct therapy in 3 dogs with myasthenia gravis and myasthenia-like syndrome. J Vet Emerg Crit Care 2021;31:106–11.
[7] Monaghan KN, Acierno MJ. Extracorporeal removal of drugs and toxins. Vet Clin North Am Small Anim Pract 2011;41(1):227–38.

[8] King JD, Kern MH, Jaar BG. Extracorporeal Removal of Poisons and Toxins. Clin J Am Soc Nephrol 2019; 14(9):1408–15.

[9] Londoño LA, Buckley GJ, Bolfer L, et al. Clearance of plasma ivermectin with single pass lipid dialysis in 2 dogs. J Vet Emerg Crit Care 2017;27:232–7.

[10] Roberts DM, Buckley NA. Pharmacokinetic considerations in clinical toxicology: Clinical applications. Clin Pharmacokinet 2007;46:897–939.

[11] Eloot S, Schneditz D, Cornelis T, et al. Protein-bound uremic toxin profiling as a tool to optimize hemodialysis. PLoS One 2016;11:e0147159.

[12] Kim Z, Goldfarb DS. Continuous renal replacement therapy does not have a clear role in the treatment of poisoning. Nephron Clin Pract 2010;115(1):c1–6.

[13] Torre DM, Labato MA, Rossi T, et al. Treatment of a dog with severe baclofen intoxication using hemodialysis and mechanical ventilation. J Vet Emerg Crit Care 2008;18: 312–8.

[14] Gabba L, Iannucci C, Vigani A. Hemodialysis as emergency treatment of a severe baclofen intoxication in a 3 kg dog. Vet Med Sci 2023;9(1):43–6.

[15] Hoffman L, Londoño LA, Martinez J. Management of severe baclofen toxicosis using hemodialysis in conjunction with mechanical ventilation in a cat with chronic kidney disease. JFMS Open Rep 2021;7(2). https://doi.org/10.1177/20551169211033770.

[16] Schweighauser A, Francey T. Ethylene glycol poisoning in three dogs: Importance of early diagnosis and role of hemodialysis as a treatment option. Schweiz Arch Tierheilkd 2016;158(2):109–14.

[17] Vitalaru BA, Balascau SB. Antifreeze acute intoxication: hemodialysis in two German Sheppard dogs. Bull UASVM Vet Med 2015;72(2):411–4.

[18] Keno LA, Langston CE. Treatment of accidental ethanol intoxication with hemodialysis in a dog. J Vet Emerg Crit Care 2011;21:363–8.

[19] Teichmann-Knorrn S, Doerfelt S, Doerfelt R. Retrospective evaluation of the use of hemodialysis in dogs with suspected metaldehyde poisoning (2012-2017): 11 cases. J Vet Emerg Crit Care 2020;30(2):194–201.

[20] Ghannoum M, Lavergne V, Gosselin S, et al. Practice trends in the use of extracorporeal treatments for poisoning in four countries. Semin Dial 2016;29:71–80.

[21] Buckley GJ, Londoño L, Grabar RD, et al. Ex-vivo evaluation of ibuprofen removal by AimaLogic V100-Atlas hemoperfusion device from canine whole blood. J Vet Emerg Crit Care 2020;30(S1):3.

[22] Ghannoum M, Bouchard J, Nolin TD, et al. Hemoperfusion for the treatment of poisoning: Technology, determinants of poison clearance, and application in clinical practice. Semin Dial 2014;27:350–61.

[23] Zmuda MJ. Resin hemoperfusion in dogs intoxicated with ethchlorvynol (Placidyl). Kidney Int 1980;17(3): 303–11.

[24] Pardo M, Lanaux T, Davy R, et al. Use of charcoal hemoperfusion and hemodialysis in the treatment of

[25] methotrexate toxicosis in a dog. J Vet Emerg Crit Care 2018;28(3):269–73.

[25] Hill JB, Palaia FL, McAdams JL, et al. Efficacy of activated charcoal hemoperfusion in removing lethal doses of barbiturates and salicylate from the blood of rats and dogs. Clin Chem 1976;22(6):754–60.

[26] Tauk BS, Foster JD. Treatment of ibuprofen toxicity with serial charcoal hemoperfusion and hemodialysis in a dog. J Vet Emerg Crit Care 2016;26:787–92.

[27] Fick ME, Messenger KM, Vigani A. Efficacy of a single session in-series hemoperfusion and hemodialysis in the management of carprofen overdose in two dogs. J Vet Emerg Crit Care 2020;30:226–31.

[28] Segev G, Cowgill LD. Treatment of acute kidney injury associated with cyclosporine overdose in a dog using hemodialysis and charcoal hemoperfusion. J Vet Emerg Crit Care 2018;28(2):163–7.

[29] Winters JL. Plasma exchange: concepts, mechanisms, and an overview of the American Society for Apheresis guidelines. Hematology Am Soc Hematol Educ Program 2012; 2012(1):7–12.

[30] Francey T, Schweighauser A. Membrane-based therapeutic plasma exchange in dogs: Prescription, anticoagulation, and metabolic response. J Vet Intern Med 2019;33:1635–45.

[31] Culler CA, Vigani A, Ripoll AZ, et al. Centrifugal therapeutic plasma exchange in dogs with immune-mediated hemolytic anemia (2016–2018): 7 cases. J Vet Emerg Crit Care 2022;32:645–52.

[32] Walton S, Ryan KA, Davis JL, et al. Treatment of ibuprofen intoxication in a dog via therapeutic plasma exchange. J Vet Emerg Crit Care 2017;27:451–7.

[33] Rosenthal MG, Labato MA. Use of therapeutic plasma exchange to treat nonsteroidal anti-inflammatory drug overdose in dogs. J Vet Intern Med 2019;33:596–602.

[34] Butty EM, Suter SE, Chalifoux NV, et al. Outcomes of nonsteroidal anti-inflammatory drug toxicosis treated with therapeutic plasma exchange in 62 dogs. J Vet Intern Med 2022;36(5):1641–7.

[35] Walton S, Ryan KA, Davis JL, et al. Treatment of meloxicam overdose in a dog via therapeutic plasma exchange. J Vet Emerg Crit Care 2017;27:444–50.

[36] Kjaergaard AB, Davis JL, Acierno MJ. Treatment of carprofen overdose with therapeutic plasma exchange in a dog. J Vet Emerg Crit Care 2018;28:356–60.

[37] Kicera-Temple K, Londoño L, Lanaux TM, et al. Treatment of a massive naproxen overdose with therapeutic plasma exchange in a dog. Clin Case Rep 2019;7(8):1529–33.

[38] Reeves HM, Winters JL. The mechanisms of action of plasma exchange. Brit J Haematol 2014;164:342–51.

[39] Padmanabhan A, Connelly-Smith L, Aqui N, et al. Guidelines on the use of therapeutic apheresis in clinical practice – evidence-based approach from the Writing Committee of the American Society for Apheresis: the eighth special issue. J Clin Apheresis 2019;34:171–354.

[40] Crump KL, Seshadri R. Use of therapeutic plasmapheresis in a case of canine immune-mediated hemolytic anemia. J Vet Emerg Crit Care 2009;19:375–80.

[41] Scagnelli AM, Walton SA, Liu CC, et al. Effects of therapeutic plasma exchange on serum immunoglobulin concentrations in a dog with refractory immune-mediated hemolytic anemia. J Am Vet Med Assoc 2018;252:1108–12.

[42] Francey T, Etter M, Schweighauser A. Evaluation of membrane-based therapeutic plasma exchange as adjunctive treatment for immune-mediated hematologic disorders in dogs. J Vet Intern Med 2021;35:925–35.

[43] Kopecny L, Palm CA, Naylor S, et al. Application of therapeutic plasma exchange in dogs with immune-mediated thrombocytopenia. J Vet Intern Med 2020;34:1576–81.

[44] Messmer AS, Zingg C, Müller M, et al. Fluid Overload and Mortality in Adult Critical Care Patients-A Systematic Review and Meta-Analysis of Observational Studies. Crit Care Med 2020;48(12):1862–70.

[45] Cavanagh AA, Sullivan LA, Hansen BD. Retrospective evaluation of fluid overload and relationship to outcome in critically ill dogs. J Vet Emerg Crit Care 2016;26(4):578–86.

[46] Prowle JR, Kirwan CJ, Bellomo R. Fluid management for the prevention and attenuation of acute kidney injury. Nat Rev Nephrol 2014;10(1):37–47.

[47] Zarbock A, Kellum JA, Schmidt C, et al. Effect of Early vs Delayed Initiation of Renal Replacement Therapy on Mortality in Critically Ill Patients With Acute Kidney Injury: The ELAIN Randomized Clinical Trial. JAMA 2016;315(20):2190–9.

[48] Ronco C, Ricci A, Brendolan A, et al. Ultrafiltration in Patients with Hypervolemia and Congestive Heart Failure. Blood Purif 2004;22(1):150–63.

[49] Keklik M, Sivgin S, Kaynar L, et al. Treatment with plasma exchange may serve beneficial effect in patients with severe hyperbilirubinemia: a single center experience. Transfus Apher Sci 2013;48(3):323–6.

[50] Tovar T, Deitschel S, Guenther C. The use of therapeutic plasma exchange to reduce serum bilirubin in a dog with kernicterus. J Vet Emerg Crit Care 2017;27:458–64.

[51] Heffner GG, Cavanagh A, Nolan B. Successful management of acute bilirubin encephalopathy in a dog with immune-mediated hemolytic anemia using therapeutic plasma exchange. J Vet Emerg Crit Care 2019;29:549–57.

[52] Culler CA, Reinhardt A, Vigani A. Successful management of clinical signs associated with hepatic encephalopathy with manual therapeutic plasma exchange in a dog. J Vet Emerg Crit Care 2020;30:312–7.

Advances in Small Animal Care 4 (2023) 71–87

ADVANCES IN SMALL ANIMAL CARE

The Use of Biomarkers to Track and Treat Critical Illness

Robert Goggs, BVSc, PhD, DACVECC, DECVECC, MRCVS

Department of Clinical Sciences, Cornell University College of Veterinary Medicine, Ithaca, NY 14850, USA

KEYWORDS

• Dogs   • Cats   • Kidney injury   • Sepsis   • Cardiac disease   • Omics   • Glycocalyx

KEY POINTS

- Biomarkers are objectively measurable parameters that provide clinicians with timely information to guide diagnosis and patient management beyond what can be obtained from routinely available data.
- Clinicians should evaluate the primary literature supporting use of a novel biomarker before using it to guide patient management.
- Biomarkers are available to help clinicians recognize acute kidney injury early, evaluate cardiac injury and dysfunction, assess the inflammatory and immune responses, and to identify damage to the endothelium.
- In the near future, omics technologies may provide us with panels of biomarkers that will substantially improve our ability to diagnose disease and to monitor critically ill patients.
- Biomarkers should ideally be measured serially to maximize diagnostic and prognostic performance and to optimize management of individual patients.

INTRODUCTION

A biomarker is defined as "a characteristic that can be objectively measured and evaluated as an indicator of normal biological processes, pathogenic processes, or pharmacologic responses to a therapeutic intervention" [1,2]. Although any physical examination parameter could, by this definition, be classified as a biomarker, "the utility of a biomarker lies in its capacity to provide timely information beyond that which is readily available from routine physiologic data and clinical examination" [3]. In 2015, the US Food and Drug Administration and the US National Institutes of Health developed the BEST (Biomarkers, EndpointS, and other Tools) Resource to codify various terms in this field in the interests of clarity and consistency [4] and defined 7 types of biomarkers: diagnostic, monitoring, pharmacodynamic, predictive, prognostic, risk (susceptibility), and safety. Optimal biomarker use

also requires understanding of some key principles of statistics and probability.

Incidence
Number of new cases of disease in a specified period in the population of interest.

Prevalence
The proportionate amount of a disease present in the population of interest at a point or period of time.

Diagnostic Pretest Probability
The probability a patient has the disease of interest before a diagnostic test result is known. This is a means to estimate prevalence in the specific population evaluated based on signalment, history, presentation, and setting. The pretest probability helps determine which,

---

E-mail address: r.goggs@cornell.edu

https://doi.org/10.1016/j.yasa.2023.07.001

if any, biomarker should be measured and aids in test interpretation.

Sensitivity
Proportion of patients with a disease that test positive (true positive proportion). Sensitivity = TP/TP + FN, where TP is true positive and FN is false negative. High sensitivity diagnostic tests are best used to rule out disease. Highly sensitive tests have low false-negative rates. If the test is sensitive and the test result is negative, then the disease is unlikely. The only exception is if the prevalence is very high.

Specificity
Proportion of patients without a disease that test negative (true negative proportion). Specificity = TN/TN + FP, where TN is true negative and FP is false positive. High-specificity tests are best used to rule in disease. Highly specific tests have low false-positive rates. If the test is specific and the test result is positive, then one can be confident of the diagnosis. The only exception is if the prevalence is very low.

Positive Predictive Value
The proportion of patients that test positive test that have the disease: positive predictive value (PPV) = TP/TP + FP.

Negative Predictive Value
The proportion of patients that test negative test that are disease free: negative predictive value (NPV) = TN/TN + FN.

The ideal biomarker is minimally invasive, sensitive, and specific; has high prognostic value; correlates with illness severity; tracks the course of disease; provides biologic insight into the disorder; and can be cheaply, easily, rapidly, and ubiquitously measured. The veterinary and human literature is littered with biomarker studies. A brief, unsystematic literature search identified 6100 articles related to biomarkers in dogs and cats in the last 25 years with 3385 in the last 10 years. Ideally, the primary literature should be critically evaluated, and biomarker performance scrutinized before new markers are used to guide patient management. Biomarkers used in clinical practice should have been extensively validated, with known characteristics and repeatable, reproducible, standardized, precise, and accurate assay performance. Few biomarkers in veterinary medicine fulfill these criteria. The following sections discuss groups of biomarkers categorized by organ system, disease process or by biomarker class. Lactate will not be discussed because although it is a vital biomarker for veterinary critical care, its utility is well established and has been thoroughly reviewed elsewhere [5,6].

ACUTE KIDNEY INJURY
Established markers of kidney function, including blood urea nitrogen, creatinine, and symmetric dimethylarginine (SDMA), are surrogate indicators of global kidney glomerular filtration rate (GFR). Following acute kidney injury (AKI), these markers take 48 hours or greater to increase and only after 20% or greater decrease in GFR; hence, none of these markers identifies AKI in its early stages. More sensitive markers that increase rapidly following AKI might enable early therapeutic intervention. Moreover, markers that pinpoint the anatomic area of injury would provide pathophysiologic and diagnostic insights. The most promising markers are neutrophil gelatinase-associated lipocalin (NGAL), cystatin C (CysC), cystatin B, clusterin, and kidney-injury molecule-1 (KIM-1) (Fig. 1). A multiplexed bead-based assay for 5 kidney-injury biomarkers has been validated for use in dogs [7] and has been used to demonstrate AKI in dogs following hemorrhagic shock and resuscitation [8,9].

Neutrophil gelatinase-associated lipocalin
NGAL is a small neutrophil protein that is also expressed at very low levels in the epithelia of the kidneys, skin, and lungs. Expression of NGAL is markedly increased in damaged epithelia, such as in patients with sepsis. Renal NGAL expression is a robust and early response to ischemic or toxic kidney injury and can be detected in blood and urine soon after AKI using commercially available enzyme linked immunosorbent assays (ELISAs). There are now multiple studies in the veterinary literature describing the use of NGAL for the detection of AKI in small animals. Serum and urine NGAL (sNGAL, uNGAL) concentrations in azotemic dogs are significantly higher than in nonazotemic dogs and correlate with serum creatinine [11,12]. Urine NGAL in dogs following surgery enables an early identification of AKI [13]. Significantly increased concentrations of plasma and urine NGAL are detectable in dogs with renal azotemia compared with healthy controls, whereas plasma NGAL concentrations are significantly higher in dogs with AKI compared with dogs with chronic kidney disease (CKD), suggesting that plasma NGAL could be helpful to differentiate these processes [14]. In dogs with CKD, sNGAL, and uNGAL concentrations were significantly greater and superior to creatinine as a negative prognostic indicator in nonsurvivors [15].

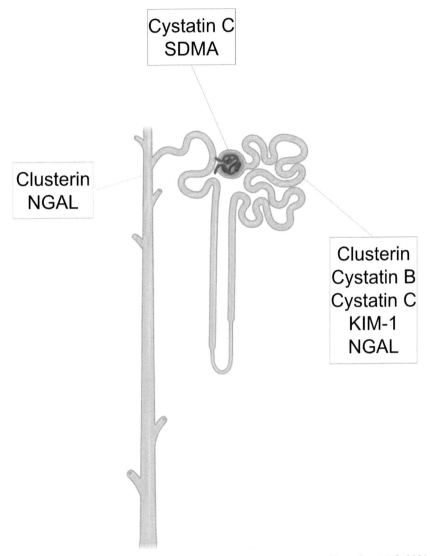

Cystatin C
SDMA

Clusterin
NGAL

Clusterin
Cystatin B
Cystatin C
KIM-1
NGAL

FIG. 1 The tissue locations of kidney injury indicated by available biomarkers. (*From* Gewin LS, 2021, 10 per Yu Ueda, NCSU. [10] - Gewin LS. Sugar or Fat? Renal Tubular Metabolism Reviewed in Health and Disease. Nutrients. May 9 2021;13(5):1580. https://doi.org/10.3390/nu13051580)

Cystatin C

Cystatin C (CysC) is a low molecular weight cysteine protease inhibitor, synthesized and released into the blood at a constant rate by all nucleated cells [16]. It is freely filtered by the glomerulus, completely reabsorbed by the proximal tubule, and not secreted, making CysC an excellent marker of GFR [17]. Urinary CysC concentrations are extremely low in healthy individuals compared with individuals with renal tubular damage [18]. Human CysC assays have been validated for urine and serum for both dogs and cats [19–22], and dogs with CKD had significantly higher CysC concentrations compared with healthy dogs [23,24], and dogs with various nonrenal diseases [20,25–28]. There is an overlap in serum CysC concentrations between dogs with nonrenal disease and healthy dogs and between healthy dogs and dogs with CKD however, which may limit the utility of serum CysC. The urinary CysC to creatinine ratio is significantly higher in dogs and in cats with renal disease compared with healthy dogs and dogs with nonrenal disease [21,24]. The effects of age, sex, and bodyweight on CysC concentrations are equivocal but it does seem that CysC should be measured on fasted samples. A recent study suggested that serum CysC may be inferior to creatinine and SDMA for the detection of decreased GFR [29]. Additional questions about assay accuracy, prognostic significance and the effect of proteinuria, inflammation, and drug therapies on CysC values remain to be answered.

Cystatin B

In contrast to CysC, which is a marker of GFR, cystatin B is a small intracellular protein released specifically from injured kidney cells. Serum and urine concentrations of cystatin B released by ruptured renal tubular epithelial cells increase early in kidney injury but are not altered in dogs with urinary tract infections [30]. In experimental models in dogs, kidney injury induced by aminoglycoside administration increased cystatin B concentrations days before an increase in serum creatinine concentration was observed [30]. This suggests serum cystatin B concentrations may provide advanced warning of kidney injury in dogs. Urinary cystatin B concentrations are also increased after envenomation by *Vipera* snakes known to have nephrotoxic venom, despite no changes in creatinine or SDMA, suggesting that cystatin B is highly sensitive to tubular injury in dogs [31].

Clusterin

Clusterin, also called apolipoprotein J, is a highly glycosylated extracellular chaperone expressed in various tissues that undergoes tissue-specific posttranslational modifications [30]. Urine clusterin concentrations are frequently undetectable in health and increase substantially following tubular damage. Serum clusterin concentrations increase in various pathologic processes but are always an order of magnitude higher than in urine. To identify AKI, it is therefore crucial that kidney-specific clusterin is measured in urine samples devoid of blood contamination. Increased urine concentrations of kidney-specific clusterin measured using a sensitive immunoassay indicate proximal tubular damage [32]. Experimental studies in dogs demonstrate dramatic increases in the concentration of this marker in response to aminoglycoside administration not accompanied by changes in serum creatinine concentration [33]. The assay has also been used to identified proximal tubular injury in dogs envenomated by European adder (*Vipera berus berus*) [31]. The assay can also

be used to measure clusterin concentrations in feline urine samples [30].

Kidney-injury molecule-1

This is a transmembrane glycoprotein primarily found on the surfaces of T cells. Following ischemic or toxic AKI, proximal tubule cells dedifferentiate and overexpress KIM-1, an increase of up to 100-fold. Proteolytic cleavage of this transmembrane protein yields a fragment that can be readily detected in urine [34–36]. Urinary concentrations of KIM-1 increase within several hours of injury and remain increased for up to 48 hours in humans, and thus may have utility as an early warning system for AKI prediction [37]. KIM-1 does not seem to be significantly affected by chronic kidney disease or urinary tract infections in people and may therefore be useful for differentiating subtypes of AKI. KIM-1 can be detected in dogs and has been demonstrated to be sensitive to nephrotoxin-induced proximal tubular damage [38]. In dogs with naturally occurring AKI, urine KIM-1 concentrations were significantly increased but this biomarker may not be ideal for the differentiation of AKI from CKD [39]. In cats, KIM-1 expression in kidney tissue is a sensitive indicator of AKI in induced and naturally occurring disease [40].

CARDIAC BIOMARKERS

Cardiac disease is a common cause of emergency admission, whereas cardiac dysfunction is an important component of the syndrome of critical illness. Cardiac biomarkers aid the identification of myocardial injury and help gauge the degree of dysfunction. The most widely used and carefully studied are the troponins and natriuretic peptides. Novel cardiac biomarkers including cytokine panels [41], galectin-3 and interleukin-1 receptor-like-1 protein [42], are being investigated. It seems likely, that veterinarians will increasingly look to proteomics and metabolomics to identify new markers that can be used to improve care of the critically ill cardiac patient [43,44].

Troponins

Cardiac troponin I (cTnI) is 1 of 3 cardiomyocyte actin/myosin binding and regulatory proteins. Myocyte damage and disruption of the contractile apparatus leads to leakage of these proteins into circulation (Fig. 2). The cardiac isoform cTnI is specific to cardiac tissue and denotes cardiomyocyte injury or necrosis. Although cTnI is specific for cardiac muscle injury, it does not help to differentiate the underlying cause such that cTnI values are increased in dogs with myocardial trauma,

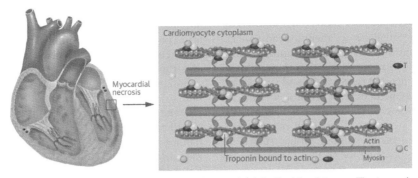

FIG. 2 Myocardial injury leads to release of troponin proteins into the bloodstream. The troponin complex consists of troponin C, troponin I, and troponin T, bound to actin or free within cardiomyocyte cytoplasm. The amino acid sequences of troponins I and T are heart specific, making them ideal cardiac injury biomarkers. (*From* Brush et al. 2016 [50]. Brush JE, Kaul S, Krumholz HM. Troponin Testing for Clinicians. Journal of the American College ofJ Am Coll Cardiology. 2016;68(21):2365-2375. https://doi.org/10.1016/j.jacc. 2016.08.066)

chronic heart disease, myocarditis, and myocardial infarction (rare) but also with systemic diseases such as sepsis, GDV syndrome, babesiosis, dirofilariasis, and following doxorubicin therapy [45]. In general, cardiac troponin concentrations reflect the severity of cardiac injury and are inversely associated with morbidity and mortality [46–48]. Sensitive laboratory assays for cTnI exist but the most frequently used cTnI assay has a limit of detection that is quite high (~ 0.2 ng/mL) providing the assay with specificity but at the expense of sensitivity [49]. As with other biomarkers such as lactate and C-reactive protein (CRP), serial cTnI measurement may be of value in charting the progress of reversible insults, including myocarditis, blunt trauma, or hypoxia. In these patients, cTnI values should fall with time and appropriate therapy. In contrast, values that remain persistently elevated or increase suggest ongoing myocardial injury and warrant further investigation, treatment intensification or both. Any patient with a history of blunt or penetrating chest trauma, a clinically relevant arrhythmia, or a history suggestive of significant cardiac disease warrants cTnI measurement. In cats, measurement of cTnI can also be considered for detection of cats with a high likelihood for hypertrophic cardiomyopathy but it is less useful for the identification of occult myocardial disease in dogs [49].

Natriuretic Peptides

The natriuretic peptides, atrial natriuretic peptide (ANP) and B-type natriuretic peptide (BNP), are produced as precursors by cardiomyocytes in response to atrial and ventricular stretch. These precursors are cleaved to N-terminal and C-terminal fragments, which bind to specific vascular and renal receptors to cause vasodilation and diuresis. Assays exist for C-ANP and C-BNP but because these peptides have short half-lives most studies have measured N-terminal pro B-type natriuretic peptide (NT-proBNP). Plasma concentrations of NT-proBNP are positively correlated to clinical, radiographic, and echocardiographic measures of disease severity [49]. As with other biomarkers, NT-proBNP concentrations should not be viewed in isolation but rather in the context of the patient's signalment, history, physical examination parameters, and combined with other diagnostic modalities including thoracic radiography [45]. In patients presenting with respiratory distress, low or normal NT-proBNP concentrations suggest a noncardiac cause of the current signs, whereas elevated NT-proBNP is more consistent with a cardiac cause including congestive heart failure [51]. Increased NT-proBNP concentrations can confound diagnosis of respiratory disease in animals with asymptomatic heart disease, however. If occult cardiac disease is a preexisting comorbidity in a patient with an intercurrent primary respiratory disease such as pneumonia, the NT-proBNP concentration may well be increased, yet therapy for heart failure in such a patient would be inappropriate. NT-proBNP performs better than cTnI for differentiation of cardiac from noncardiac causes of respiratory signs in dogs and cats [45,49]. It is also worth remembering that NT-proBNP can be measured in pleural effusion, and this may enhance the diagnostic value of this test for the identification of the cause of the fluid [52–54]. Although it may be reasonable to initiate therapy based on information including an NT-proBNP assay, there are no studies that have evaluated biomarker based treatment selection to guide your therapeutic selection. Any primary or secondary disorder that causes atrial and ventricular stretch or wall stress might increase NT-proBNP concentrations. Thus, high concentrations are not diagnostic of any one disease. Moreover, NT-proBNP release from myocytes can be triggered without cardiac stretch in sepsis, further complicating the picture in critically ill animals [55,56].

SEPSIS AND INFLAMMATION

Two review articles of biomarkers of sepsis in humans [57,58] documented an increase of 5367 articles within the intervening 10-year period, with more than 8700 articles identified across the 2 reviews. However, of the 258 biomarkers identified, most had been evaluated in less than 5 studies, with a third assessed in only 1. Only 28 biomarkers (10.9%) had been assessed in clinical studies involving more than 300 participants. In sepsis, for example, the ideal biomarker can be measured at the point-of-care, accurately differentiates infectious from noninfectious causes of inflammation, predicts outcome, identifies response to therapy, and warns of the onset of organ dysfunction. No veterinary biomarker can clear such a high bar.

Acute Phase Proteins

C-reactive protein is a highly conserved plasma protein that binds specific damage and pathogen-associated molecular patterns and functions as a soluble pattern recognition receptor [59]. As such, CRP is an innate immune response component that is synthesized rapidly following tissue injury or infection. It is this rapid synthesis and correlation with the degree of inflammation that has made CRP an attractive biomarker in critical illness. Serum concentrations of CRP increase rapidly in dogs with babesiosis, leishmaniosis, leptospirosis, parvoviral enteritis, and sepsis [60]. CRP is very sensitive and offers biologic insight but it cannot differentiate infectious from noninfectious causes of inflammation, and although it parallels disease severity, it is typically not prognostic. Alpha-1 acid glycoprotein is a recognized biomarker of inflammation in cats, with increased concentrations reported in feline infectious peritonitis [61], and neoplasia [62], although it too is not prognostic. Serum amyloid A may also be a useful marker in the cat because it is rapidly responsive to a variety of inflammatory and infectious conditions

[63,64]. CRP is not a useful biomarker in the cat, and although haptoglobin is increased during the feline acute phase response, additional work will be needed to determine its potential diagnostic utility in feline sepsis specifically [65–69].

Inflammatory biomarkers are now widely used in humans to guide antimicrobial administration in sepsis [70] and to support decisions to discontinue antimicrobial therapy while minimizing risk [71–74]. Various inflammatory biomarkers have been evaluated to aid identification of the appropriate time to safely discontinue antimicrobials. Retrospective and prospective studies using absolute or relative changes in procalcitonin (PCT) concentrations have shown that patients in whom antimicrobials were discontinued based on PCT values received shorter courses of treatment with no difference in outcome [73]. The acute phase reactant C-reactive protein has also been evaluated as part of a decision-making algorithm for antimicrobial therapy in patients suffering from sepsis [75]. CRP-guided antimicrobial therapy in humans is associated with shorter antimicrobial administration without changes in patient outcome [76], whereas a pilot study in canine pyometra suggests that novel postoperative increases in CRP may help identify postoperative complications such as surgical wound infections [77]. The optimal duration of antimicrobial in dogs with sepsis is unknown but data from humans suggest it may be possible to safely reduce the duration of antimicrobials for those diseases. Veterinarians typically rely on clinical, clinicopathologic, and radiographic criteria to discontinue therapy. For instance, it is commonly recommended that antimicrobials be continued for a least 1 week after radiographic resolution of pneumonia. Biomarkers of the inflammatory response might provide superior guidance [78–82].

Cytokines

Recently, the importance of sepsis-induced immunoparalysis in the morbidity and mortality of sepsis has been recognized [83]. In human medicine, there is a huge potential for precision medicine through immunophenotyping to provide targeted interventions specific to the patient's underlying pathologic condition. For instance, those patients with a hyperactive immune response may benefit from anti-inflammatory therapies, whereas those with suppressed and inadequate immune responses may benefit from immunostimulatory therapies. Achieving a better understanding of the nature of the inflammatory and immune responses to sepsis is a crucial first step in this endeavor in veterinary medicine. Accordingly, profiling cytokines and chemokines may provide a snapshot of the current immunologic state that could be used to tailor treatment [84,85]. Cytokines have the potential to be ideal biomarkers for inflammatory and infectious diseases by providing sensitivity, specificity, and biological insight. Dogs with parvoviral enteritis have increased concentrations of tumor necrosis factor-α (TNF-α) [86]. Proinflammatory cytokines have also been documented in other inflammatory disease states including pyometra and non-infectious systemic inflammatory response syndrome (SIRS) [87]. In a study of dogs with immune-mediated hemolytic anemia (IMHA), cytokines associated with macrophage activity and recruitment were prognostic and seem to provide insight into the nature of this disease process [88]. Immunophenotyping data characterizing sepsis are now available for both dogs [89,90] and cats [91,92]. This may be particularly valuable given the challenges recognizing and characterizing sepsis in cats [93,94].

Procalcitonin

In humans, PCT is a valuable biomarker for sepsis diagnosis and is also used as a therapeutic guide. In sepsis, PCT originates from stimulated mononuclear leukocytes [95], and its release occurs within hours of an endotoxin challenge before returning to baseline within 48 hours [96]. Although the exact role of PCT in patients with sepsis is still unknown, it has been shown to increase inducible nitric oxide synthase-mediated nitric oxide release and therefore may play a role in amplification of the inflammation [97]. Studies in humans suggest PCT may be able to differentiate bacterial sepsis from noninfectious SIRS and may be used as a guide to initiate antimicrobial therapy [98]. In some studies, PCT levels correlate with disease severity and may have prognostic value in humans with sepsis and septic shock [99,100]. There is evidence of PCT gene expression in both thyroidal and extrathyroidal tissues in dogs with SIRS; whereas in contrast, normal dogs only express PCT in the thyroid [101]. Although early attempts to measure PCT were unsuccessful [102], several more recent studies have demonstrated that PCT is increased in dogs with endotoxemia [96] and sepsis [103,104], and that PCT is prognostic in canine sepsis [105]. Development of a veterinary point-of-care assay for PCT will be necessary to maximize the potential of this biomarker.

Cell-free DNA and Nucleosomes

Neutrophil extracellular trap formation or NETosis has now been described in several diseases and syndromes in critically ill humans including those with sepsis,

acute respiratory distress syndrome, burns, cancer, and trauma [106–110]. This cell-free DNA (cfDNA) may originate from apoptotic cells, necrotic tissue, or neutrophil extracellular traps (NETs) (Fig. 3) [111,112]. Increased cfDNA has been shown to have prognostic significance in human patients with severe sepsis and those with bacteremia [113,114]. As such, cfDNA has the potential to provide biologic insight into the extent and nature of the innate immune response to infection and inflammation. In addition to being an indicator of nature of the disease process and its severity, it has been demonstrated that NET formation may directly contribute to pathogenesis in sepsis through the phenomenon of immunothrombosis [115], whereas cfDNA can inhibit plasmin-mediated fibrinolysis [116]. Increased cfDNA concentrations have also been detected in dogs with sepsis [103,117], and that these concentrations may have prognostic utility [118].

Nucleosomes are complexes formed by DNA and histone proteins that are released into circulation during cell death and cellular damage such as apoptosis and necrosis [119]. They can also be due to the process of NET formation [120]. As such, cfDNA and nucleosomes share potential origins but are distinct entities [121], with differential potential for immune cell activation through pattern recognition receptors [119]. Measuring both biomarkers may provide better insights into the disease process than either alone [121]. Humans with septic shock have significantly higher nucleosome concentrations than patients with sepsis, noninfectious SIRS, or fever [119]. In humans, plasma nucleosome concentrations distinguish septic from nonseptic critically ill patients and correlate with the severity of immunosuppression and with organ dysfunction [122]. Nucleosome concentrations are increased in dogs with sepsis [123] and may have prognostic utility in some conditions [124].

OMICS

Technological advancements have made it possible and inexpensive to evaluate the whole biologic makeup of individual patients through analysis of their genes (genomics), the RNA messages derived from these genes (transcriptomics), the proteins that these messages are translated into (proteomics) and the results of myriad cellular biochemical processes (metabolomics) (Fig. 4).

In humans, epidemiologic data and candidate gene investigations suggest that genetic risk factors increase susceptibility to and severity of sepsis [126,127]. A brief literature search reveals more than 2000 publications investigating polymorphisms in humans with sepsis

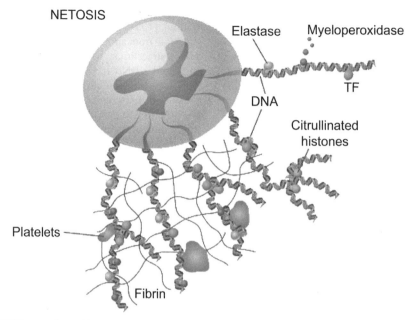

FIG. 3 NETs are released in a process termed NETosis. Detection of NETs can be performed using microscopy and immunocytochemistry, whereas quantitation of NETs can be undertaken by measurement of cell-free DNA, nucleosomes (histones with DNA), and citrullinated histones. (*Modified from* Hazzard M, in Li and Smyth 2019 [125])

conducted over several decades. These studies have identified genomic biomarkers that might aid sepsis diagnosis, that are associated with outcome, and that might be used to guide therapeutic decision-making [128]. Presently, there are no reports of genetic polymorphisms in dogs or cats with sepsis, however.

Evaluation of host gene expression is known as transcriptomics and involves measurement of messenger RNA (mRNA) in blood or circulating leucocytes [129]. This approach has been widely studied in human sepsis but there are few publications in veterinary medicine to date [130–132]. Transcriptomics offers the potential for rapid diagnosis of sepsis and for patient stratification for prognostic or therapeutic purposes. From a diagnostic perspective, transcriptomics offers the tantalizing possibility of differentiation of severe infections from noninfectious inflammation [133,134]. Experimental studies using lipopolysaccharide infusion in dogs have identified alterations in mRNA levels for the inflammatory cytokines interleukin-6 (IL-6) and TNF-α [135,136]. Transcriptomic studies of canine leukocytes stimulated with lipopolysaccharide ex vivo have identified novel drug effects [136], with intriguing pharmacologic links to NETosis [137].

Several studies have also investigated both proteomics and metabolomics to discover new diagnostic and prognostic biomarkers for sepsis in humans [138,139]. Proteomics evaluates the array of translated proteins and offers a distinct picture than the underlying transcriptome profile because of differences in the timing and extent of translation, the influence of post-translational modifications, and the half-lives of proteins relative to those of mRNA. For veterinary medicine, proteomics also offers advantages over traditional protein assays such as ELISAs, where the applicability and diagnostic accuracy of the assay depends on immunologic reagent availability and efficacy. Several studies have recently been published using proteomics to study veterinary patients with sepsis [140,141]. Dogs with pyometra had numerous downregulated proteins including transthyretin, antithrombin, retinol-binding protein, and vitamin D binding protein. Upregulated proteins included haptoglobin light chain, alpha-1-acid glycoprotein, C-reactive protein precursor, and lipopolysaccharide-binding protein [140]. These studies provide insight into the complex pathophysiology of inflammation associated with sepsis in dogs and will likely aid identification of novel predictive biomarkers.

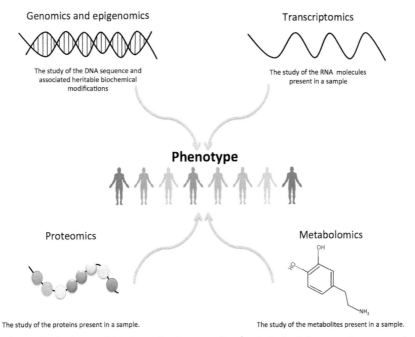

Genomics and epigenomics

The study of the DNA sequence and associated heritable biochemical modifications

Transcriptomics

The study of the RNA molecules present in a sample

Phenotype

Proteomics

The study of the proteins present in a sample.

Metabolomics

The study of the metabolites present in a sample.

FIG. 4 Omics technologies use high-throughput approaches to study the influence of genes, environmental influences, protein expression, and metabolic networks on phenotype and responses to disease. (Functional genomics An introduction to EMBL-EBI resources. What is functional genomics? © EMBL 2023. *Retrieved from*: https://www.ebi.ac.uk/training/online/courses/functional-genomics-introduction-embl-ebi-resource/ what-is-functional-genomics/)

Metabolomics is the most recent of the high-throughput screening technologies and uses high-performance chromatography and tandem mass spectrometry to simultaneously identify, quantify, and characterize large numbers of metabolites in complex biological samples [142]. The metabolic derangements in sepsis are myriad [143], and metabolomics allows blood concentrations of nucleic acids, amino acids, carbohydrates, and lipids in addition to microbial components to be evaluated simultaneously. Panels of metabolites can differentiate patients with humans with sepsis from healthy subjects [144] and predict adverse events and mortality in sepsis [145]. Nutritional treatments can improve clinical outcomes by attenuating the metabolic response to stress, reducing oxidative injury, and modulating the immune response [146]. In humans with sepsis, targeted nutritional support reduces organ dysfunction, hospital-acquired infections, and death [147,148], whereas in dogs with sepsis, early enteral nutrition can decrease length of hospitalization [149] and improve survival rates [150]. Metabolomics has recently been applied to dogs with sepsis [151]. Pathway analysis identified multiple enriched metabolic pathways including pyruvaldehyde degradation, ketone body metabolism, the glucose-alanine cycle, vitamin-K metabolism, amino acid biosynthesis, and metabolism of glutamine/glutamate. The study also identified various prognostic factors including 3-(2-hydroxyethyl) indole, indoxyl sulfate, and xanthurenic acid [151].

ENDOTHELIAL FUNCTION AND THE GLYCOCALYX

The endothelium is a monolayer of epithelial cells that forms the inner cellular lining of all blood vessels and the lymphatic system and hence is in direct contact with both blood and lymph; it helps to regulate blood flow, vascular tone, immune responses, inflammation, hemostasis, and angiogenesis [152]. Measurement of von Willebrand factor and endothelin can aid in the assessment of endothelial activation or injury. The endothelial glycocalyx is a complex matrix of proteins, proteoglycans, and glycosaminoglycans, particularly heparan sulfate, hyaluronan, and syndecan-1 that covers the luminal surface of endothelial cells (Fig. 5).

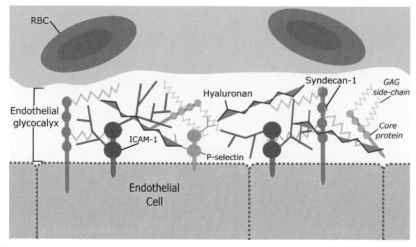

FIG. 5 The endothelial glycocalyx. Key structural components include hyaluronan, syndecan-1, and the glycosaminoglycans (GAGs). Abbreviations: ICAM-1, intercellular adhesion molecule-1; RBC, red blood cell. (*Reproduced from* Lawrence-Mills et al. 2022 [153])

It is now apparent that the endothelial glycocalyx plays critical homeostatic roles in health and is readily injured by disease and potentially by iatrogenic harms including overzealous crystalloid resuscitation. The endothelial glycocalyx is integral to the maintenance of normal vascular permeability, mechanotransduction of shear stress, and the regulation of blood cell interactions with the endothelium [153]. Measurements of shed structural glycocalyx components in plasma are used to infer injury to the glycocalyx but a lack of species-specific reagents and challenges with assay validation has limited progress [154,155]. Hyaluronan [156–159] and endothelial cell-specific molecule-1 (ESM-1) [155,160] are presently the only viable endothelial glycocalyx biomarkers for dogs. Imaging techniques, such as sidestream dark field microscopy [161], are a valid means to assess the health of the glycocalyx but are not typically considered biomarkers and will not be further discussed.

Von Willebrand Factor

Von Willebrand factor (VWF) is essential for platelet arrest, adhesion, and activation adjacent to endothelial defects. Increased plasma VWF is consistently seen in people with endothelial dysfunction, such that VWF can be used as a biomarker of endothelial damage or dysfunction [162–165]. Although VWF has been proposed as a marker of endothelial function in dogs [166], there are relatively few reports of the use of VWF to assess endothelial function in small animals

[167]. Short-term exercise significantly increased canine plasma VWF concentrations. There were breed-related and "white coat" effects on this marker, however, which may limit its usefulness in dogs [168]. VWF antigen concentration was used as a marker of endothelial injury in cats with cardiac disease. Cats with cardiac disease were divided into mild atrial enlargement, moderate atrial enlargement, and those with spontaneous echocardiographic contrast or atrial thrombi and those with a thromboembolic event. Only cats with thrombi had evidence of arterial thrombi had significantly higher median VWF antigen concentrations than did the other groups. The authors attributed this to downstream endothelial injury following thrombus occlusion. This study also suggests VWF is not a sensitive marker of endothelial dysfunction in cats with cardiac disease [169].

Endothelin-1

Endothelin-1 is a small peptide vasoconstrictor molecule with additional cardiovascular effects including renin-angiotensin-aldosterone system activation, sympathetic stimulation, and positive inotropy and chronotropy [170]. For clinical purposes, measurement of its precursor molecule, big ET-1, is favored because ET-1 has a very short half-life. Big ET-1 circulates longer and is the predominant fraction of ET immunoreactivity in patients with heart failure [171]. Big ET-1 is potentially a stronger indicator of prognosis in human heart failure than other clinical data including other neurohormones [172,173]. A recent study of dogs with DCM found that affected dogs had significantly higher concentrations of big ET-1, and increasing big ET-1 concentrations were also associated with shorter survival times [174]. ET-1 is not specific for cardiopulmonary disease however; dogs with hemangiosarcoma, adenocarcinoma, histiocytic sarcoma, osteosarcoma, and hepatocellular carcinoma also have significantly increased levels of ET-1 compared with healthy dogs. At this point, the optimal role for ET-1 in the evaluation of dogs with cancer or cardiopulmonary disease remains to be determined.

Hyaluronan

The endothelial glycocalyx plays crucial roles in regulation of vascular permeability and tone, and glycocalyx injury is an early feature of sepsis in humans [175]. Shedding of endothelial glycocalyx components might contribute to sepsis pathophysiology and are prognostic [176]. Shed components act as damage-associated molecular patterns that can perpetuate and augment inflammation through cytokine release from monocytes [177]. Furthermore, the degradation of the endothelial glycocalyx might also contribute to the increased thrombotic risk seen in sepsis [178]. In dogs, increased serum hyaluronan concentration is observed in a variety of disease processes that may predispose to thrombosis [158]. Plasma hyaluronan concentrations increase in dogs with septic peritonitis within 3 days of hospitalization and then decrease as animals recover [179]. Blood concentrations of IL-6 and hyaluronan were correlated, suggesting an association between inflammation and glycocalyx injury.

Endothelial glycocalyx injury as indicated by increased plasma hyaluronan concentrations can also occur secondary to therapeutic interventions including rapid crystalloid fluid administration [159]. In experimental hemorrhagic shock models in dogs, rapid crystalloid administration increased plasma hyaluronan concentrations, suggesting that endothelial glycocalyx component shedding occurred because of bolus fluid resuscitation [156].

Endothelial Cell-specific Molecule-1

In dogs with parvoviral enteritis, circulating ESM-1 concentrations are increased compared with controls suggesting endothelial cell injury [155] but the authors could not identify alterations in plasma syndecan-1 or heparan sulfate concentrations, likely due to poor assay performance. Increased ESM-1 concentrations have also been documented in dogs with decompensated heart failure associated with mitral valve disease [160],

although biomarker concentrations did not correlate with cardiac disease severity grades in dogs with stable disease. In this study, ESM-1 concentrations were prognostic and did improve with intensification of treatment in some dogs.

CLINICS CARE POINTS

- All biomarkers need to be evaluated in the context of findings from anamnesis, physical examination, and other diagnostic testing.
- In general, serial quantitation of biomarkers is superior to single time point measurement.
- Presently, NGAL may be the best novel biomarker for kidney injury.
- cTnI is a sensitive but nonspecific marker of myocardial injury.
- NT-proBNP is a specific marker for myocardial stretch but can be nonspecifically increased in sepsis.
- Be aware that preexisting cardiac disease may increase NT-proBNP in patients with other causes of respiratory disease.
- Acute phase proteins are highly sensitive but nonspecific for inflammation.
- Serial measurement of acute phase proteins can aid antimicrobial stewardship.
- Many biomarkers of NET formation are not specific for NETs.
- Hyaluronan is presently the most reliable biomarker for the endothelial glycocalyx.

REFERENCES

[1] Biomarkers Definitions Working Group. Biomarkers and surrogate endpoints: preferred definitions and conceptual framework. Clin Pharmacol Ther 2001;69(3):89–95.
[2] Puntmann VO. How-to guide on biomarkers: biomarker definitions, validation and applications with examples from cardiovascular disease. Postgrad Med J 2009;85(1008):538–45.
[3] Marshall JC, Reinhart K. Biomarkers of sepsis. Crit Care Med 2009;37(7):2290–8.
[4] FDA-NIH. BEST (Biomarkers, EndpointS, and other Tools) Resource. Food and Drug Administration (US) National Institutes of Health (US). Available at: https://www.ncbi.nlm.nih.gov/books/NBK326791/. Accessed June 20, 2023, 2023.
[5] Rosenstein PG, Tennent-Brown BS, Hughes D. Clinical use of plasma lactate concentration. Part 1: physiology,

pathophysiology, and measurement. J Vet Emerg Crit Care 2018;28(2):85–105.

[6] Rosenstein PG, Tennent-Brown BS, Hughes D. Clinical use of plasma lactate concentration. Part 2: prognostic and diagnostic utility and the clinical management of hyperlactatemia. J Vet Emerg Crit Care 2018;28(2):106–21.

[7] Davis J, Raisis AL, Miller DW, et al. Analytical validation and reference intervals for a commercial multiplex assay to measure five novel biomarkers for acute kidney injury in canine urine. Res Vet Sci 2021;139:78–86.

[8] Boyd CJ, Claus MA, Raisis AL, et al. Evaluation of biomarkers of kidney injury following 4% succinylated gelatin and 6% hydroxyethyl starch 130/0.4 administration in a canine hemorrhagic shock model. J Vet Emerg Crit Care 2019;29(2):132–42.

[9] Boyd CJ, Sharp CR, Claus MA, et al. Prospective randomized controlled blinded clinical trial evaluating biomarkers of acute kidney injury following 6% hydroxyethyl starch 130/0.4 or Hartmann's solution in dogs. J Vet Emerg Crit Care 2021;31(3):306–14.

[10] Gewin LS. Sugar or fat? Renal tubular metabolism reviewed in health and disease. Nutrients 2021;13(5):1580.

[11] Segev G, Palm C, LeRoy B, et al. Evaluation of neutrophil gelatinase-associated lipocalin as a marker of kidney injury in dogs. J Vet Intern Med 2013;27(6):1362–7.

[12] Palm CA, Segev G, Cowgill LD, et al. Urinary neutrophil gelatinase-associated lipocalin as a marker for identification of acute kidney injury and recovery in dogs with gentamicin-induced nephrotoxicity. J Vet Intern Med 2016;30(1):200–5.

[13] Lee YJ, Hu YY, Lin YS, et al. Urine neutrophil gelatinase-associated lipocalin (NGAL) as a biomarker for acute canine kidney injury. BMC Vet Res 2012;8:248.

[14] Steinbach S, Weis J, Schweighauser A, et al. Plasma and urine neutrophil gelatinase-associated lipocalin (NGAL) in dogs with acute kidney injury or chronic kidney disease. J Vet Intern Med 2014;28(2):264–9.

[15] Hsu WL, Lin YS, Hu YY, et al. Neutrophil gelatinase-associated lipocalin in dogs with naturally occurring renal diseases. J Vet Intern Med 2014;28(2):437–42.

[16] Abrahamson M, Olafsson I, Palsdottir A, et al. Structure and expression of the human cystatin C gene. Biochem J 1990;268(2):287–94.

[17] Seronie-Vivien S, Delanaye P, Pieroni L, et al. Cystatin C: current position and future prospects. Clin Chem Lab Med 2008;46(12):1664–86.

[18] Conti M, Moutereau S, Zater M, et al. Urinary cystatin C as a specific marker of tubular dysfunction. Clin Chem Lab Med 2006;44(3):288–91.

[19] Ghys L, Paepe D, Smets P, et al. A new renal marker and its potential use in small animal medicine. J Vet Intern Med 2014;28(4):1152–64.

[20] Jensen AL, Bomholt M, Moe L. Preliminary evaluation of a particle-enhanced turbidimetric immunoassay (PETIA) for the determination of serum cystatin C-like immunoreactivity in dogs. Vet Clin Pathol 2001;30(2):86–90.

[21] Monti P, Benchekroun G, Berlato D, et al. Initial evaluation of canine urinary cystatin C as a marker of renal tubular function. J Small Anim Pract 2012;53(5):254–9.

[22] Ghys LF, Meyer E, Paepe D, et al. Analytical validation of a human particle-enhanced nephelometric assay for cystatin C measurement in feline serum and urine. Vet Clin Pathol 2014;43(2):226–34.

[23] Almy FS, Christopher MM, King DP, et al. Evaluation of cystatin C as an endogenous marker of glomerular filtration rate in dogs. J Vet Intern Med 2002;16(1):45–51.

[24] Miyagawa Y, Takemura N, Hirose H. Evaluation of the measurement of serum cystatin C by an enzyme-linked immunosorbent assay for humans as a marker of the glomerular filtration rate in dogs. J Vet Med Sci 2009;71(9):1169–76.

[25] Antognoni MT, Siepi D, Porciello F, et al. Use of serum cistatin C determination as a marker of renal function in the dog. Vet Res Commun 2005;29(Suppl 2):265–7.

[26] Braun JP, Perxachs A, PéChereau D, et al. Plasma cystatin C in the dog: reference values and variations with renal failure. Comp Clinical Pathol 2002;11(1):44–9.

[27] Wehner A, Hartmann K, Hirschberger J. Utility of serum cystatin C as a clinical measure of renal function in dogs. J Am Anim Hosp Assoc 2008;44(3):131–8.

[28] Antognoni MT, Siepi D, Porciello F, et al. Serum cystatin-C evaluation in dogs affected by different diseases associated or not with renal insufficiency. Vet Res Commun 2007;31(Suppl 1):269–71.

[29] Pelander L, Häggström J, Larsson A, et al. Comparison of the diagnostic value of symmetric dimethylarginine, cystatin C, and creatinine for detection of decreased glomerular filtration rate in dogs. J Vet Intern Med 2019;33(2):630–9.

[30] Yerramilli M, Farace G, Quinn J, et al. Kidney disease and the nexus of chronic kidney disease and acute kidney injury: the role of novel biomarkers as early and accurate diagnostics. Vet Clin North Am Small Anim Pract 2016;46(6):961–93.

[31] Gordin E, Gordin D, Viitanen S, et al. Urinary clusterin and cystatin B as biomarkers of tubular injury in dogs following envenomation by the European adder. Res Vet Sci 2021;134:12–8.

[32] García-Martínez JD, Tvarijonaviciute A, Cerón JJ, et al. Urinary clusterin as a renal marker in dogs. J Vet Diagn Invest 2012;24(2):301–6.

[33] Zhou X, Ma B, Lin Z, et al. Evaluation of the usefulness of novel biomarkers for drug-induced acute kidney injury in beagle dogs. Toxicol Appl Pharmacol 2014;280(1):30–5.

[34] Ichimura T, Bonventre JV, Bailly V, et al. Kidney injury molecule-1 (KIM-1), a putative epithelial cell adhesion molecule containing a novel immunoglobulin domain,

is up-regulated in renal cells after injury. J Biol Chem 1998;273(7):4135–42.

[35] Ichimura T, Hung CC, Yang SA, et al. Kidney injury molecule-1: a tissue and urinary biomarker for nephrotoxicant-induced renal injury. Am J Physiol Renal Physiol 2004;286(3):F552–63.

[36] Han WK, Bailly V, Abichandani R, et al. Kidney Injury Molecule-1 (KIM-1): a novel biomarker for human renal proximal tubule injury. Kidney Int 2002;62(1):237–44.

[37] Han WK, Waikar SS, Johnson A, et al. Urinary biomarkers in the early diagnosis of acute kidney injury. Kidney Int 2008;73(7):863–9.

[38] Burt D, Crowell SJ, Ackley DC, et al. Application of emerging biomarkers of acute kidney injury in development of kidney-sparing polypeptide-based antibiotics. Drug Chem Toxicol 2014;37(2):204–12.

[39] Lippi I, Perondi F, Meucci V, et al. Clinical utility of urine kidney injury molecule-1 (KIM-1) and gamma-glutamyl transferase (GGT) in the diagnosis of canine acute kidney injury. Vet Res Commun 2018;42(2):95–100.

[40] Bland SK, Schmiedt CW, Clark ME, et al. Expression of kidney injury molecule-1 in healthy and diseased feline kidney tissue. Vet Pathol 2017;54(3):490–510.

[41] Fonfara S, Hetzel U, Tew SR, et al. Myocardial cytokine expression in dogs with systemic and naturally occurring cardiac diseases. Am J Vet Res 2013;74(3):408–16.

[42] Klein S, Nolte I, Granados-Soler JL, et al. Evaluation of new and old biomarkers in dogs with degenerative mitral valve disease. BMC Vet Res 2022;18(1):256.

[43] Ibrahim NE, Januzzi JL Jr. Established and emerging roles of biomarkers in heart failure. Circ Res 2018;123(5):614–29.

[44] Rešetar Maslov D, Farkaš V, Rubić I, et al. Serum proteomic profiles reflect the stages of myxomatous mitral valve disease in dogs. Int J Mol Sci 2023;12(8):24.

[45] Smith KF, Quinn RL, Rahilly LJ. Biomarkers for differentiation of causes of respiratory distress in dogs and cats: Part 1–Cardiac diseases and pulmonary hypertension. J Vet Emerg Crit Care 2015;25(3):311–29.

[46] Ljungvall I, Hoglund K, Tidholm A, et al. Cardiac troponin I is associated with severity of myxomatous mitral valve disease, age, and C-reactive protein in dogs. J Vet Intern Med 2010;24(1):153–9.

[47] Hezzell MJ, Boswood A, Chang YM, et al. The combined prognostic potential of serum high-sensitivity cardiac troponin I and N-terminal pro-B-type natriuretic peptide concentrations in dogs with degenerative mitral valve disease. J Vet Intern Med 2012;26(2):302–11.

[48] Oyama MA, Sisson DD. Cardiac troponin-I concentration in dogs with cardiac disease. J Vet Intern Med 2004;18(6):831–9.

[49] Oyama MA. Using cardiac biomarkers in veterinary practice. Clin Lab Med 2015;35(3):555–66.

[50] Brush JE, Kaul S, Krumholz HM. Troponin testing for clinicians. J Am Coll Cardiol 2016;68(21):2365–75.

[51] de Lima GV, Ferreira FDS. N-terminal-pro brain natriuretic peptides in dogs and cats: a technical and clinical review. Vet World 2017;10(9):1072–82.

[52] Wurtinger G, Henrich E, Hildebrandt N, et al. Assessment of a bedside test for N-terminal pro B-type natriuretic peptide (NT-proBNP) to differentiate cardiac from non-cardiac causes of pleural effusion in cats. BMC Vet Res 2017;13(1):394.

[53] Hezzell MJ, Rush JE, Humm K, et al. Differentiation of cardiac from noncardiac pleural effusions in cats using second-generation quantitative and point-of-Care NT-proBNP measurements. J Vet Intern Med 2016;30(2):536–42.

[54] Humm K, Hezzell M, Sargent J, et al. Differentiating between feline pleural effusions of cardiac and non-cardiac origin using pleural fluid NT-proBNP concentrations. J Small Anim Pract 2013;54(12):656–61.

[55] Piechota M, Banach M, Irzmanski R, et al. N-terminal brain natriuretic propeptide levels correlate with procalcitonin and C-reactive protein levels in septic patients. Cell Mol Biol Lett 2007;12(2):162–75.

[56] Maeder M, Fehr T, Rickli H, et al. Sepsis-associated myocardial dysfunction: diagnostic and prognostic impact of cardiac troponins and natriuretic peptides. Chest 2006;129(5):1349–66.

[57] Pierrakos C, Vincent JL. Sepsis biomarkers: a review. Crit Care 2010;14(1):R15.

[58] Pierrakos C, Velissaris D, Bisdorff M, et al. Biomarkers of sepsis: time for a reappraisal. Crit Care 2020;24(1):287.

[59] Black S, Kushner I, Samols D. C-reactive protein. J Biol Chem 2004;279(47):48487–90.

[60] Ceron JJ, Eckersall PD, Martynez-Subiela S. Acute phase proteins in dogs and cats: current knowledge and future perspectives. Vet Clin Pathol 2005;34(2):85–99.

[61] Giordano A, Spagnolo V, Colombo A, et al. Changes in some acute phase protein and immunoglobulin concentrations in cats affected by feline infectious peritonitis or exposed to feline coronavirus infection. Vet J 2004;167(1):38–44.

[62] Correa SS, Mauldin GN, Mauldin GE, et al. Serum alpha 1-acid glycoprotein concentration in cats with lymphoma. J Am Anim Hosp Assoc 2001;37(2):153–8.

[63] Kajikawa T, Furuta A, Onishi T, et al. Changes in concentrations of serum amyloid A protein, alpha(1)-acid glycoprotein, haptoglobin, and C-reactive protein in feline sera due to induced inflammation and surgery. Vet Immunol Immunopathol 1999;68(1):91–8.

[64] Troia R, Gruarin M, Foglia A, et al. Serum amyloid A in the diagnosis of feline sepsis. J Vet Diagn Invest 2017;29(6):856–9.

[65] Petini M, Drigo M, Zoia A. Prognostic value of systemic inflammatory response syndrome and serum concentrations of acute phase proteins, cholesterol, and total thyroxine in cats with panleukopenia. J Vet Intern Med 2020;34(2):719–24.

[66] Vilhena H, Tvarijonaviciute A, Cerón JJ, et al. Acute phase proteins response in cats naturally infected with Hepatozoon felis and Babesia vogeli. Vet Clin Pathol 2017;46(1):72–6.

[67] Hazuchova K, Held S, Neiger R. Usefulness of acute phase proteins in differentiating between feline infectious peritonitis and other diseases in cats with body cavity effusions. J Feline Med Surg 2017;19(8):809–16.

[68] Silvestre-Ferreira AC, Vieira L, Vilhena H, et al. Serum acute phase proteins in Dirofilaria immitis and Wolbachia seropositive cats. J Feline Med Surg 2017;19(6):693–6.

[69] Ottenjann M, Weingart C, Arndt G, et al. Characterization of the anemia of inflammatory disease in cats with abscesses, pyothorax, or fat necrosis. J Vet Intern Med 2006;20(5):1143–50.

[70] Quenot JP, Luyt CE, Roche N, et al. Role of biomarkers in the management of antibiotic therapy: an expert panel review II: clinical use of biomarkers for initiation or discontinuation of antibiotic therapy. Ann Intensive Care 2013;3(1):21.

[71] Bouadma L, Luyt CE, Tubach F, et al. Use of procalcitonin to reduce patients' exposure to antibiotics in intensive care units (PRORATA trial): a multicentre randomised controlled trial. Lancet 2010;375(9713): 463–74.

[72] Albrich WC, Dusemund F, Bucher B, et al. Effectiveness and safety of procalcitonin-guided antibiotic therapy in lower respiratory tract infections in "real life": an international, multicenter poststudy survey (ProREAL). Arch Intern Med 2012;172(9):715–22.

[73] Maseda E, Suarez-de-la-Rica A, Anillo V, et al. Procalcitonin-guided therapy may reduce length of antibiotic treatment in intensive care unit patients with secondary peritonitis: a multicenter retrospective study. J Crit Care 2015;30(3):537–42.

[74] Hochreiter M, Kohler T, Schweiger AM, et al. Procalcitonin to guide duration of antibiotic therapy in intensive care patients: a randomized prospective controlled trial. Crit Care 2009;13(3):R83.

[75] Han JH, Nachamkin I, Coffin SE, et al. Use of a combination biomarker algorithm to identify medical intensive care unit patients with suspected sepsis at very low likelihood of bacterial infection. Antimicrobial Agents Chemother 2015;59(10):6494–500.

[76] Oliveira CF, Botoni FA, Oliveira CR, et al. Procalcitonin versus C-reactive protein for guiding antibiotic therapy in sepsis: a randomized trial. Crit Care Med 2013; 41(10):2336–43.

[77] Dabrowski R, Kostro K, Lisiecka U, et al. Usefulness of C-reactive protein, serum amyloid A component, and haptoglobin determinations in bitches with pyometra for monitoring early post-ovariohysterectomy complications. Theriogenology 2009;72(4):471–6.

[78] Viitanen SJ, Lappalainen AK, Christensen MB, et al. The utility of acute-phase proteins in the assessment of treatment response in dogs with bacterial pneumonia. J Vet Intern Med 2017;31(1):124–33.

[79] Goggs R, Robbins SN, LaLonde-Paul DM, et al. Serial analysis of blood biomarker concentrations in dogs with pneumonia, septic peritonitis, and pyometra. J Vet Intern Med 2022;36(2):549–64.

[80] Menard J, Porter I, Lerer A, et al. Serial evaluation of thoracic radiographs and acute phase proteins in dogs with pneumonia. J Vet Intern Med 2022;36(4):1430–43.

[81] Fernandes Rodrigues N, Giraud L, Bolen G, et al. Antimicrobial discontinuation in dogs with acute aspiration pneumonia based on clinical improvement and normalization of C-reactive protein concentration. J Vet Intern Med 2022;36(3):1082–8.

[82] Fernandes Rodrigues N, Giraud L, Bolen G, et al. Comparison of lung ultrasound, chest radiographs, C-reactive protein, and clinical findings in dogs treated for aspiration pneumonia. J Vet Intern Med 2022;36(2):743–52.

[83] Sriskandan S, Altmann DM. The immunology of sepsis. J Pathol 2008;214(2):211–23.

[84] Peters van Ton AM, Kox M, Abdo WF, et al. Precision Immunotherapy for Sepsis. Front Immunol 2018;9: 1926.

[85] Pickkers P, Kox M. Towards precision medicine for sepsis patients. Crit Care 2017;21(1):11.

[86] Otto CM, Drobatz KJ, Soter C. Endotoxemia and tumor necrosis factor activity in dogs with naturally occurring parvoviral enteritis. J Vet Intern Med 1997;11(2):65–70.

[87] Karlsson I, Hagman R, Johannisson A, et al. Cytokines as immunological markers for systemic inflammation in dogs with pyometra. Reprod Domest Anim 2012; 47(Suppl 6):337–41.

[88] Kjelgaard-Hansen M, Goggs R, Wiinberg B, et al. Use of serum concentrations of interleukin-18 and monocyte chemoattractant protein-1 as prognostic indicators in primary immune-mediated hemolytic anemia in dogs. J Vet Intern Med 2011;25(1):76–82.

[89] Karlsson I, Hagman R, Johannisson A, et al. Multiplex cytokine analyses in dogs with pyometra suggest involvement of KC-like chemokine in canine bacterial sepsis. Vet Immunol Immunopathol 2016;170:41–6.

[90] Johnson V, Burgess B, Morley P, et al. Comparison of cytokine responses between dogs with sepsis and dogs with immune-mediated hemolytic anemia. Vet Immunol Immunopathol 2016;180:15–20.

[91] Declue AE, Delgado C, Chang CH, et al. Clinical and immunologic assessment of sepsis and the systemic inflammatory response syndrome in cats. J Am Vet Med Assoc 2011;238(7):890–7.

[92] Troia R, Mascalzoni G, Agnoli C, et al. Cytokine and chemokine profiling in cats with sepsis and septic shock. Front Vet Sci 2020;7:305.

[93] Brady CA, Otto CM, Van Winkle TJ, et al. Severe sepsis in cats: 29 cases (1986-1998). J Am Vet Med Assoc 2000;217(4):531–5.

[94] Babyak JM, Sharp CR. Epidemiology of systemic inflammatory response syndrome and sepsis in cats hospitalized in a veterinary teaching hospital. J Am Vet Med Assoc 2016;249(1):65–71.

[95] Oberhoffer M, Stonans I, Russwurm S, et al. Procalcitonin expression in human peripheral blood mononuclear cells and its modulation by lipopolysaccharides and sepsis-related cytokines in vitro. J Lab Clin Med 1999; 134(1):49–55.

[96] Easley F, Holowaychuk MK, Lashnits EW, et al. Serum procalcitonin concentrations in dogs with induced endotoxemia. J Vet Intern Med 2020;34(2):653–8.

[97] Hoffmann G, Totzke G, Seibel M, et al. In vitro modulation of inducible nitric oxide synthase gene expression and nitric oxide synthesis by procalcitonin. Crit Care Med 2001;29(1):112–6.

[98] Assicot M, Gendrel D, Carsin H, et al. High serum procalcitonin concentrations in patients with sepsis and infection. Lancet 1993;341(8844):515–8.

[99] Jekarl DW, Lee SY, Lee J, et al. Procalcitonin as a diagnostic marker and IL-6 as a prognostic marker for sepsis. Diagn Microbiol Infect Dis 2013;75(4): 342–7.

[100] Georgopoulou AP, Savva A, Giamarellos-Bourboulis EJ, et al. Early changes of procalcitonin may advise about prognosis and appropriateness of antimicrobial therapy in sepsis. J Crit Care 2011;26(3):331 e1-7.

[101] Giunti M, Peli A, Battilani M, et al. Evaluation of CALC-I gene (CALCA) expression in tissues of dogs with signs of the systemic inflammatory response syndrome. J Vet Emerg Crit Care 2010;20(5):523–7.

[102] Floras AN, Holowaychuk MK, Hodgins DC, et al. Investigation of a commercial ELISA for the detection of canine procalcitonin. J Vet Intern Med 2014;28(2):599–602.

[103] Martiny P, Goggs R. Biomarker guided diagnosis of septic peritonitis in dogs. Front Vet Sci 2019;6:208.

[104] Goggs R, Milloway M, Troia R, et al. Plasma procalcitonin concentrations are increased in dogs with sepsis. Vet Rec Open 2018;5(1):e000255.

[105] Troia R, Giunti M, Goggs R. Plasma procalcitonin concentrations predict organ dysfunction and outcome in dogs with sepsis. BMC Vet Res 2018;14(1):111.

[106] Chiu TW, Young R, Chan LYS, et al. Plasma cell-free DNA as an indicator of severity of injury in burn patients. Clin Chem Lab Med 2006;44(1):13–7.

[107] Johnson PJ, Lo YMD. Plasma nucleic acids in the diagnosis and management of malignant disease. Clin Chem 2002;48(8):1186–93.

[108] Lo YMD, Rainer TH, Chan LYS, et al. Plasma DNA as a prognostic marker in trauma patients. Clin Chem 2000; 46(3):319–23.

[109] Saukkonen K, Lakkisto P, Varpula M, et al. Association of cell-free plasma DNA with hospital mortality and organ dysfunction in intensive care unit patients. Intensive Care Med 2007;33(9):1624–7.

[110] Saukkonen K, Lakkisto P, Pettila V, et al. Cell-free plasma DNA as a predictor of outcome in severe sepsis and septic shock. Clin Chem 2008;54(6):1000–7.

[111] Lichtenstein AV, Melkonyan HS, Tomei LD, et al. Circulating nucleic acids and apoptosis. Ann N Y Acad Sci 2001;945(1):239–49.

[112] Hamaguchi S, Akeda Y, Yamamoto N, et al. Origin of circulating free DNA in sepsis: analysis of the CLP mouse model. Mediators Inflamm 2015;2015:614518.

[113] Huttunen R, Kuparinen T, Jylhava J, et al. Fatal outcome in bacteremia is characterized by high plasma cell free DNA concentration and apoptotic DNA fragmentation: a prospective cohort study. PLoS One 2011;6(7):e21700.

[114] Dwivedi DJ, Toltl LJ, Swystun LL, et al. Prognostic utility and characterization of cell-free DNA in patients with severe sepsis. Crit Care 2012;16(4):R151.

[115] Gould TJ, Lysov Z, Liaw PC. Extracellular DNA and histones: double-edged swords in immunothrombosis. J Thromb Haemost 2015;13(Suppl 1):S82–91.

[116] Liaw PC, Ito T, Iba T, et al. DAMP and DIC: The role of extracellular DNA and DNA-binding proteins in the pathogenesis of DIC. Blood Rev 2016;30(4):257–61.

[117] Letendre JA, Goggs R. Measurement of plasma cell-free DNA concentrations in dogs with sepsis, trauma, and neoplasia. J Vet Emerg Crit Care 2017;27(3):307–14.

[118] Letendre JA, Goggs R. Determining prognosis in canine sepsis by bedside measurement of cell-free DNA and nucleosomes. J Vet Emerg Crit Care 2018;28(6): 503–11.

[119] Zeerleder S, Zwart B, Wuillemin WA, et al. Elevated nucleosome levels in systemic inflammation and sepsis. Crit Care Med 2003;31(7):1947–51.

[120] Goggs R, Jeffery U, LeVine DN, et al. Neutrophil-extracellular traps, cell-Free DNA, and immunothrombosis in companion animals: a review. Vet Pathol 2020; 57(1):6–23.

[121] Marsman G, Zeerleder S, Luken BM. Extracellular histones, cell-free DNA, or nucleosomes: differences in immunostimulation. Cell Death Dis 2016;7(12):e2518.

[122] Chen Q, Ye L, Jin Y, et al. Circulating nucleosomes as a predictor of sepsis and organ dysfunction in critically ill patients. Int J Infect Dis 2012;16(7):e558–64.

[123] Letendre J-A, Martiny P, Goggs R. Determining prognosis in canine sepsis by bedside measurement of cell-free DNA. J Vet Emerg Crit Care 2016;26(S1):S7.

[124] Letendre JA, Goggs R. Concentrations of plasma nucleosomes but Not Cell-Free DNA Are prognostic in dogs following trauma. Front Vet Sci 2018;5:180.

[125] Li Z, Smyth SS. Interactions between platelets, leukocytes, and the endothelium. In: Michelson AD, editor. Platelets. 4th edition. London, UK: Academic Press, Elsevier; 2019. p. 295–310, chap 16.

[126] Cooke GS, Hill AVS. Genetics of susceptibitlity to human infectious disease. Nat Rev Genet 2001;2(12): 967–77.

[127] Srinivasan L, Kirpalani H, Cotten CM. Elucidating the role of genomics in neonatal sepsis. Semin Perinatol 2015;39(8):611–6.

[128] Russell JA. Genomics and pharmacogenomics of sepsis: so close and yet so far. Crit Care 2016;20(1):185.

[129] Langley RJ, Wong HR. Early diagnosis of sepsis: is an integrated omics approach the way forward? Mol Diagn Ther 2017;21(5):525–37.

[130] Li J, D'Annibale-Tolhurst MA, Adler KB, et al. A myristoylated alanine-rich C kinase substrate-related peptide suppresses cytokine mRNA and protein expression in LPS-activated canine neutrophils. Am J Respir Cell Mol Biol 2013;48(3):314–21.

[131] Hagman R, Ronnberg E, Pejler G. Canine uterine bacterial infection induces upregulation of proteolysis-related genes and downregulation of homeobox and zinc finger factors. PLoS One 2009;4(11):e8039.

[132] Frangogiannis NG, Mendoza LH, Smith CW, et al. Induction of the synthesis of the C-X-C chemokine interferon-gamma-inducible protein-10 in experimental canine endotoxemia. Cell Tissue Res 2000; 302(3):365–76.

[133] McHugh L, Seldon TA, Brandon RA, et al. A molecular host response assay to discriminate between sepsis and infection-negative systemic inflammation in critically ill patients: discovery and validation in independent cohorts. PLoS Med 2015;12(12):e1001916.

[134] Sweeney TE, Shidham A, Wong HR, et al. A comprehensive time-course-based multicohort analysis of sepsis and sterile inflammation reveals a robust diagnostic gene set. Sci Transl Med 2015;7(287):287ra71.

[135] Song R, Kim J, Yu D, et al. Kinetics of IL-6 and TNF-alpha changes in a canine model of sepsis induced by endotoxin. Vet Immunol Immunopathol 2012;146(2): 143–9.

[136] Song R, Yu D, Yoon J, et al. Valproic acid attenuates the expression of pro-inflammatory cytokines lipopolysaccharide-treated canine peripheral blood mononuclear cells (in vitro) and in a canine endotoxemia model (in vivo). Vet Immunol Immunopathol 2015;166(3–4):132–7.

[137] Poli V, Pui-Yan Ma V, Di Gioia M, et al. Zinc-dependent histone deacetylases drive neutrophil extracellular trap formation and potentiate local and systemic inflammation. iScience 19 2021;24(11):103256.

[138] Průcha M, Zazula R, Russwurm S. Sepsis diagnostics in the era of "omics" technologies. Prague Med Rep 2018; 119(1):9–29.

[139] Ng S, Strunk T, Jiang P, et al. Precision medicine for neonatal sepsis. Front Mol Biosci 2018;5:70.

[140] Kuleš J, Horvatić A, Guillemin N, et al. The plasma proteome and the acute phase protein response in canine pyometra. J Proteomics 2020;223:103817.

[141] Franco-Martínez L, Horvatić A, Gelemanović A, et al. Changes in the salivary proteome associated with canine pyometra. Front Vet Sci 2020;7:277.

[142] Van Wyngene L, Vandewalle J, Libert C. Reprogramming of basic metabolic pathways in microbial sepsis: therapeutic targets at last? EMBO Mol Med 2018; 10(8):e8712.

[143] Wasyluk W, Zwolak A. Metabolic Alterations in Sepsis. J Clin Med 2021;10(11):2412.

[144] Beloborodova NV, Olenin AY, Pautova AK. Metabolomic findings in sepsis as a damage of host-microbial metabolism integration. J Crit Care 2018;43:246–55.

[145] Eckerle M, Ambroggio L, Puskarich MA, et al. Metabolomics as a driver in advancing precision medicine in sepsis. Pharmacotherapy 2017;37(9):1023–32.

[146] Englert JA, Rogers AJ. Metabolism, metabolomics, and nutritional support of patients with sepsis. Clin Chest Med 2016;37(2):321–31.

[147] Pontes-Arruda A, Martins LF, de Lima SM, et al. Enteral nutrition with eicosapentaenoic acid, gamma-linolenic acid and antioxidants in the early treatment of sepsis: results from a multicenter, prospective, randomized, double-blinded, controlled study: the INTERSEPT study. Crit Care 2011;15(3):R144.

[148] Galban C, Montejo JC, Mesejo A, et al. An immune-enhancing enteral diet reduces mortality rate and episodes of bacteremia in septic intensive care unit patients. Crit Care Med 2000;28(3):643–8.

[149] Liu DT, Brown DC, Silverstein DC. Early nutritional support is associated with decreased length of hospitalization in dogs with septic peritonitis: a retrospective study of 45 cases (2000-2009). J Vet Emerg Crit Care 2012;22(4):453–9.

[150] Hoffberg JE, Koenigshof A. Evaluation of the safety of early compared to late enteral nutrition in canine septic peritonitis. J Am Anim Hosp Assoc 2017;53(2):90–5.

[151] Montague B, Summers A, Bhawal R, et al. Identifying potential biomarkers and therapeutic targets for dogs with sepsis using metabolomics and lipidomics analyses. PLoS One 2022;17(7):e0271137.

[152] Balistreri CR. Promising strategies for preserving adult endothelium health and reversing its dysfunction: from liquid biopsy to new omics technologies and noninvasive circulating biomarkers. Int J Mol Sci 2022;23(14). https://doi.org/10.3390/ijms23147548.

[153] Lawrence-Mills SJ, Hughes D, Hezzell MJ, et al. The microvascular endothelial glycocalyx: an additional piece of the puzzle in veterinary medicine. Vet J 2022; 285:105843.

[154] Yini S, Heng Z, Xin A, et al. Effect of unfractionated heparin on endothelial glycocalyx in a septic shock model. Acta Anaesthesiol Scand 2015;59(2):160–9.

[155] Naseri A, Gulersoy E, Ider M, et al. Serum biomarkers of endothelial glycocalyx injury in canine parvoviral infection. Austral J Vet Sci 2020;52(3):95–101.

[156] Smart L, Boyd CJ, Claus MA, et al. Large-volume crystalloid fluid is associated with increased hyaluronan shedding and inflammation in a canine hemorrhagic shock model. Inflammation 2018;41(4): 1515–23.

[157] Turner K, Boyd C, Rossi G, et al. Allergy, inflammation, hepatopathy and coagulation biomarkers in dogs with suspected anaphylaxis due to insect envenomation. Front Vet Sci 2022;9:875339.

[158] Lawrence-Mills SJ, Hezzell MJ, Adamantos SE, et al. Circulating hyaluronan as a marker of endothelial glycocalyx damage in dogs with myxomatous mitral valve disease and dogs in a hypercoagulable state. Vet J 2022; 285:105845.

[159] Beiseigel M, Simon BT, Michalak C, et al. Effect of peri-operative crystalloid fluid rate on circulating hyaluronan in healthy dogs: a pilot study. Vet J 2021;267: 105578.

[160] Hong HJ, Oh YI, Park SM, et al. Evaluation of endothelial cell-specific molecule-1 as a biomarker of glycocalyx damage in canine myxomatous mitral valve disease. BMC Vet Res 2022;18(1):261.

[161] Yozova ID, Londoño LA, Millar KK, et al. Rapid patient-side evaluation of endothelial glycocalyx thickness in healthy sedated cats using glycocheck® software. Front Vet Sci 2022;8:727063.

[162] Blann AD. Endothelial cell activation, injury, damage and dysfunction: separate entities or mutual terms? Blood Coagul Fibrinolysis 2000;11(7):623–30.

[163] Blann AD. Plasma von Willebrand factor, thrombosis, and the endothelium: the first 30 years. Thromb Haemost 2006;95(1):49–55.

[164] Felmeden DC, Blann AD, Spencer CG, et al. A comparison of flow-mediated dilatation and von Willebrand factor as markers of endothelial cell function in health and in hypertension: relationship to cardiovascular risk and effects of treatment: a substudy of the Anglo-Scandinavian Cardiac Outcomes Trial. Blood Coagul Fibrinolysis 2003;14(5):425–31.

[165] Schumacher A, Seljeflot I, Sommervoll L, et al. Increased levels of endothelial haemostatic markers in patients with coronary heart disease. Thromb Res 2002;105(1):25–31.

[166] Huang LF, Guo FQ, Liang YZ, et al. Simultaneous determination of L-arginine and its mono- and dimethylated metabolites in human plasma by high-performance liquid chromatography-mass spectrometry. Anal Bioanal Chem 2004;380(4):643–9.

[167] Tarnow I, Kristensen AT, Olsen LH, et al. Assessment of changes in hemostatic markers in cavalier king charles spaniels with myxomatous mitral valve disease. Am J Vet Res 2004;65(12):1644–52.

[168] Moesgaard SG, Holte AV, Mogensen T, et al. Effects of breed, gender, exercise and white-coat effect on markers of endothelial function in dogs. Article. Res Vet Sci 2007;82(3):409–15.

[169] Stokol T, Brooks M, Rush JE, et al. Hypercoagulability in cats with cardiomyopathy. J Vet Intern Med 2008;22(3): 546–52.

[170] Giannessi D, Del Ry S, Vitale RL. The role of endothelins and their receptors in heart failure. Pharmacol Res 2001;43(2):111–26.

[171] Wei CM, Lerman A, Rodeheffer RJ, et al. Endothelin in human congestive heart failure. Circulation 1994; 89(4):1580–6.

[172] Pacher R, Stanek B, Hulsmann M, et al. Prognostic impact of big endothelin-1 plasma concentrations compared with invasive hemodynamic evaluation in severe heart failure. J Am Coll Cardiol 1996;27(3): 633–41.

[173] Frey B, Pacher R, Locker G, et al. Prognostic value of hemodynamic vs big endothelin measurements during long-term IV therapy in advanced heart failure patients. Chest 2000;117(6):1713–9.

[174] O'Sullivan ML, O'Grady MR, Minors SL. Plasma big endothelin-1, atrial natriuretic peptide, aldosterone, and norepinephrine concentrations in normal Doberman Pinschers and Doberman Pinschers with dilated cardiomyopathy. J Vet Intern Med 2007;21(1):92–9.

[175] Martin L, Koczera P, Zechendorf E, et al. The endothelial glycocalyx: new diagnostic and therapeutic approaches in sepsis. BioMed Res Int 2016;2016: 3758278.

[176] Nelson A, Berkestedt I, Schmidtchen A, et al. Increased levels of glycosaminoglycans during septic shock: relation to mortality and the antibacterial actions of plasma. Shock 2008;30(6):623–7.

[177] Goodall KJ, Poon IK, Phipps S, et al. Soluble heparan sulfate fragments generated by heparanase trigger the release of pro-inflammatory cytokines through TLR-4. PLoS One 2014;9(10):e109596.

[178] Hoppensteadt D, Tsuruta K, Hirman J, et al. Dysregulation of inflammatory and hemostatic markers in sepsis and suspected disseminated intravascular coagulation. Clin Appl Thromb Hemost 2015;21(2):120–7.

[179] Shaw KE, Bersenas AM, Bateman SW, et al. Use of serum hyaluronic acid as a biomarker of endothelial glycocalyx degradation in dogs with septic peritonitis. Am J Vet Res 2021;82(7):566–73.

Advances in Small Animal Care 4 (2023) 89–100

ADVANCES IN SMALL ANIMAL CARE

Controversies of and Indications for Use of Glucocorticoids in the Intensive Care Unit and the Emergency Room

Yekaterina Buriko, DVM, DACVECC[a],*, Ashlei Tinsley, VMD[a]

[a]Department of Clinical Sciences and Advanced Medicine, University of Pennsylvania School of Veterinary Medicine, 3900 Delancey Street, Philadelphia, PA 19104, USA

KEYWORDS
- Glucocorticoids • Anti-inflammatory • CIRCI • ARDS • Infection • Anaphylaxis • Inflammation

KEY POINTS

- Glucocorticoids (GC) have variable GC and mineralocorticoid activity, onset of action, and biological half-life, which makes individual drug selection important.
- There is evidence that GC may be useful for treatment of certain infectious diseases, such as severe pneumonia and infectious meningitis.
- Evidence for GC use in traumatic brain injury, spinal injury, and as a first-line treatment of anaphylaxis is lacking—consideration should be given to not using GC for these conditions unless an alternate clear indication for their use exists.
- GC can be considered for conditions such as acute respiratory distress syndrome and pancreatitis in a specific subset of patients, using certain doses and duration of treatment.
- The recommendations for most of the potential indications for GC use were derived from human literature—veterinary studies are urgently needed for an evidence-based approach to the use of GC.

ENDOGENOUS AND EXOGENOUS CORTICOSTEROID FORMULATIONS

Corticosteroids are hormones that are synthesized in the zona fasciculata and zona glomerulosa of the adrenal cortex [1]. Cortisol and aldosterone are the main endogenous compounds synthesized, with cortisol stimulating both glucocorticoid (GC) and mineralocorticoid receptors, and aldosterone having only mineralocorticoid effects. Cholesterol is the precursor for adrenocortical hormones. The structure (21 carbon ring skeleton) of these steroids is the foundation for the generation of synthetic GC [2]. Throughout this article, we will refer to cortisol and cortisol-associated and derived synthetic corticosteroid compounds as

GC, even though they have variable GC and mineralocorticoid properties.

GC production is regulated by the hypothalamic-pituitary-adrenal (HPA) axis. Corticotropin-releasing hormone (CRH) in the hypothalamus stimulates the secretion of adrenocorticotropic hormone (ACTH) from the pituitary gland. ACTH is then released into circulation, stimulating the synthesis and secretion of cortisol. Through negative feedback, cortisol inhibits the release of CRH and ACTH as the cortisol level rises. In healthy dogs and humans, ACTH and CRH are secreted in a pulsatile manner. In humans, the secretion has a circadian rhythm and peaks before awakening, but this has not been found in dogs [1]. Stress and other

---

*Corresponding author, *E-mail address:* buriko@vet.upenn.edu

https://doi.org/10.1016/j.yasa.2023.04.001

factors including exercise, infection, trauma, and pain induce CRH release [2].

The cortisol molecule has been chemically changed to create various steroids with different duration of action, potency and mineralocorticoid and GC effects. Typically, manipulation of the cortisol molecule to produce subsequent steroids has diminished their mineralocorticoid properties and enhanced the GC effects, as the anti-inflammatory properties and potency have grown [1]. Cortisol is arbitrarily assigned a potency of one and all of the other preparations are compared to cortisol in potency, as well as GC and mineralocorticoid effects (Table 1). The relative potency of GC in relation to cortisol is also considered in choosing the dosing regimen for individual drugs, with higher doses of lower potency GC producing the same effect as lower doses of more potent drugs. The cellular and molecular effects of steroid compounds depend on their GC and mineralocorticoid activity, relative potency, and dose administered, as well as the duration of action. It is important to consider the biological half-life as opposed to plasma half-life, as the former is key to the pharmacological effects in the patients receiving steroids. Typically, GC are divided as short acting, intermediate acting, and long acting based on their biological half-life (see Table 1). Some GC like prednisone and cortisone are biologically inactive when administered and need to be converted to the active compounds prednisolone and cortisol in the liver to exert their effects. Cats require three to five times the amount of prednisone compared to prednisolone for an equivalent effect, which may be due to the inferior absorption or conversion to prednisolone in the liver. Cats and dogs with liver disease may benefit from the administration of prednisolone to optimize the GC dosing [1].

Further modifications to the steroid compounds can be made by esterification to affect their water solubility, which will further determine their onset and duration of action. For example, water-soluble esters, sodium phosphate and sodium succinate, will ensure immediate release after intravenous administration. Some esters such as acetate, pivalate, or dipropionate are insoluble, and result in sustained long-term release of days to months, and are typically administered intramuscularly or intralesionally. The insoluble ester preparations do not allow for dose titration and have variable blood concentrations, in addition to suppressing the HPA axis for extended periods. Furthermore, one formulation of dexamethasone for veterinary use exists as a free alcohol solution compounded with polyethylene glycol, with onset of action of minutes to hours [1].

Molecular Effects of Glucocorticoids

GC activity can be divided into genomic and nongenomic effects. A cytoplasmic glucocorticoid receptor (GR) within the nuclear receptor superfamily mediates the genomic effect. GR are widely dispersed throughout cells in the body and remain inactive until bound to a GC ligand [1]. In the resting state, GR is located in the

TABLE 1				
Duration of Action and Relative Potencies of Commonly Used Steroid Formulations in Veterinary Medicine				
Drug	Half-Life (Hours)	Anti-inflammatory Activity	Equivalent Dosage	Mineralocorticoid Activity
Hydrocortisone	8–12	1	20	2
Cortisone	8–12	0.8	25	2
Prednisone	12–36	4	5	1
Prednisolone	12–36	4	5	1
Methylprednisolone	12–36	5	4	0
Triamcinolone	12–36	5	4	0
Betamethasone	36–72	20–30	0.6	0
Dexamethasone	36–72	20–30	0.75	0
Fludrocortisone	18–36	10	2	125–200
Desoxycorticosterone (DOCP)	17 d[a]	0		200–1000

[a] DOCP half-life is 17 d when administered subcutaneously; if administered intramuscularly, it is 8 d.

cytoplasm as a multiprotein complex. GC enter cells by passive diffusion via the cell membrane and bind to the GR. After binding, a conformation change occurs, and the GC–GR complex is translocated into the nucleus. Once in the nucleus, the complex activates or represses target gene transcription. The GC–GR complex binds specific DNA sites called glucocorticoid response elements (GRE) [1,3]. When the complex is bound to positive GRE, gene activation and synthesis of anti-inflammatory proteins and regulator proteins important for metabolism occur. This process is called transactivation and likely contributes to the adverse effects of GC. Binding of the complex to negative GRE results in the inhibition of gene transcription of the prolactin gene and the precursor of ACTH (pro-opiomelanocortin) known as transrepression [1]. Binding to negative GRE also leads to suppression of inflammatory genes, including interleukin (IL)-1β and IL-2. Target gene suppression can also occur via direct protein-to-protein interaction with pro-inflammatory transcription factors (ie, activation protein-1, nuclear factor kappa B [NF-κB]). The duration from activation of the GR to initiation of transcription and translation is about 30 minutes; however, cellular and tissue changes become evident within hours to days [3]. A smaller portion of GC effects can also be mediated by the mineralocorticoid receptor, depending on the relative mineralocorticoid effects of the individual drug.

Non-genomic actions contribute to the rapid onset of cellular effects seen with GC, and are classified as nonspecific interactions of GC with cell membranes, effects mediated by cytosolic GR, or specific interactions with membrane-bound GR [1,3]. The GR does not need to be translocated into the nucleus to influence transcription. GC can insert into membranes which alter the membrane activity and physiologic properties. This leads to reduced calcium and sodium cycling across immune cell membranes, resulting in immuno-suppression and reduced inflammatory processes [1]. In addition, membrane-bound GR play a role in T cell receptor-mediated signal transduction and apoptosis [1,3]. Binding of GC to cytosolic GR results in the dissociation of proteins from the cytosolic GR multiprotein complex. The released proteins are proposed to be responsible for the rapid GC effects. GC can also inhibit arachidonic acid which mediates cell growth, and metabolic and inflammatory reactions.

Biologic Effects of Glucocorticoids

The activity of GC is dose-dependent and is categorized as physiologic, anti-inflammatory, and immunosuppressive. Prednisone and prednisolone are commonly used

as a reference for calculating the relative doses to result in various biologic effects. The goal of physiologic dosing is to replace GC in amounts that are similar to what the adrenal gland releases under normal conditions. Under physiologic conditions, GC help maintain serum glucose levels by increasing hepatic gluconeogenesis and decreasing the uptake of glucose in peripheral tissues. They also stimulate collagen production [1]. Renal effects include increased glomerular filtration rate, water diuresis, and sodium transport in the proximal tubule. GCs have an inhibitory effect on antidiuretic hormone. Cardiac effects include positive chronotropic and inotropic actions. GC play a role in catecholamine sensitivity and contribute to the maintenance of normal vascular tone [1]. A physiologic prednisolone dose range of 0.1 to 0.25 mg/kg daily is recommended.

Anti-inflammatory and immunologic effects occur due to decreased recruitment of inflammatory cells, inhibition of arachidonic acid release, decreased vascular permeability, and transcription modulation [4]. GC repress transcription of genes encoding cell adhesion molecules, pro-inflammatory cytokines, and chemokines. This inhibits proliferation, differentiation, adhesion, migration, and chemotaxis of neutrophils, T cells, and macrophages [1]. Anti-inflammatory doses are used to combat signs associated with inflammatory and allergic conditions. In dogs, a prednisolone dose of 0.5 to 1 mg/kg per day is recommended, while in cats, the dose can range from 1 to 2 mg/kg. Immunosuppressive dosing can be used to obtain disease remission, prevent organ rejection post-transplantation, and treat immune-mediated disease by reducing immunological reactions. Prednisolone dosages can range from 2 to 4 mg/kg. It is recommended that large dogs (over 25 kg) receive the low range of the immunosuppressive dose [1], as dosing per body weight in large breed dogs frequently overestimates the required dose [5]. Some advocate not to exceed 60 to 80 mg prednisone/prednisolone daily dose for large dogs. Dosing of GC in large dogs based on the body surface area has been recommended at 50 to 60 mg/m^2 once daily to provide an immunosuppressive dose [6]. A study evaluating the pharmacokinetics of immunosuppressive doses of prednisolone in small and large healthy dogs concluded that the pharmacologic effect of a 2 mg/kg dose of prednisolone is significantly higher in large dogs compared to small dogs, and that dosing on the body surface area at 40 mg/m^2 twice daily resulted in the lowest plasma drug concentration of the groups [5]. Further studies are necessary to achieve optimal dosing of GC in large dogs. Recommendations to divide the daily amount of prednisone into twice daily dosing have been made to minimize gastrointestinal effects [1]; however, no clear evidence exists for once daily or twice daily dosing. The dose should be titrated to the lowest amount needed to control clinical signs.

Adverse Effects Associated with Glucocorticoid Administration

Adverse effects are not uncommon with GC use. They can range from cosmetic effects to life-threatening alterations in homeostasis and should be heavily weighed when considering treatment with GC. The type of medication, the dose, and duration of action should all play a role in the decision-making process.

Signs consistent with iatrogenic hyperadrenocorticism can be seen within the first 1 to 2 weeks of administration of GC, and include polydipsia, polyuria, polyphagia, and panting [1]. Additional signs with longer durations of therapy (weeks to months) include thin hair coat, alopecia, muscle atrophy, and poor wound healing. Increased susceptibility to infections can occur due to alterations in phagocytes, leukocytes, and cell-mediated immunity [1]. Patients receiving anti-inflammatory and immunosuppressive doses can exhibit these clinical features, but they can also be seen with physiologic doses in sensitive dogs. GC sensitivity varies among dogs, while cats are thought to be more resistant to the development of iatrogenic hyperadrenocorticism. In cats, signs typically occur after recurrent injections of long-acting GC. Affected cats may also exhibit spontaneous sloughing and tearing of the skin [1].

Synthetic GC suppress the HPA axis and CRH and ACTH secretion [1,2]. Over time, atrophy of the adrenal glands occurs and affected animals lose the ability to adequately secrete cortisol in response to stress, leading to signs of adrenal insufficiency if the GC therapy is withdrawn acutely [1]. The greater the anti-inflammatory potency of the administered GC, the more substantial the effect on the HPA axis. Topical administration in addition to systemic administration can result in HPA axis suppression. Gradual weaning of GC therapy is therefore recommended when GC duration of therapy exceeds 2 weeks [1].

GC can lead to hyperglycemia, increased insulin resistance in muscles and tissues, and increased hepatic glucose production leading to diabetes mellitus. They can also negatively impact glycemic control in diabetic patients. Hyperglycemia can contribute to inhibition of the immune response, altered innate immunity, and increased pro-inflammatory cytokine production. GC use can result in decreased cell turnover, increased protein breakdown, and impaired fibroblasts and collagen formation, resulting in delayed wound healing

[1]. Doses above the physiologic range can alter mucus production, decrease mucosal cell turnover, and impair mucosal blood flow in the gastrointestinal (GI) tract, resulting in ulceration and hemorrhage [1].

Glucocorticoid Use in Specific Disease Conditions

GC have been utilized to treat a great number of conditions in companion animals. The below-listed indications are some of the pathologies where steroid use is considered in the veterinary emergency and intensive care setting. The use of steroids in hypoadrenocorticism, inflammatory diseases like asthma or vasculitis, immune-mediated diseases, as well as neoplastic conditions is well established and will not be discussed in this article.

Acute Respiratory Distress Syndrome

Acute respiratory distress syndrome (ARDS) results in hypoxemic respiratory failure caused by an insult such as pneumonia, trauma, inhaled toxicants, sepsis, or pancreatitis. In humans, it is defined as respiratory failure within a week of insult not explained by cardiac function or volume overload and acute hypoxemia (Pao_2/Fio_2 <300 mm Hg) on at least positive end expiratory pressure (PEEP) of 5 cm H_2O [7]. In veterinary medicine, Vet ARDS has been defined as severe hypoxemia with Pao_2/Fio_2 ratio of less than 200 without the necessity for PEEP, that is acute in onset and secondary to a precipitating cause with no evidence of left atrial hypertension and one recommended criterion of documented pulmonary inflammation via sampling of the airway [8]. During these disease states, there is dysregulated systemic inflammation and coagulation pathways in response to injury. Due to increased lung permeability and diffuse alveolar capillary membrane injury, protein-rich fluid enters the alveoli, impairing gas exchange and lung compliance [7,9]. Over time, the lung can develop areas of fibrosis.

Treatment of ARDS is multifactorial and is dependent on the underlying cause. Therapies can include antibiotics, oxygen supplementation, positive pressure ventilation with lung protective strategies, and GC therapy. GC therapy is associated with a progressive increase in GR-mediated activities, resulting in reductions in NF-κB DNA binding and transcription of tumor necrosis factor (TNF)-α and IL-1β [9,10]. Additional anti-inflammatory effects include inhibition of neutrophil degranulation and macrophage superoxide anion production. Various randomized control trials in humans reported an association between improvement in systemic markers of inflammation and reduction in duration of mechanical ventilation, development of multi-organ dysfunction, and intensive care unit stay [9,11]. In humans with ARDS, the suggested GC is methylprednisolone, as it has greater penetration into the lung tissue [11].

Timing of initiation of GC treatment, doses and type of GC, and the duration of treatment have all been a topic of debate and investigation in human medicine. Prophylactic treatment to prevent ARDS in high-risk populations is not recommended and has been shown to increase mortality [12,13]. Similarly, high doses of GC are not recommended due to increased risk of infectious complications [11]. The current recommendation for initiation of GC therapy can range from early (within 72 hours) after onset of ARDS to 7 days after onset of ARDS with some sources recommending monitoring response to conventional therapy for up to 7 days before election of GC treatment [12], and other sources advocating for earlier GC treatment, as it might be associated with faster disease resolution [11,13]. GC therapy is not recommended after 2 weeks of onset of ARDS and has been associated with increased mortality [10,11].

Dosing and duration of treatment with GC in patients with ARDS have varied as well. The 2021 ARDS clinical practice guidelines recommend a daily intravenous dose of methylprednisolone of 1 to 2 mg/kg for at least 7 days [13]. The Society of Critical Care Medicine (SCCM) and the European Society of Intensive Care Medicine (ESICM) recommend an intravenous methylprednisolone dose of 1 mg/kg/day in patients within 7 days of ARDS onset; and a dose of 2 mg/kg/day in patients in which GC treatment is initiated after day 6 of ARDS development, followed by a 13-day taper [11]. Other sources recommend a methylprednisolone taper of 2 to 4 weeks [10]. If tapered too quickly or stopped abruptly, decompensation can occur due to recurrent inflammatory response [11,12].

There is a paucity of veterinary literature regarding the management of ARDS and the role of GC in the treatment regimen. A case report of a dog with acute lung injury or ARDS secondary to anaphylactic shock caused by bee envenomation has been described. The dog received prednisone (0.5 mg/kg/day) after 7 days of supportive care to prevent pulmonary fibrosis [14]. Another case report described the use of dexamethasone in a dog with ARDS due to an unknown cause [15]. Studies are needed to investigate GC utility in the treatment of ARDS in the veterinary species.

Critical Illness-Related Corticosteroid Insufficiency

Adrenal insufficiency is a common cause of mortality in the emergency and critical care setting. Guidelines for the diagnosis and management of critical illness-related corticosteroid insufficiency (CIRCI) are ever changing. As previously mentioned, GC play an important role in stress response and homeostasis. Adrenocortical function is altered in the critically ill populations. These patients have a normal to high basal cortisol concentration, but a blunted response to ACTH stimulation [16,17]. During periods of marked stress, normal functions including cardiac contractility, immune function, vascular tone, and permeability are altered in CIRCI patients [16–18]. Alterations in these functions play a role in patient mortality.

CIRCI is commonly found in cases of systemic inflammatory response syndrome (SIRS) and sepsis [11,16,17]. In these disease states, the release of inflammatory mediators can suppress CRH and ACTH [19]. Cytokines and hemorrhage can also damage the hypothalamus, pituitary, or adrenal glands resulting in deficient cortisol production and/or inadequate response to exogenous ACTH. The diagnosis of CIRCI can be difficult to obtain. Baseline cortisol concentrations, ACTH stimulation testing, response to treatment, and measurement of total and free cortisol have been used to identify patients with CIRCI. In humans, a delta cortisol < 9 µg/dL or a random plasma cortisol <10 µg/dL may be used, but no single test has been found to reliably diagnose CIRCI [11]. The Surviving Sepsis Campaign guidelines have not found plasma cortisol levels useful and suggest not using ACTH stimulation test to select which septic shock patients may be treated with hydrocortisone [11]. Dogs with a delta cortisol (ACTH-stimulated cortisol minus basal cortisol) of less than or equal to 3 ug/dL had an increased mortality in comparison to dogs with a cortisol increase > 3 ug/dL[17]. In one study, basal cortisol >5 µg/dL was associated with increased mortality [16]. The diagnosis of CIRCI in cats has been difficult to achieve, and previous studies have not found a significant difference in baseline cortisol, delta cortisol, or post-ACTH stimulation cortisol between survivors and non-survivors [17].

Treatment of CIRCI consists of fluid resuscitation, treatment of the underlying disease process, and GC therapy [1,9]. Indication for the use of GC therapy in humans with suspicion of CIRCI includes fluid-resuscitated septic shock that is not responsive to vasopressors [16–18]. Hydrocortisone is used in these cases [11,17,19]. The dose and duration of hydrocortisone vary, and additional studies are needed to determine the ideal duration of therapy and taper course of GC in CIRCI. The SCCM and ESICM guidelines recommend IV hydrocortisone at less than 400 mg/day for 3 days or longer [11]. A consensus statement by the American

College of Critical Care Medicine recommended stress dose corticosteroid treatment (hydrocortisone IV 200 mg/day) divided into four doses or as a 100 mg bolus followed by a 10 mg/hour constant rate infusion (CRI) for 24 hours [11,17]. The Surviving Sepsis Campaign recommends a hydrocortisone CRI to help avoid hyperglycemic episodes [17]. In dogs and cats, hydrocortisone doses of 0.5 to 1 mg/kg IV every 6 hours, as well as bolus administration (1 mg/kg) followed by a CRI (0.08–0.16 mg/kg/h IV) have been reported [16,17,20,21]. Hydrocortisone therapy duration can range from 1 to 5 days depending on the response to therapy, followed by a gradual taper, which is variable and frequently not specified in the available literature, but generally consists of 4 to 6 days [16,17,20]. Several case reports of GC treatment and favorable outcomes in suspected or confirmed CIRCI in veterinary patients have been described [16,20,21]. One study reported hydrocortisone treatment of dogs with SIRS, some of which also were documented to have CIRCI based on a delta cortisol level <3 ug/dL. No difference in survival between hydrocortisone-treated and not treated dogs, or between dogs with and without CIRCI was documented in this small study [16]. Another retrospective study evaluated hydrocortisone therapy in dogs diagnosed with septic shock and suspected CIRCI [22]. This study did not find a difference in survival between GC-treated and not treated dogs; however, the treated dogs were significantly sicker, introducing bias into the results.

It is reasonable to consider hydrocortisone therapy in patients with a suspicion of CIRCI who are suffering from shock with vasopressor refractory hypotension, and consideration should be given to a CRI as opposed to intermittent boluses. A gradual taper should be considered instead of an abrupt withdrawal, but the ideal timing of the taper is unknown. Additional veterinary studies are needed to determine the ideal dose, timing, and weaning protocols.

Neurologic disease

Traumatic brain injury. Traumatic brain injury (TBI) is a sequela of head trauma and a cause of mortality in human and veterinary species. Common inciting events include vehicular incidents, high-rise syndrome, and bite wound trauma [23]. The injuries are categorized as either primary or secondary. Primary injuries such as contusions and lacerations are the result of physical damage to the brain and occur at the time of insult. Secondary injuries occur in the days following the trauma due to biochemical changes such as ATP depletion, cytokine production, and free radical production [23].

The development of cerebral edema and increased intracranial pressure contribute to mortality.

Although GC have been used for the treatment of edema and for their anti-inflammatory effects in cases of trauma, they are contraindicated in TBI [23]. Corticosteroids have been shown to worsen mortality in cases of TBI [2,23]. Administration of GC can lead to hyperglycemia and insulin resistance [2,23]. Hyperglycemia is thought to worsen brain injury by increasing free radical production, excitatory amino acid release, and increased cerebral edema [23].

Stress doses of GC may be beneficial in patients with concurrent CIRCI and TBI [2]. These patients may develop a form of CIRCI due to direct trauma to the pituitary gland and the hypothalamus resulting in acute secondary adrenal insufficiency [2,24]. Apoptosis of the neurons in the paraventricular nucleus (PVN) also plays a role, as CRH is secreted in these neurons. CIRCI has been shown to increase mortality after severe TBI due to its association with hemodynamic instability [2,25]. In an experimental model using male rats with TBI, the use of low-dose methylprednisolone, high-dose methylprednisolone, or low-dose corticosterone was evaluated. The effect of these medications on intracellular signaling pathways important for neuronal apoptosis and survival was assessed. In this study, the number of CRH-positive neurons was reduced after TBI, while the number of apoptotic cells in the PVN was increased [25]. High-dose methylprednisolone was associated with an increased mortality and affected hypothalamic activity by increasing neuronal apoptosis and downregulating CRH expression. This effect was not present in the low-dose methylprednisolone group. Low-dose corticosterone exhibited a protective effect by inhibiting neuronal apoptosis and improving the survival of CRH-positive neurons [25].

The use of GC in a dog with damage to the pituitary and hypothalamus following a TBI was discussed in a case report [24]. The patient exhibited signs of intermittent hypotension, hypothermia, and electrolyte abnormalities, and mentation changes due to HPA axis damage. Dexamethasone sodium phosphate at 0.06 mg/kg IV was administered daily in addition to aggressive supportive care; ultimately, euthanasia was elected due to concerns for long-time prognosis despite initial improvement. The use of low-dose GC could be considered in patients with documented TBI-related adrenal insufficiency.

Spinal cord injury. Spinal cord injury (SCI) due to trauma or intravertebral disk disease (IVDD) can be a significant source of morbidity in veterinary patients.

Steroid utilization in SCI has been investigated for years, with some human data indicating that high-dose infusions of methylprednisolone given within 3 to 8 hours and up to 48 hours post-injury improve neurologic recovery scores. However, the degree of improvement was modest, and major complications such as significantly more episodes of pneumonia and sepsis in the steroid-treated group were documented. Guidelines on SCI by Hulbert and colleagues published in 2013 recommended against the use of methylprednisolone in SCI [26]. Heterogeneous veterinary studies utilizing various types and doses of GC have not found significant beneficial effects of steroid administration in dogs with SCI; however, a number of substantial adverse effects were reported, such as gastrointestinal signs including vomiting, diarrhea, ulceration, and bleeding, as well as urinary tract infections [2]. One retrospective study evaluating medical management of presumptive IVDD in dogs found that GC use was not associated with management success or quality of life in this patient population [27]. Routine administration of GC in this setting cannot be recommended, and prospective placebo-controlled studies with standardized type and dose of GC are necessary to draw meaningful conclusions about the use of GC in SCI.

Pancreatitis. Pancreatitis occurs by the inappropriate binding of lysosome to zymogens within the acinar cells of the pancreas, resulting in conversion of trypsinogen to trypsin, which activates other pancreatic proenzymes [28–30]. Changes in acinar intracellular pH, increases in intracellular calcium, and signal transduction changes are also associated with its development [29,30]. Calcium is a second messenger in stimulus-secretion coupling in exocrine pancreatic cells, and disruption of intracellular calcium signaling plays a role in cell injury [29]. The severity of pancreatitis can range from mild to life-threatening. Common clinical signs include abdominal discomfort, vomiting, anorexia, and diarrhea. In its more severe form, SIRS, sepsis, multi-organ failure, and death can occur. Pancreatic hemorrhage, necrosis, increased capillary permeability, cytokine stimulation, alterations in coagulation and inflammation play important roles in the development of severe pancreatitis.

Diagnosis of pancreatitis is made by a combination of physical examination findings, clinical signs, abdominal imaging, and laboratory tests such as biochemistry panels and species-specific serum pancreatic lipase testing [28,30]. In addition, markers of inflammation including IL-8, IL-6, and C-reactive protein (CRP) are useful in determining the degree of severity and response to treatment in people; CRP has been used in dogs for diagnosis, severity assessment, and treatment monitoring in pancreatitis [30]. Treatment of pancreatitis consists of fluid resuscitation, analgesia, gastroprotectants, anti-emetics, adequate nutrition, and treatment of comorbidities such as diabetes mellitus, when present [28,30]. Mortality rates for acute pancreatitis range from 27% to 58% in dogs [30].

GC have been used in cases of pancreatitis that do not appropriately respond to standard treatments. Whereas GC administration was initially thought of as a risk factor for pancreatitis, the anti-inflammatory effects provided by GC have been shown to be protective against pancreatic inflammation [28,30]. In cases of acute pancreatitis, GC use was associated with improved survival times in dogs and humans [31]. In a study of 65 dogs with acute pancreatitis (AP), the response to treatment with and without subcutaneous prednisolone therapy was evaluated [28]. CRP was measured and was significantly lower in dogs who received prednisolone therapy (1 mg/kg/day subcutaneously) beginning on day 3 of hospitalization. Prednisolone was administered until discharge with a median stay of 5 days. These patients also had shorter hospitalization periods, quicker resolution of clinical signs, and improved survival [28].

A review evaluating GC use in cases of experimental and naturally occurring pancreatitis in dogs, rodents, and humans showed improvement in some aspects of pancreatitis with corticosteroid use [31]. GC reduced CRP levels when given early (within 1 hour) in the disease course. Patients who received steroids had a shorter length of hospitalization. Unlike the previous study, the effect of corticosteroids on mortality showed conflicting results. In some studies, there was no significant difference in survival between the GC and control group, while others supported improved survival with GC therapy. In this review, the types of steroids varied and included hydrocortisone, prednisolone, methylprednisolone, cortisone acetate, and dexamethasone. The dose, route, and timing of initiation of therapy also varied with the majority of doses in the anti-inflammatory range. Overall, the use of GC may benefit patients in cases of acute pancreatitis. It should be considered in cases of severe pancreatitis who are nonresponsive to supportive therapy [32]. Further investigation is needed to determine the optimal dose, timing, duration of therapy, and type of GC with the most benefit.

Community acquired pneumonia. Systemic GC administration in patients with pneumonia might be attractive for a number of reasons. The anti-inflammatory effects of GC could be beneficial in exuberant cytokine release, thus, protecting the lung from inflammatory damage. In addition, if a high organism burden is present, steroids might be protective in massive endotoxin and cytokine release due to bacterial die-off when antibiotic therapy is initiated. In patients with septic shock due to pneumonia, GC could be beneficial in case of relative adrenal insufficiency [33].

There is considerable evidence that steroids, specifically dexamethasone, may be of benefit in severe COVID pneumonia with moderate to severe ARDS [34]. One systematic review evaluating adults and children with pneumonia concluded that GC reduced mortality in severe but not non-severe pneumonia, and reduced early clinical failure and clinical failure rates (death from any cause, radiographic worsening during hospitalization) and days in the hospital for severe and non-severe pneumonia without a significantly increased risk of secondary infections [3]. Several pneumonia severity scoring systems exist [35], and this review utilized the Pneumonia Severity Index which considers demographics and extrapulmonary body functions in addition to lung disease scoring. The benefit of GC in this study was independent of their effects in septic shock. The doses of steroids used in the study were equivalent to 40 to 50 mg of prednisone per patient once daily for 5 to 10 days [33]. Hyperglycemia was the main adverse event associated with GC administration. This is in line with a number of clinical studies and meta-analyses demonstrating a consistent but variable magnitude benefit of GC in pneumonia patients [33,36]. However, a recent study evaluating IV tapering dose infusion of methylprednisolone for severe pneumonia in a blinded placebo-controlled study did not confer a mortality benefit in using GC and did not appreciate any difference in multiple morbidity outcomes evaluated [37]. Guidelines on treatment of community acquired pneumonia (CAD) by the American Thoracic Society and Infectious Diseases Society of America established in 2019 currently recommend against the use of GC in patients with CAD unless they require them for treatment of septic shock [38]. Currently, no studies in veterinary medicine evaluate the use of GC treatment in pneumonia and, therefore, a recommendation for or against the use of GC in veterinary patients with pneumonia cannot be made.

Infectious meningitis. Infectious meningitis refers to inflammation of the meninges covering the brain and the spinal cord (dura mater, arachnoid and subarachnoid space, and pia mater) and cerebrospinal fluid (CSF) secondary to an invading pathogen. Meningitis results in pathology ranging from pain to variable neurologic dysfunction commiserate with anatomic location of infection and severity of the lesion [39]. Meningitis may occur due to direct inoculation of the central nervous system (CNS) from penetrating bite wounds or foreign bodies, infection of tissues in proximity to the CNS, such as the middle and inner ear, nasal cavity, vertebrae or the intervertebral disks, or hematogenous spread. Multiple pathogens have been reported as causative agents of infectious meningitis, such as viruses (distemper, feline infectious peritonitis, West Nile, etc.); bacteria (*Escherichia coli*, *Streptococcus*, *Nocardia*, *Actinomyces*, *Brucella*, *Borrelia*, *Anaplasma*, etc.); fungi (*Cryptococcus*, *Aspergillus*, etc.), algae (protothecosis) and protozoal organisms (*Toxoplasma*, *Neospora*, *Babesia*, etc.) among others [40]. Listeriosis is associated with immunocompromise in people and is an important cause of meningitis. There is a relative lack of inflammatory and phagocytic cells in the CSF enabling the pathogens to multiply unaffected before the defensive immune response by the body [39].

Definitive diagnosis of infectious meningitis relies on evaluation of the CSF typically indicating neutrophilic, lymphocytic, or eosinophilic pleocytosis, increased protein concentration and may include direct visualization of the inciting organisms. Advanced imaging such as CT and MRI before the CSF sampling is a valuable diagnostic tool to support the diagnosis of meningitis. Cerebrospinal fluid culture and sensitivity, PCR assays for variable infectious agents should be performed based on the index of suspicion for a certain inciting agent, and additional diagnostic tests may include serologic testing of the blood or the CSF.

Treatment of infectious meningitis includes supportive care depending on the neurologic status and comfort of the patient and includes antimicrobial agents to address the underlying infectious process, as well as surgical debridement of abscessation whenever possible. Anti-inflammatory doses of GC have been utilized to manage the inflammatory process associated with the host response to the infection, as well as the exuberant inflammatory reaction that can happen shortly after starting antibiotics which may exacerbate the neuronal injury and worsen clinical signs. Their benefit has been evaluated extensively in people, and steroid administration with bacterial meningitis has been reported in a dog [41], but no studies evaluating the efficacy of GC in the treatment of infectious meningitis in veterinary species are available. Dexamethasone at 0.15 mg/kg IV every 6 hours initiated before or with the first dose of antibiotics and administered for 4 days has been described as a recommended protocol, as dexamethasone has a longer half-life and superior CNS penetration [42]. GC are indicated in adults and children with community acquired bacterial meningitis, where it improves survival in *Streptococcal* infections, which is the leading cause of acute bacterial meningitis in people [42–44]. GC use in patients with meningitis due to Listeriosis is not recommended as it appears to be associated with increased mortality [2,43,45]. Most evidence for use of GC in bacterial meningitis exists in people from high-income countries where the incidence of human immunodeficiency virus (HIV) and malnutrition is lower and where it lowers morbidity associated with meningitis, such as hearing loss after the infection [42,44,46].

In other causes of infectious meningitis, steroid use has been variably reported. Currently, no compelling evidence exists for use of GC in viral meningitis [47]. Routine use of steroids in cryptococcal meningitis with HIV has been associated with increased mortality in people and is not recommended [48]. Steroid use has been described in humans with chronic meningitis due to tuberculosis [49]. More studies are necessary for veterinary medicine to evaluate the efficacy of GC in the treatment of infectious meningitis. The use of anti-inflammatory doses of dexamethasone might be reasonable as adjunct treatment of confirmed bacterial meningitis to prevent worsening of clinical signs associated with bacterial killing by antibiotic therapy.

Anaphylaxis. Anaphylaxis refers to an acute severe systemic potentially fatal allergic reaction that requires immediate medical attention. Allergic reaction is most frequently due to a type I hypersensitivity which implies previous exposure to the antigen and is IgE mediated. Additionally, other immunologic (IgG) and non-immunologic (exercise, cold) mechanisms have been described as a cause of anaphylaxis.

GC continue to be commonly used for the management of anaphylaxis in human and veterinary patients. Currently, the main indications for usage of GC in anaphylaxis is treatment of protracted symptoms associated with anaphylaxis, as well as mitigation of the possible biphasic response associated with acute anaphylaxis [50]. Biphasic reaction in anaphylaxis consists of initial resolution of pathological manifestations of anaphylaxis followed by recrudescence of symptoms without further exposure to the offending agent, most commonly within 10 hours (1–78 hours) of the initial event [51]—they are yet to be described in veterinary patients. Compelling evidence on the use of GC in the treatment of allergic reactions is lacking despite widespread use [50,52,53], but high-quality randomized

trials investigating the use of GC in anaphylaxis are lacking. Studies investigating GC as agents administered for prevention of anaphylaxis have not demonstrated a clear benefit of steroids in preventing reactions due to contrast agents, snake antivenom administration, and allergen immunotherapy [54], although some positive effects were observed with mitigating reactions to certain chemotherapy agents [55]. GC should not be used as a first line of treatment in acute anaphylaxis—epinephrine remains the drug of choice [51,53,55]. The evidence for or against the routine use of GC as an adjunct treatment of anaphylaxis is lacking in human and veterinary medicine due to the paucity of high-quality studies. Recent guidelines on anaphylaxis recommended against the use of GC in acute anaphylaxis, as well as to prevent the biphasic response [55]. However, a systematic review investigating GC in anaphylaxis concluded that they may reduce the length of hospital stay and GC administration is not associated with increased adverse outcomes [56]. Whereas GC should not be prioritized in place of epinephrine for acute stabilization of a patient with anaphylaxis, their use at anti-inflammatory doses can be considered to mitigate long-term effects of anaphylaxis.

Edema/inflammation of upper airways. Anti-inflammatory effects of GC are relied on in a number of clinical situations associated with upper and large airway inflammation, including laryngeal edema associated with long-term intubation or repeated re-intubation; upper airway swelling associated with complications from brachycephalic airway syndrome; surgery associated with upper airways (BAOS, laryngeal paralysis, mass removal); infectious or inflammatory laryngitis, trauma of the upper airways, and medical management of collapsing trachea. The main rationale for using GC in these situations is reduction of inflammation which will lead to reduction in swelling and discomfort, thus preserving the airway patency and function. The maximum efficacy of GC when given for airway swelling and edema is likely hours after administration, although non-genomic effects on edema may be more rapid. No studies exist in veterinary medicine investigating the effects of GC in these situations in veterinary medicine, even though their use is widespread. In human patients, the use of GC has primarily been investigated in relation to their effect after intubation, as well as steroid administration in children with croup.

Children with infectious laryngotracheobronchitis, most commonly due to a parainfluenza virus (croup), suffer virus-induced inflammatory upper airway inflammation and edema that frequently results in airway obstruction. A single dose of dexamethasone at 0.6 mg/kg administered orally or parenterally is highly effective at treating the upper airway signs associated with croup in children [57]. A recent meta-analysis concluded that dexamethasone was the preferred steroid for reduction of croup-associated clinical signs, and that a lower dose of 0.15 mg/kg might be as effective [58]. The closest correlation of this pathology is likely the upper respiratory infection (URI) complex in cats, where laryngeal inflammation associated with the viral infection may result in airway obstruction. Further studies are indicated to evaluate the efficacy of GC in cats with laryngeal edema secondary to URI.

Laryngeal edema is reported to occur in 4% to 50% of children and adults undergoing intubation and mechanical ventilation [59]. Intubation and presence of the tube traumatize the airway mucosa and cause an inflammatory response, which is evident as early as 24 hours after intubation [59,60]. Children are particularly vulnerable to laryngeal edema due to their airway anatomy and looser connective tissue in the subglottic area, allowing for more edema accumulation [61]. The laryngeal edema contributes to airway obstruction and increases the rate of re-intubation, thus increasing morbidity, hospital stay, and mortality. Several studies have concluded that GC administration decreases the morbidity associated with intubation and decreases laryngeal edema as well as the need for re-intubation in adults and children who have experienced prolonged intubation and mechanical ventilation [60,61]. Prophylactic GC administration in a patient population at high risk of adverse events associated with extubation, as well as administration of GC for known laryngeal edema seem to have a benefit [60]. The risk level associated with airway obstruction after extubation is commonly assessed by the cuff leak test, where a lower cuff volume to occlude the leak is associated with increased risk of re-intubation [60]. There is some evidence that higher cumulative doses and earlier steroid administration (12–24 hours before planned extubation) are beneficial [61]. The dosing regimens and the types of steroids administered vary widely, and there is not a clear answer on which one is superior to the others. Generally, anti-inflammatory doses of steroids are administered either as single or several doses (up to four) within 12 to 24 hours before intubation. The main adverse events associated with steroid use in this patient population included hyperglycemia and GI bleeding [60]. Placebo-controlled studies evaluating the benefit of GC in commonly used scenarios (tracheal collapse, BAOS surgery) are necessary to make strong

recommendations regarding the benefit, timing, and dose of GC in these scenarios.

CLINICS CARE POINTS

- GC administration is associated with a plethora of significant and potentially life-threatening effects that should be weighed before their administration, especially in cases where the evidence for their use is lacking.
- GC administration could be considered in cases of severe community acquired pneumonia, pancreatitis, critical illness-related adrenal insufficiency, and infectious meningitis.
- GC can potentially be useful in treatment of upper airway swelling and inflammation, and consideration should be given to early GC administration, which may be beneficial to increase the chances of successful airway extubation.
- There is no evidence to recommend routine use of GC in anaphylaxis and in spinal cord or traumatic brain injury.

DISCLOSURE

The authors have nothing to disclose.

REFERENCES

[1] Reusch CE. Glucocorticoid therapy. In: Feldman EC, Nelson RW, Reusch CE, editors. et al., Canine and feline endocrinology. 4th edition. St. Louis, MO: W.B. Saunders; 2015. p. 555–70.
[2] Aharon MA, Prittie JE, Buriko K. A review of associated controversies surrounding glucocorticoid use in emergency and critical care. J Vet Emerg Crit Care 2017;27(3):267–77.
[3] Stahn C, Buttgereit F. Genomic and nongenomic effects of glucocorticoids. Nat Clin Pract Rheumatol 2008;4(10):525–33.
[4] Gupta P, Bhatia V. Corticosteroid physiology and principles of therapy. Indian J Pediatr 2008;75(10):1039–44.
[5] Nam A, Kim SM, Jeong JW, et al. Comparison of body surface area-based and weight-based dosing format for oral prednisolone administration in small and large-breed dogs. Pol J Vet Sci 2017;20(3):611–3.
[6] Prednisone/prednisolone monograph. In: Plumb, D, ed. Plumb's Veterinary Drug Handbook,. Available at: https://academic-plumbs-com.proxy.library.upenn.edu/drug-monograph/sShl11M9aPPROD Assessed 8 March, 2023

[7] Meyer NJ, Gattinoni L, Calfee CS. Acute respiratory distress syndrome. Lancet 2021;398(10300):622–37.

[8] Wilkins PA, Otto CM, Baumgardner JE, et al. Acute lung injury and acute respiratory distress syndromes in veterinary medicine: consensus definitions: The Dorothy Russell Havemeyer Working Group on ALI and ARDS in Veterinary Medicine. J Vet Emerg Crit Care 2007;17(4):333–9.

[9] Meduri G, Siemieniuk R, Ness R, et al. Prolonged low-dose methylprednisolone treatment is highly effective in reducing duration of mechanical ventilation and mortality in patients with ARDS. J Intensive Care Med 2018;6:53.

[10] Djillai A. Glucocorticoids for ARDS: Just Do It. Chest 2007;131(4):945–6.

[11] Annane D, Pastores SM, Rochwerg B, et al. Guidelines for the diagnosis and management of critical illness-related corticosteroid insufficiency (CIRCI) in critically ill patients (Part I): Society of Critical Care Medicine (SCCM) and European Society of Intensive Care Medicine (ESICM) 2017. Intensive Care Med 2017;43(12):1751–63.

[12] Chan ED, Chan MM, Chan MM, et al. Use of glucocorticoids in the critical care setting: Science and clinical evidence. Pharmacol Ther 2020;206:107428.

[13] Tasaka S, Ohshimo S, Takeuchi M, et al. ARDS Clinical Practice Guideline 2021. J Intensive Care 2022;10(1):32.

[14] Walker T, Tidwell AS, Rozanski EA, et al. Imaging diagnosis: acute lung injury following massive bee envenomation in a dog. Vet Radiol Ultrasound 2005;46(4):300–3.

[15] Hunter TL. Acute respiratory distress syndrome in a 10-year-old dog. Can Vet J Rev Veterinaire Can 2001;42(9):727–9.

[16] Marchetti M, Pierini A, Favilla G, et al. Critical illness-related corticosteroid insufficiency in dogs with systemic inflammatory response syndrome: A pilot study in 21 dogs. Vet J 2021;273:105677.

[17] Burkitt-Creedon J. Controversies surrounding critical illness-related corticosteroid insufficiency in animals. J Vet Emerg Crit Care 2015;25(1):107–12.

[18] Marik PE. Critical illness-related corticosteroid insufficiency. Chest 2009;135(1):181–93.

[19] Martin L, Groman RP. Relative adrenal insufficiency in critical illness. J Vet Emerg Crit Care 2004;14(3):149–57.

[20] Pisano SRR, Howard J, Posthaus H, et al. Hydrocortisone therapy in a cat with vasopressor-refractory septic shock and suspected critical illness-related corticosteroid insufficiency. Clin Case Rep 2017;5(7):1123–9.

[21] Peyton JL, Burkitt JM. Critical illness-related corticosteroid insufficiency in a dog with septic shock. J Vet Emerg Crit Care 2009;19(3):262–8.

[22] Summers AM, Culler C, Yaxley PE, et al. Retrospective evaluation of the use of hydrocortisone for treatment of suspected critical illness-related corticosteroid insufficiency (CIRCI) in dogs with septic shock (2010-2017): 47 cases. J Vet Emerg Crit Care 2021;31(3):371–9.

[23] Sande A, West C. Traumatic brain injury: a review of pathophysiology and management. J Vet Emerg Crit Care 2010;20(2):177–90.

[24] Foley C, Bracker K, Drellich S. Hypothalamic-pituitary axis deficiency following traumatic brain injury in a dog. J Vet Emerg Crit Care 2009;19(3):269–74.

[25] Zhang B, Bai M, Xu X, et al. Corticosteroid receptor rebalancing alleviates critical illness-related corticosteroid insufficiency after traumatic brain injury by promoting paraventricular nuclear cell survival via Akt/CREB/BDNF signaling. J Neuroinflammation 2020;17(1):318.

[26] Hurlbert RJ, Hadley MN, Walters BC, et al. Pharmacological Therapy for Acute Spinal Cord Injury. Neurosurgery 2013;72(Suppl 2):93–105.

[27] Levine JM, Levine GJ, Johnson SI, et al. Evaluation of the success of medical management for presumptive cervical intervertebral disk herniation in dogs. Vet Surg VS 2007;36(5):492–9.

[28] Okanishi H, Nagata T, Nakane S, et al. Comparison of initial treatment with and without corticosteroids for suspected acute pancreatitis in dogs. J Small Anim Pract 2019;60(5):298–304.

[29] Halangk W, Lerch MM. Early events in acute pancreatitis. Clin Lab Med 2005;25(1):1–15.

[30] Mansfield C. Acute pancreatitis in dogs: advances in understanding, diagnostics, and treatment. Top Companion Anim Med 2012;27(3):123–32.

[31] Bjørnkjær-Nielsen KA, Bjørnvad CR. Corticosteroid treatment for acute/acute-on-chronic experimental and naturally occurring pancreatitis in several species: a scoping review to inform possible use in dogs. Acta Vet Scand 2021;63(1):28.

[32] Mansfield C, Beths T. Management of acute pancreatitis in dogs: a critical appraisal with focus on feeding and analgesia. J Small Anim Pract 2015;56(1):27–39.

[33] Stern A, Skalsky K, Avni T, et al. Corticosteroids for pneumonia. Cochrane Database Syst Rev 2017;2017(12):CD007720.

[34] Tomazini BM, Maia IS, Cavalcanti AB, et al. Effect of dexamethasone on days alive and ventilator-free in patients with moderate or severe acute respiratory distress syndrome and COVID-19: the CoDEX randomized clinical trial. JAMA 2020;324(13):1307–16.

[35] Morgan A, Glossop A. Severe community-acquired pneumonia. Br J Addiction 2016;16(5):167–72.

[36] Torres A, Sibila O, Ferrer M, et al. Effect of corticosteroids on treatment failure among hospitalized patients with severe community-acquired pneumonia and high inflammatory response: a randomized clinical trial. JAMA 2015;313(7):677–86.

[37] Meduri GU, Shih MC, Bridges L, et al. Low-dose methylprednisolone treatment in critically ill patients with severe community-acquired pneumonia. Intensive Care Med 2022;48(8):1009–23.

[38] Metlay JP, Waterer GW, Long AC, et al. Diagnosis and treatment of adults with community-acquired pneumonia. an official clinical practice guideline of the

American thoracic society and infectious diseases society of America. Am J Respir Crit Care Med 2019;200(7): e45–67.

[39] C.E. Greene, Bacterial meningitis, in: J.E. Sykes (Ed.), Canine and feline infectious diseases. St. Louis, Mo, W.B. Saunders, 2014, pp. 886–892.

[40] Buhmann G, Wielaender F, Rosati M, et al. Canine meningoencephalitis and meningitis: retrospective analysis of a veterinary hospital population. Tierarztl Prax Ausg K Klientiere Heimtiere 2020;48(4):233–44.

[41] Song RB, Vitullo CA, da Costa RC, et al. Long-term survival in a dog with meningoencephalitis and epidural abscessation due to Actinomyces species. J Vet Diagn Invest 2015;27(4):552–7.

[42] Brouwer MC, McIntyre P, Prasad K, et al. Corticosteroids for acute bacterial meningitis. Cochrane Database Syst Rev 2015;2015(9):CD004405.

[43] Hasbun R. Progress and Challenges in Bacterial Meningitis: A Review. JAMA 2022;328(21):2147–54.

[44] Aksamit AJJ, Berkowitz AL. Meningitis. Continuum 2021; 27(4):836.

[45] Swanson D. Meningitis. Pediatr Rev 2015;36(12):514–26.

[46] van de Beek D, Brouwer MC, Koedel U, et al. Community-acquired bacterial meningitis. Lancet Lond Engl 2021;398(10306):1171–83.

[47] Kohil A, Jemmieh S, Smatti MK, et al. Viral meningitis: an overview. Arch Virol 2021;166(2):335–45.

[48] Spec A, Powderly WG. Cryptococcal meningitis in AIDS. Handb Clin Neurol 2018;152:139–50.

[49] Bystritsky RJ, Chow FC. Infectious meningitis and encephalitis. Neurol Clin 2022;40(1):77–91.

[50] Cardona V, Ansotegui IJ, Ebisawa M, et al. World allergy organization anaphylaxis guidance 2020. World Allergy Organ J 2020;13(10):100472.

[51] Shmuel DL, Cortes Y. Anaphylaxis in dogs and cats. J Vet Emerg Crit Care 2013;23(4):377–94.

[52] Gabrielli S, Clarke A, Morris J, et al. Evaluation of prehospital management in a canadian emergency department anaphylaxis cohort. J Allergy Clin Immunol Pract 2019; 7(7):2232–8.e3.

[53] Navalpakam A, Thanaputkaiporn N, Poowuttikul P. Management of anaphylaxis. Immunol Allergy Clin North Am 2022;42(1):65–76.

[54] Sheikh A. Glucocorticosteroids for the treatment and prevention of anaphylaxis. Curr Opin Allergy Clin Immunol 2013;13(3):263–7.

[55] Shaker MS, Wallace DV, Golden DBK, et al. Anaphylaxis-a 2020 practice parameter update, systematic review, and Grading of Recommendations, Assessment, Development and Evaluation (GRADE) analysis. J Allergy Clin Immunol 2020;145(4):1082–123.

[56] Liyanage CK, Galappatthy P, Seneviratne SL. Corticosteroids in management of anaphylaxis; a systematic review of evidence. Eur Ann Allergy Clin Immunol 2017;49(5): 196–207.

[57] Ortiz-Alvarez O. Acute management of croup in the emergency department. Paediatr Child Health 2017; 22(3):166–73.

[58] Aregbesola A, Tam CM, Kothari A, et al. Glucocorticoids for croup in children. Cochrane Database Syst Rev 2023; 1(1):CD001955.

[59] Lewis K, Culgin S, Jaeschke R, et al. Cuff leak test and airway obstruction in mechanically ventilated intensive care unit patients: a pilot randomized controlled clinical trial. Ann Am Thorac Soc 2022;19(2):238–44.

[60] Kuriyama A, Umakoshi N, Sun R. Prophylactic corticosteroids for prevention of postextubation stridor and reintubation in adults: a systematic review and meta-analysis. Chest 2017;151(5):1002–10.

[61] Kimura S, Ahn JB, Takahashi M, et al. Effectiveness of corticosteroids for post-extubation stridor and extubation failure in pediatric patients: a systematic review and meta-analysis. Ann Intensive Care 2020;10(1):155.

Advances in Small Animal Care 4 (2023) 101–112

ADVANCES IN SMALL ANIMAL CARE

The Microbiome in Critical Illness

Melanie Werner, Dr med vet, Dipl. ECVIM-CA (Internal Medicine)*,
Alessio Vigani, Dr med vet, PhD, Dipl.ACVECC & ECVECC, ACVAA
Clinic for Small Animal Internal Medicine, Vetsuisse Faculty, Winterthurerstrasse 260, Zurich 8057, Switzerland

KEYWORDS
• Microbiota • Critical care • Dysbiosis • Antimicrobials • Parvovirus • Fecal microbiota transplantation

KEY POINTS
- Evidence suggests that the intestinal microbiome may play an important role in the pathogenesis and progression of acute critical illness in humans and other mammals, although evidence in small animal medicine is scarce. Moreover, the intestinal microbiota plays many important metabolic roles (production of short-chain fatty acids, trimethylamine-N-oxide, and normal bile acid metabolism) and is crucial for immunity as well as defense against enteropathogens.
- Multiple changes can occur as a result of critical illness (ie, hypoperfusion, shock, inflammation, impaired immunity, dietary changes, medication, and decreased intestinal motility), which can make the cat or dog prone to the development of dysbiosis.
- The use of probiotics and fecal microbiota transplantation as instruments to modulate the intestinal microbiota seems to be safe and effective in studies on critically ill dogs with acute gastrointestinal diseases.

INTRODUCTION–WHY THE INTESTINAL MICROBIOTA IS IMPORTANT IN CRITICAL ILLNESS

Throughout the intestinal tract, there is an abundance of microorganisms that are constantly communicating with each other and symbiotically interacting with their hosts on an ongoing basis. As well as playing a major role in health, the microorganisms are also a significant contributor to the development of many diseases, such as inflammatory, cardiovascular, and metabolic disorders in cases when dysbiosis occurs (ie, when the composition of the intestinal microbiota is altered) [1–4]. The term "acute critical illness" (ACI) refers to conditions that demand immediate medical attention in order to preserve vital organ functions. There are several diseases that cause ACI in companion animals, including sepsis, trauma, respiratory failure, cardiovascular failure, and acute pancreatitis. Although knowledge about special microbial changes in critically ill dogs and cats is lacking, evidence suggests that the

intestinal microbiome may play an important role in the pathogenesis and progression of organ damage and dysfunction. Critically ill dogs and cats undergo a state of major stress that is mediated by endocrine, immunological, neuronal, and inflammatory mechanisms [5]. There are several factors that can adversely affect the intestinal microbiota, including medication, critical illnesses, and fasting [6].

More recently, the intestinal microbiota has been identified as a dynamic system, and its dysfunction, exemplified by dysbiosis, is increasingly being considered as a form of organ failure [6–9]. The mechanism of dysbiosis and its involvement in the outcome of critical illness is therefore imperative to implement better therapeutic strategies. The most recent studies on the intestinal microbiota were conducted on either animal models or from human studies. Both have substantially different intestinal physiology and microbiota composition compared with those of companion animals, so direct extrapolation of data to dogs and cats is

*Corresponding author, *E-mail address:* melanie.werner@uzh.ch

challenging [10–13]. The data, however, allow us to improve our understanding of the intestinal microbiota and the changes it undergoes in a dynamic manner. With a better understanding of the role of the microbiome in critically ill animals, therapeutic strategies such as the use of probiotics and fecal microbiota transplantation can be used more effectively in critically ill dogs and cats. The aim of this review is to present the current state of knowledge from human and veterinary medicine with regard to the role of the intestinal microbiota in critical illness and the possible effect of specific therapeutic options on it.

COMPOSITION OF THE NORMAL INTESTINAL MICROBIOTA AND ITS CHANGE IN CRITICALLY ILL INDIVIDUALS

Physiologic Composition of the Intestinal Microbiota

The intestinal microbiota is known as a complex system of microorganisms (in the form of bacteria, archaea, fungi, viruses) and their genomes. There are many parts to this ecosystem, but each of them contributes to the stability of the whole and the interaction with the host on a regular basis. Most of the research that is available focuses on bacterial microorganisms. There is no longer any need to use the term intestinal flora, and it should be replaced with the term intestinal microbiota. In addition to suppressing specific pathogens, this resident microbiota also plays a significant role in sensitizing the immune system as well as having proinflammatory and antiinflammatory effects on the intestinal tract and forming important metabolites, commonly referred to as the metabolome, which are essential for the health of the organism. There is no single microbiome that is the same for every individual. However, these individual differences are minimal compared with those caused by animal species, gastrointestinal diseases, or drug administration [4,14–16]. The microbiota is mostly affected by dietary change, caused in turn by major changes in substrates and macronutrient distributions (eg, switching from a commercial diet to a raw meat diet) [17]. There is an increase in the number of bacteria in the intestinal tract as one travels distally, with the large intestine containing more bacteria than the small intestine. It has been estimated that the total number of bacteria in the large intestine is approximately 10^{12} to 10^{14} CFU/gram of content [4]. Most of the bacteria found in the colon are anaerobes. Because fecal microbiomes are more readily accessible than intraluminal microbiomes,

most research today is focused on the fecal microbiome. The 4 dominant phyla of bacteria in the digestive tract of dogs and cats are Firmicutes, Fusobacteria, Bacteroidetes, and Proteobacteria. Among these, Firmicutes is the most important family. All dogs share a common list of core bacterial groups that include Clostridia as a dominant class, Bacilli (Lactobacillales, which includes *Streptococcus* species and *Lactobacillus* species), and Erysipelotrichia (*Turicibacter* species, *Catenibacter* species, and *Coprobacillus* species) [4,15,16]. Clostridia have 3 different familial clusters: IV (eg, Ruminococcaceae, *Faecalibacterium prausnitzii*), XI (eg, Peptostreptococcaceae), and XIVa (eg, Lachnospiraceae, *Blautia* spp). Despite the minor differences between individuals, the basic microbiota of each dog or cat is generally considered stable after having reached its adulthood [4,15,18].

Metabolic Functions of the Intestinal Microbiota

The intestinal microbiota plays many important roles in the body. As part of the degradation process, anaerobic bacteria ferment food polysaccharides into various metabolites such as short-chain fatty acids (SCFAs) such as butyrate, acetate, and propionate, all of which are vital substrates for enterocyte function [19]. Also, the intestine plays a role in the defense against infectious diseases of the gastrointestinal tract by acting as a competitive agent between commensal and pathogenic bacteria, as well as in the development of a local immune system. In addition, the intestinal microbiota contributes to the normal functioning of organs and is closely related to them [20,21]. This latter point led to the development of the concept of the gut-organ axis.

It is thought that *Clostridium hiranonis* is one of the bacterial species that is included in the Dysbiosis Index and represents an important aspect of the bile acid metabolism as a key metabolic pathway in dogs. The presence of an appropriate number of *C hiranonis* seems to have major beneficial effects on the dog's or cat's health. Primary bile acids, which have been secreted into the intestinal lumen, must be converted into secondary bile acids using the 7-alpha-hydroxylase enzyme provided by the microbiota [22]. A strong correlation between the abundance of *C hiranonis* and the concentration of secondary bile acids in the feces has been demonstrated [23]. It is essential to maintain the proper levels of secondary bile acids in the intestinal tract so that an antiinflammatory environment is maintained, which inhibits the growth of potentially pathogenic bacteria (eg, *Clostridioides difficile*) [24]. When primary bile acids are not converted to secondary bile acids in the feces, the primary bile acids accumulate in the feces and can cause an osmotic type of diarrhea known as "bile acid diarrhea" [25].

Assessment of the Intestinal Microbiota

Different methods can be used to examine the intestinal microbiota, of which the 3 most commonly used are described later. Molecular profiling of 16S ribosomal RNA can provide a taxonomic overview of the bacteria present in a sample and can provide information on microbial richness and diversity of the sample, among other factors [6]. There are many benefits to this method, such as its simplicity and speed. A limitation of this method is that it does not provide information on gene functions, and it is possible that 2 organisms with the same sequence of the 16S rRNA gene might be misclassified as one organism [26–28]. In addition, the results are only relevant in the context of the samples measured in the same run, because reproducibility is not available. It is possible to obtain a more precise picture of the microbial composition of a sample by unbiased sequencing of all DNA present in the sample (shotgun metagenomics) [26]. In spite of the fact that this higher resolution approach is more expensive, it gives information on richness, diversity, and gene functions up to species level and can be used to identify bacteria on a species level [26,27,29]. There are several ways in which these approaches can be further advanced by incorporating them with the profiling of proteins (metaproteomics) and small molecules (metabolomics). Lastly, these methods produce results that are complex to interpret. Correct interpretation must be related to a particular research question [30]. 16s-rRNA sequencing, as well as shotgun metagenomics are not available in clinical practice and are reserved for scientific investigations. A newer approach to dysbiosis detection available in clinical practice is the polymerase chain reaction (PCR)-based Dysbiosis Index (DI). In dogs, the DI is a numeric quantity based on the abundance of bacteria from 7 different groups, that is, *Turicibacter, Streptococcus, Escherichia coli, Blautia, Fusobacterium, C hiranonis*, as well as the total number of bacteria found within the sample. In cats it is based on the total bacteria and the abundance of Bacteroides, *Bifidobacterium, C hiranonis, E coli, Faecalibacterium, Streptococcus*, and *Turicibacter*. As a result of the administration of antibiotics (metronidazole, tylosin) and other drugs such as proton pump inhibitors, about half of the animals suffering from inflammatory bowel disease were found to have altered DI, indicating dysbiosis [17,31–34]. As routine fecal cultures do not represent the anaerobic microbiota in dogs and cats,

they are not suitable for evaluating fecal bacterial composition. Possible enteropathogens (eg, *C difficile* and Salmonella spp) can be found as part of the normal microbiota in dogs [35]. It may be possible for a positive culture to be interpreted as a sign that the physiologic microbiome has been altered, and the dysbiosis has enabled these pathogens to proliferate (eg, the suppression of the protective microbiota by antimicrobial administration) [35,36].

COMPOSITION OF THE INTESTINAL MICROBIOTA IN CRITICAL ILLNESS

Critical illnesses, regardless of their underlying cause, are characterized by pathophysiologic features that can affect all major organ systems, including the gastrointestinal tract. It is common for dogs and cats with acute critical illness to experience ischemia, tissue injury, and systemic inflammation, with possible adverse effects on the intestinal microbiota composition as well as function.

In one study in critically ill humans, commensal intestinal bacteria such as Firmicutes (with Ruminococcaceae and Veillonellaceae) or Bacteroidetes (with Bacteroidaceae and Prevotellaceae) were of decreased abundance, and potentially pathogenic bacteria (pathobionts) such as Proteobacteria (especially Enterobacteriaceae) became more prevalent [37]. According to qPCR analysis of fecal samples (the Dysbiosis Index) in dogs with intestinal dysbiosis, *Blautia* spp, *Faecalibacterium* spp, and *Turicibacter* spp abundances were significantly decreased [38,39]. A further decrease was observed in *Fusobacterium* spp and *C hiranonis*, and an increase was observed in *Streptococcus* spp and *E coli* [38].

There is both a decrease in diversity as well as a change in the ratio of pathogenic bacteria to "health-promoting" commensal bacteria that contributes to dysbiosis (Fig. 1). The presence of an overgrowth (>50% relative abundance) of pathogenic genera, such as *E coli*, *C difficile*, and *Staphylococcus* spp, may be evident in some instances [37]. Intestinal microbiota and homeostasis may change within the first 48 hours following a critical illness [40,41]. A study comparing the microbiota on intensive care unit (ICU) admission and discharge of 115 critically ill human patients revealed that Firmicutes and Bacteroidetes had decreased, whereas Proteobacteria and taxa with pathogenic bacteria had increased [40]. It was also found that during the course of a mechanically ventilated ICU stay by people, the proportion of Bacteroidetes and Firmicutes varied. In this study, the Bacteroidetes/Firmicutes

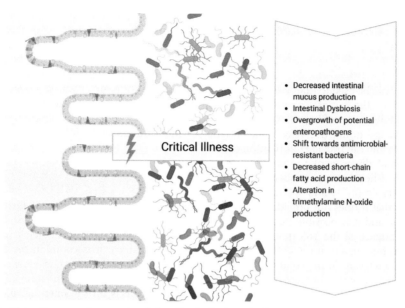

- Decreased intestinal mucus production
- Intestinal Dysbiosis
- Overgrowth of potential enteropathogens
- Shift towards antimicrobial-resistant bacteria
- Decreased short-chain fatty acid production
- Alteration in trimethylamine N-oxide production

Critical Illness

FIG. 1 Identifying the causative agents of alteration in the intestinal microbiota of critically ill individuals. Created with BioRender.com.

ratio was also a predictor of mortality [8]. It has been also demonstrated that an intestinal dysbiosis may contribute to the risk of nosocomial infections, sepsis, and distant organ failure [13,42–45].

DETERMINANTS AND EFFECTS OF INTESTINAL DYSBIOSIS IN CRITICALLY ILL INDIVIDUALS

Change in Intestinal Mucous Production
Goblet cells of the intestinal mucosa continuously produce hydrophobic mucus to cover the intestinal wall. The mucus serves as a barrier against the translocation of bacteria and toxins into the vascular system and protects enterocytes and colonocytes from digestive enzymes [37,42]. Mucous production and mucous hydrophobicity decrease in critically ill patients with splanchnic hypoperfusion or fasting, resulting in enterocyte injury that leads to cell apoptosis and pathogen spread [37,46]. As a result, nutrients are not absorbed, and SCFAs are not produced, which leads to diarrhea [37].

The Role of Short-Chain Fatty Acids
Currently, most of the knowledge about SCFAs comes from in vitro bench studies on human or mouse feces, as well as from interventional studies using prebiotics and from dogs with chronic enteropathies [38,47–49]. During the fermentation of dietary fibers in the

intestinal tract, the anaerobic microbiota produces metabolites such as SCFAs, which are essential for maintaining the integrity of the intestinal barrier and promoting the immune response of the host [50]. The colonic epithelium relies on SCFAs for energy and maintaining functional intercellular junctions. In mice, SCFAs also play a role in gastrointestinal immunity by regulating T-helper cells, regulatory T cells (Treg), antibodies, and cytokines that have mainly anti-inflammatory properties. As well as enhancing cell viability under stress conditions, SCFAs also induced cytoprotective proteins [42,51]. As a result of dysbiosis, critically ill patients exhibit a decrease in anaerobic bacteria, which has been linked to cellular apoptosis, malabsorption, diarrhea, and bacterial translocation [52–54].

Alteration in Trimethylamine N-Oxide Production
As another important metabolite, trimethylamine N-oxide (TMAO) is produced both by the intestinal microbiota as well as the liver [55]. Triethylamine (TMA) is produced by the intestinal microbiota from choline, lecithin, and carnitine [56]. TMA is then absorbed and translocated to the liver through portal circulation [55], where it is converted directly into TMAO [56]. Composition and diversity of the intestinal microbiota play a major role in the production of TMAO, and in

dysbiosis, TMAO levels were elevated [56,57]. Trimethylamine N-oxide was suppressed by broad-spectrum antibiotics in humans [58], but reappeared after discontinuation of the antibiotics, supporting the hypothesis that the intestinal microbiota is crucial for TMAO production. There has been evidence linking high levels of TMAO to heart failure, atherosclerosis, and thrombosis in humans [56,59,60].

Adaptation of the Intestinal Immunity
During the development of the immune system, the intestinal microbiota plays an important role [61]. The microbiota promotes and adapts the immune system to certain conditions; however, the immune system also needs to tolerate the presence of the gut microbiota while also being able to respond to potential threats. One of the ways the immune system achieves this balance is by developing tolerance to nonharmful commensal bacteria while retaining the ability to mount an effective response to pathogens. In order to accomplish this, the Toll-like receptor as well as other immunocompetence systems are involved and recognize microbe-associated molecular patterns through the release of proinflammatory cytokines [62], secretion of mucus, and the production of SCFAs that activate Treg cells [19,63]. A "mucosal firewall" that consists of the epithelial wall, immunoglobulin A (IgA) secretion, antimicrobial peptides, and immune cell function limits the contact between the microbiota and epithelial cells to reduce the translocation of bacteria [64]. Dysregulation of the microbiota can lead to a decrease in IgA and T cell levels, favoring the growth of bacteria, leading to dysbiosis and increased risk of infection [6,65].

KEY ASPECTS OF INTESTINAL DYSBIOSIS IN THE CRITICAL CARE SETTING
An overview on the potential beneficial and harmful modulators of the intestinal microbiota is shown in Fig. 2. The gastrointestinal environment undergoes multiple changes during critical illness due to the combination of hypoperfusion, hypoxia, inflammation, impaired immunity, dietary changes, medications, and impaired intestinal motility [30,43,66]. Although currently little knowledge about the influence of the effect of each of these factors is present in veterinary medicine, it is clear that they often coexist in the course of ACI.

Factors Triggering Dysbiosis in the Critical Care Setting
Gastrointestinal dysmotility and prolonged intestinal transit time during critical illness can be associated with a reduction in bacterial density, which in humans is known to lead to dysbiosis [7,67]. Electrolyte fluctuations, fasting, and use of sedatives and opiates in the ICU may contribute to gastrointestinal dysmotility [68]. Medications such as antimicrobials or proton pump inhibitors commonly prescribed in critical care setting affect the composition of the intestinal microbiota [17,69-72]. In particular, proton pump inhibitors lead to an increase in gastric pH, which leads to a decreased selection pressure on bacteria and massive changes in intestinal biodiversity [71]. Dysbiosis caused by proton pump inhibitors, especially in conjunction with nonsteroidal antiinflammatory drugs, was also suspected of disrupting intestinal barrier function and triggering intestinal inflammation [34,73].

Antibiotics have multiple effects on the intestinal microbiota, depending on their class and mechanism of action. Generally, antibiotics alter commensal microbiota and its biodiversity and are capable of selecting and/or promoting the growth of organisms that are or become resistant [74]. Based on previous study findings, there is an interspecies variability of the effect of antimicrobials on the intestinal microbiota. Cats seemed to be much more sensitive to the effects of antibiotics on their intestinal microbiome than dogs [72,74]. Examples of antibiotics that had been demonstrated to affect the intestinal microbiota are tylosin, metronidazole, amoxicillin-clavulanic acid, and enrofloxacin [17,33,69,70,75].

Lastly, altered feeding patterns or fasting are other important factors that can trigger dysbiosis. In general, it is known that highly altered diets with significant compositional changes significantly affect the composition of the intestinal microbiome. There is evidence that nutritional therapy has a significant impact on the intestinal microbiota. Enteral nutrition is considered to be protective for the intestinal microbiota, whereas periods of starvation or total parenteral nutrition should be avoided, as they may adversely affect the intestinal microbiota [76].

The effects of enteral versus parenteral nutrition in critical illness on the human intestinal microbiota suggest that exclusive parenteral nutrition contributes to significant dysbiosis [77,78], whereas assisted enteral nutrition is advantageous and promotes the growth of beneficial microbiota.

The Development of Pathogenic Bacteria
The density and diversity of specific bacteria in the environment are assumed to be sensed by other bacteria [42]. It has been demonstrated that intestinal bacteria are either able to colonize or become pathogenic based

The microbiome in critical illness

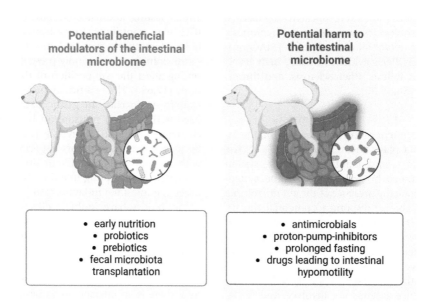

Potential beneficial modulators of the intestinal microbiome

Potential harm to the intestinal microbiome

- early nutrition
- probiotics
- prebiotics
- fecal microbiota transplantation

- antimicrobials
- proton-pump-inhibitors
- prolonged fasting
- drugs leading to intestinal hypomotility

FIG. 2 Potential harmful and beneficial modulators of the intestinal microbiota in dogs and cats. Created with BioRender.com.

on the intestinal environment. Virulence factors are expressed by many bacteria through a process called quorum sensing [42]. As a result of this system, virulence genes are expressed only when a certain bacterial density is reached that may overwhelm the host and when a negative environmental shift, such as lack of nutrients, loss of other bacteria groups, or treatment with opiates, occurs. Studies have shown that, in human patients with long stays in the ICU, "normal" microbiota were replaced by low-diversity communities of resistant pathogens whose virulence is determined by the local environment, for example, opiate exposure [79]. A study has shown that when intestinal ischemia and reperfusion leads to acute stress, the production of dynorphin, a natural human opioid, was increased. In this study, *Pseudomonas aeruginosa* was exposed to dynorphin, resulting in activation of the quorum sensing system, which allowed bacteria to recognize stress in the host, became pathogenic, and exploited host weaknesses [80]. Another example is the overgrowth of *C difficile* in the absence of a benign intestinal microbiota and bile acid–metabolizing *C hiranonis* [81]. This relationship has also been demonstrated in dogs [23]. In addition, electrolyte levels seemed to affect the composition of the intestinal microbiota in mice.

There is evidence that local phosphate levels influence the virulence of intestinal microbiota [82,83]. Hypophosphatemia caused *Pseudomonas aeruginosa* and other pathogens to develop a lethal phenotype in mice [82,84].

Intestinal Microbiota and Sepsis/Systemic Inflammatory Response Syndrome

There are many dogs and cats in the ICU that suffer from severe infections. Even though the specific mechanisms underlying sepsis/systemic inflammatory response syndrome have not yet been fully identified, the intestinal microbiota seemed to be involved in its pathophysiology [85,86]. Several factors contribute to this, including how critically ill individuals are often prescribed a wide variety of medications, which affect the microbiota diversity within the intestinal tract [86]. Critically ill individuals are also in a precarious condition, which may result in lesions due to hypoxia, inflammation, disruption of epithelial barrier, dysmotility, changes in intraluminal pH, and impaired immune function. In different studies sepsis was associated with specific patterns of intestinal microbiota. A multicenter study found that ICU patients with sepsis had an increased number of bacteria, such as Parabacteroides, Fusobacterium, and Bilophila, associated with inflammation. According to other studies, the intestinal tract has lost several important bacterial genera, including *Faecalibacterium* spp, *Prevotella* spp, *Blautia* spp. and *Ruminococcaceae* spp, which are known to produce SCFAs [8,19,79,87]. In addition, certain antibiotic-resistant species, including Enterococcus species, have been linked to sepsis [5]. In addition to bacterial translocation and the prevention of the colonization of multiresistant pathogens by the intestinal microbiota, the intestinal microbiota may also influence sepsis by regulating immune function [88–90]. As compared with healthy mice, germ-free mice exhibited greater bacterial spread, more severe levels of inflammation and organ dysfunction, as well as higher mortality during sepsis [90].

MODULATION OF THE INTESTINAL MICROBIOTA

The most evaluated specific treatments for modulating intestinal microbiota include prebiotics, probiotics, synbiotics, and fecal microbiota transplantation (FMT).

A prebiotic is an undigested food substrate, such as fiber, inulin, or oligosaccharides, that provides health benefits on ingestion by the commensal intestinal microbiota [91]. Several studies have shown that prebiotics can improve dysbiosis, increase SCFA production, and reduce hospitalization time in human ICU patients [92,93], although other studies have obtained contradictory results [94,95]. Studies on the impact of prebiotics on the intestinal microbiota in critically ill dogs and cats are lacking. One study on the usage of psyllium in acute colitis showed promising results on restoration of the intestinal microbiota due to this treatment strategy [96].

A probiotic is a living microorganism composition that maintains the balance of the intestinal microbiota in order to improve the health of the host. The term "symbiotic" refers to the simultaneous administration of prebiotics and probiotics [91]. Probiotics have been shown to reduce the incidence of ventilator-associated pneumonia (VAP) in humans [97]. There have, however, been conflicting results regarding the benefit of probiotics in critical ill individuals from subsequent randomized controlled trials [98,99]. As a result of the variable dosages and probiotics used in these studies, the findings of these studies cannot be generalized.

Studies on the usage of probiotics in feline and canine critically ill individuals are rare. One study in dogs with acute hemorrhagic diarrhea syndrome

(AHDS) described the beneficial impact of a *Lactobacilli* and *Bifidobacteria* combination on restoration of the intestinal microbiota and recurrence of *Blautia* spp [100]. Dogs with parvovirus receiving a probiotic combination of various *Lactobacilli* and *Bifidobacteria* showed more rapid clinical improvement and higher lymphocyte counts at day 5 of treatment compared with the placebo group [101]. However, the microbiome was not examined in the latter. Although cases of adverse reactions to probiotics have been seen in human medicine, especially in critically ill individuals, they are not currently known to occur in veterinary medicine and are considered safe for use even under intensive care conditions.

Recent studies have shown an increasing focus on FMT, which involves transplanting an autologous or donor stool through rectal enema and/or oral capsules in order to restore a healthy microbiota. As an example, FMT is the alternative treatment of severe or recurrent *C difficile* colitis in humans [102]. The use of FMT in septic patients with multiple organ failure and suspected dysbiosis has been reported in case reports in the ICU of humans [103,104]. In veterinary medicine one promising study in puppies with parvovirus showed better clinical scores and shorter hospitalization time in dogs that were treated with rectal fecal transplants in addition to standard treatment [105]. Moreover, rectal fecal microbiota transplantation led to a more rapid restoration of healthy microbiota in dogs with AHDS [106]. Based on physiopathologic hypotheses, FMT may increase SCFA-producing bacteria, which could assist in restoring the systemic immune response and allowing the clearance of the sepsis pathogen [107]. Instructions on how to perform an FMT in dogs and cats can be found in Fig. 3. Knowledge concerning intestinal microbiota continues to grow at an impressive rate, and we may soon be able to define the value and use of specific treatments that modulate intestinal microbiota.

SUMMARY AND FUTURE DIRECTIONS

As well as playing a major role in health, the intestinal microbiota plays a significant role in the development of inflammatory, cardiovascular, and metabolic disorders. Evidence suggests that the intestinal microbiome may play an important role in pathogenesis and progression of acute critical illness in humans and other mammals, although evidence in small animal medicine remains sparse. Moreover, the intestinal microbiota plays many important metabolic roles. Food polysaccharides are broken down by anaerobic bacteria into

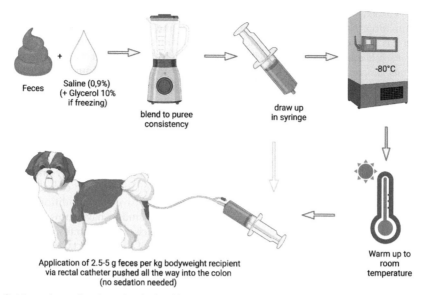

FIG. 3 Guidance for performing a fecal microbiota transplantation in dogs and cats. Created with BioRender. com.

SCFAs or in trimethylamine-N-oxide. These metabolites are vital substrates for cell function. Another microbe-driven metabolic pathway is the intestinal bile acid pathway, which can be altered in dysbiosis, leading to proinflammatory stages and overgrowth of pathogens. In addition, the intestinal microbiota plays a crucial role in the development of a local immune system as well as in the defense against enteropathogens. Following a critical illness, intestinal microbiota may change. It has been reported that the environment undergoes multiple changes in critically ill individuals, such as hypoperfusion, shock, inflammation, impaired immunity, dietary changes, medication, and decreased intestinal motility. These conditions can cause intestinal dysbiosis. Veterinary medicine currently knows little about the influence of these various factors other than the influence of drugs. In humans, prolonged transit time in ill individuals causes bacterial excretion to decrease, which results in dysbiosis. Proton pump inhibitors can lead to dysbiosis but are also suspected to disrupt intestinal barrier function and trigger intestinal inflammatory response when used together with nonsteroidal antiinflammatory drugs. Different antibiotics have different effects on microbiota depending on their class and species. Studies have found that sepsis is not only associated with specific microbiota patterns but is also linked to antibiotic-resistant bacterial species.

Prebiotics, probiotics, synbiotics, and FMT are the most evaluated specific treatments for modulating intestinal microbiota. The use of prebiotics has been shown to improve dysbiosis, increase SCFA production, and reduce hospitalization time in human ICU patients. The use of psyllium in canine acute colitis restored the intestinal microbiota with promising results but the impact of prebiotics in critically ill dogs and cats is unknown. There have been few studies of probiotics in feline and canine critical illness. It has been shown that a *Lactobacilli* spp and *Bifidobacteria* spp combination improves intestinal microbiota restoration and *Blautia* spp restoration in dogs with AHDS. Puppies with parvovirus receiving a probiotic combination improved more rapidly. In humans with multiple organ failure and suspected dysbiosis, FMT has been reported in case reports. In veterinary medicine one promising study in puppies with parvovirus showed better clinical scores and shorter hospitalization time in dogs that were treated with rectal fecal transplants in addition to standard treatment. Moreover, rectal fecal microbiota transplantation restored healthy microbiota more rapidly in dogs with acute hemorrhagic diarrhea. Future studies should primarily describe the microbiome in critically ill dogs and cats. In a second step, more information can be obtained on the use of prebiotics and fecal transplants in cats and dogs in the critical care setting.

CLINICS CARE POINTS

- Different drugs used in the critical care setting can alter the intestinal microbiota. Examples are antimicrobials and proton pump inhibitors. Usage should be guided by the clinical indication for these drug classes to avoid unnecessary overusage.
- In human medicine there is evidence that motility disorders can alter microbial diversity in richness. Drugs that can induce intestinal hypomotility (ie, opioids) should be used only when necessary and should be deescalated as soon as possible.
- Prolonged fasting should be avoided, and enteral feeding is superior in comparison to parenteral nutrition when it comes to the health of the intestinal microbiota.
- Prebiotics and probiotics are safe adjunctive in the therapy for critically ill dogs and cats that are able to receive enteral nutrition.
- Fecal microbiota transplantation seems to be a safe adjunctive in dogs with gastrointestinal disease and critical illness (parvovirus infection, AHDS).

DISCLOSURE

The authors have nothing to disclose.

REFERENCES

[1] Thursby E, Juge N. Introduction to the human gut microbiota. Biochem J 2017;474(11):1823–36.

[2] Wischmeyer P, McDonald D, Knight R. Role of the microbiome, probiotics, and 'dysbiosis therapy' in critical illness. Curr Opin Crit Care 2016;22(4):347–53.

[3] Manor O, Dai CL, Kornilov SA, et al. Health and disease markers correlate with gut microbiome composition across thousands of people. Nat Commun 2020; 11(1):5206.

[4] Suchodolski J. Diagnosis and interpretation of intestinal dysbiosis in dogs and cats. Vet J 2016;215:30–7.

[5] Agudelo-Ochoa GM, Valdés-Duque BE, Giraldo-Giraldo NA, et al. Gut microbiota profiles in critically ill patients, potential biomarkers and risk variables for sepsis. Gut Microb 2020;12(1):1707610.

[6] Szychowiak P, Villageois-Tran K, Patrier J, et al. The role of the microbiota in the management of intensive care patients. Ann Intensive Care 2022;12(1):3.

[7] Dickson R. The microbiome and critical illness. Lancet Respir Med 2016;4(1):59–72.

[8] Ojima M, Shimizu K, Motooka D, et al. Gut Dysbiosis Associated with Antibiotics and Disease Severity and Its Relation to Mortality in Critically Ill Patients. Dig Dis Sci 2021;67(6):2420–32.

[9] Lankelma JM, van Vught LV, Belzer C, et al. Critically ill patients demonstrate large interpersonal variation in intestinal microbiota dysregulation: a pilot study. Intensive Care Med 2016;43(1):59–68.

[10] Gonzalez LM, Moeser AJ, Blikslager AT. Porcine models of digestive disease: the future of large animal translational research. Transl Res 2015;166(1):12–27.

[11] Nejdfors P, Ekelund M, Jeppsson B, et al. Mucosal in vitro permeability in the intestinal tract of the pig, the rat, and man: species- and region-related differences. Scand J Gastroenterol 2000;35(5):501–7.

[12] Buchman AL, Mestecky J, Moukarzel A, et al. Intestinal immune function is unaffected by parenteral nutrition in man. J Am Coll Nutr 1995;14(6):656–61.

[13] Pilla R, Suchodolski J. The Role of the Canine Gut Microbiome and Metabolome in Health and Gastrointestinal Disease. Front Vet Sci 2020;6:498.

[14] Moreno PS, Wagner J, Mansfield CS, et al. Characterisation of the canine faecal virome in healthy dogs and dogs with acute diarrhoea using shotgun metagenomics. PLoS One 2017;12(6):e0178433.

[15] Suchodolski J, Camacho J, Steiner J. Analysis of bacterial diversity in the canine duodenum, jejunum, ileum, and colon by comparative 16S rRNA gene analysis. FEMS Microbiol Ecol 2008;66(3):567–78.

[16] Woo PCY, Lau SKP, Teng JLL, et al. Then and now: use of 16S rDNA gene sequencing for bacterial identification and discovery of novel bacteria in clinical microbiology laboratories. Clin Microbiol Infect Off Publ Eur Soc Clin Microbiol Infect Dis 2008;14(10):908–34.

[17] Pilla R, Gaschen FP, Barr JW, et al. Effects of metronidazole on the fecal microbiome and metabolome in healthy dogs. J Vet Intern Med 2020;34(5):1853–66.

[18] Garrigues Q, Apper E, Chastant S, et al. Gut microbiota development in the growing dog: A dynamic process influenced by maternal, environmental and host factors. Front Vet Sci 2022;9:964649.

[19] Rajilić-Stojanović M, de Vos WM. The first 1000 cultured species of the human gastrointestinal microbiota. FEMS Microbiol Rev 2014;38(5):996–1047.

[20] Sekirov I, Russell SL, Antunes LCM, et al. Gut microbiota in health and disease. Physiol Rev 2010;90(3):859–904.

[21] D'Argenio V, Salvatore F. The role of the gut microbiome in the healthy adult status. Clin Chim Acta Int J Clin Chem 2015;451(Pt A):97–102.

[22] Blake AB, Guard BC, Honneffer JB, et al. Altered microbiota, fecal lactate, and fecal bile acids in dogs with gastrointestinal disease. PLoS One 2019;14(10):e0224454.

[23] Blake AB, Cigarroa A, Klein HL, et al. Developmental stages in microbiota, bile acids, and clostridial species in healthy puppies. J Vet Intern Med 2020;34(6):2345–56.

[24] Allegretti JR, Kearney S, Li N, et al. Recurrent Clostridium difficile infection associates with distinct bile

acid and microbiome profiles. Aliment Pharmacol Ther 2016;43(11):1142–53.

[25] Duboc H, Rajca S, Rainteau D, et al. Connecting dysbiosis, bile-acid dysmetabolism and gut inflammation in inflammatory bowel diseases. Gut 2012;62:531–9.

[26] Durazzi F, Sala C, Castellani G, et al. Comparison between 16S rRNA and shotgun sequencing data for the taxonomic characterization of the gut microbiota. Sci Rep 2021;11(1):3030.

[27] Ashe EC, Comeau AM, Zejdlik K, et al. Characterization of Bacterial Community Dynamics of the Human Mouth Throughout Decomposition via Metagenomic, Metatranscriptomic, and Culturing Techniques. Front Microbiol 2021;12:689493.

[28] Hilton SK, Castro-Nallar E, Pérez-Losada M, et al. Metataxonomic and Metagenomic Approaches vs. Culture-Based Techniques for Clinical Pathology. Front Microbiol 2016;7:484.

[29] Quince C, Walker AW, Simpson JT, et al. Shotgun metagenomics, from sampling to analysis. Nat Biotechnol 2017;35(9):833–44.

[30] Wolff NS, Hugenholtz F, Wiersinga WJ. The emerging role of the microbiota in the ICU. Crit Care 2018;22:78.

[31] AlShawaqfeh MK, Wajid B, Minamoto Y, et al. A dysbiosis index to assess microbial changes in fecal samples of dogs with chronic inflammatory enteropathy. FEMS Microbiol Ecol 2017;93(11). https://doi.org/10.1093/femsec/fix136.

[32] Sung CH, Marsilio S, Chow B, et al. Dysbiosis index to evaluate the fecal microbiota in healthy cats and cats with chronic enteropathies. J Feline Med Surg 2022;24(6):e1–12.

[33] Manchester AC, Webb CB, Blake AB, et al. Long-term impact of tylosin on fecal microbiota and fecal bile acids of healthy dogs. J Vet Intern Med 2019;33(6):2605–17.

[34] Jones SM, Gaier A, Enomoto H, et al. The effect of combined carprofen and omeprazole administration on gastrointestinal permeability and inflammation in dogs. J Vet Intern Med 2020;34(5):1886–93.

[35] Werner M, Suchodolski JS, Lidbury JA, et al. Diagnostic value of fecal cultures in dogs with chronic diarrhea. J Vet Intern Med 2021;35(1):199–208.

[36] Wetterwik KJ, Trowald-Wigh G, Fernström LL, et al. Clostridium difficile in faeces from healthy dogs and dogs with diarrhea. Acta Vet Scand 2013;55(1):23.

[37] Moron R, Galvez J, Colmenero M, et al. The Importance of the Microbiome in Critically Ill Patients: Role of Nutrition. Nutrients 2019;11(12):3002.

[38] Minamoto Y, Minamoto T, Isaiah A, et al. Fecal short-chain fatty acid concentrations and dysbiosis in dogs with chronic enteropathy. J Vet Intern Med 2019;33(4):1608–18.

[39] Minamoto Y, Otoni C, Steelman S, et al. Alteration of the fecal microbiota and serum metabolite profiles in dogs with idiopathic inflammatory bowel disease. Gut Microb 2015;6:33–47.

[40] McDonald D, Ackermann G, Khailová L, et al. Extreme Dysbiosis of the Microbiome in Critical Illness. mSphere 2016;1(4):00199–e00216.

[41] Aardema H, Lisotto P, Kurilshikov A, et al. Marked Changes in Gut Microbiota in Cardio-Surgical Intensive Care Patients: A Longitudinal Cohort Study. Front Cell Infect Microbiol 2019;9:467.

[42] Alverdy JC, Chang EB. The re-emerging role of the intestinal microflora in critical illness and inflammation: why the gut hypothesis of sepsis syndrome will not go away. J Leukoc Biol 2008;83(3):461–6.

[43] Latorre M, Krishnareddy S, Freedberg DE. Microbiome as mediator: Do systemic infections start in the gut? World J Gastroenterol 2015;21(37):10487–92.

[44] Albrich WC, Ghosh TS, Ahearn-Ford S, et al. A high-risk gut microbiota configuration associates with fatal hyperinflammatory immune and metabolic responses to SARS-CoV-2. Gut Microb 2022;14(1):2073131.

[45] Yeoh YK, Zuo T, Lui GC, et al. Gut microbiota composition reflects disease severity and dysfunctional immune responses in patients with COVID-19. Gut 2021;70(4):698–706.

[46] Qin X, Caputo FJ, Xu DZ, et al. Hydrophobicity of mucosal surface and its relationship to gut barrier function. Shock 2008;29(3):372–6.

[47] El Kaoutari A, Armougom F, Gordon JI, et al. The abundance and variety of carbohydrate-active enzymes in the human gut microbiota. Nat Rev Microbiol 2013;11(7):497–504.

[48] Belenguer A, Holtrop G, Duncan SH, et al. Rates of production and utilization of lactate by microbial communities from the human colon. FEMS Microbiol Ecol 2011;77(1):107–19.

[49] Morrison DJ, Mackay WG, Edwards CA, et al. Butyrate production from oligofructose fermentation by the human faecal flora: what is the contribution of extracellular acetate and lactate? Br J Nutr 2006;96(3):570–7.

[50] Hamer HM, Jonkers D, Venema K, et al. Review article: the role of butyrate on colonic function. Aliment Pharmacol Ther 2008;27(2):104–19.

[51] Shimizu K, Ogura H, Goto M, et al. Altered gut flora and environment in patients with severe SIRS. J Trauma 2006;60(1):126–33.

[52] Shimizu K, Ogura H, Asahara T, et al. Probiotic/synbiotic therapy for treating critically ill patients from a gut microbiota perspective. Dig Dis Sci 2013;58(1):23–32.

[53] Osuka A, Shimizu K, Ogura H, et al. Prognostic impact of fecal pH in critically ill patients. Crit Care 2012;16(4):R119.

[54] Yamada T, Shimizu K, Ogura H, et al. Rapid and Sustained Long-Term Decrease of Fecal Short-Chain Fatty Acids in Critically Ill Patients With Systemic Inflammatory Response Syndrome. JPEN J Parenter Enteral Nutr 2015;39(5):569–77.

[55] Coutinho-Wolino KS, de F Cardozo LFM, de Oliveira Leal V, et al. Can diet modulate trimethylamine N-

oxide (TMAO) production? What do we know so far? Eur J Nutr 2021;60(7):3567–84.

[56] Liu Y, Dai M. Trimethylamine N-Oxide Generated by the Gut Microbiota Is Associated with Vascular Inflammation: New Insights into Atherosclerosis. Mediators Inflamm 2020;2020:4634172.

[57] Velasquez MT, Ramezani A, Manal A, et al. Trimethylamine N-Oxide: The Good, the Bad and the Unknown. Toxins 2016;8(11):326.

[58] Tang WHW, Wang Z, Levison BS, et al. Intestinal microbial metabolism of phosphatidylcholine and cardiovascular risk. N Engl J Med 2013;368(17):1575–84.

[59] Zhu W, Gregory JC, Org E, et al. Gut Microbial Metabolite TMAO Enhances Platelet Hyperreactivity and Thrombosis Risk. Cell 2016;165(1):111–24.

[60] Bu J, Wang Z. Cross-Talk between Gut Microbiota and Heart via the Routes of Metabolite and Immunity. Gastroenterol Res Pract 2018;2018:6458094.

[61] Rooks MG, Garrett WS. Gut microbiota, metabolites and host immunity. Nat Rev Immunol 2016;16(6): 341–52.

[62] Kamada N, Seo SU, Chen GY, et al. Role of the gut microbiota in immunity and inflammatory disease. Nat Rev Immunol 2013;13(5):321–35.

[63] Berger MM, Appelberg O, Reintam-Blaser A, et al. Prevalence of hypophosphatemia in the ICU - Results of an international one-day point prevalence survey. Clin Nutr 2021;40(5):3615–21.

[64] Macpherson AJ, Uhr T. Induction of protective IgA by intestinal dendritic cells carrying commensal bacteria. Science 2004;303(5664):1662–5.

[65] Honda K, Littman DR. The microbiota in adaptive immune homeostasis and disease. Nature 2016; 535(7610):75–84.

[66] Francino MP. Antibiotics and the Human Gut Microbiome: Dysbioses and Accumulation of Resistances. Front Microbiol 2015;6:1543. https://doi.org/10.33 89/fmicb.2015.01543.

[67] Ladopoulos T, Giannaki M, Alexopoulou C, et al. Gastrointestinal dysmotility in critically ill patients. Ann Gastroenterol 2018;31(3):273–81.

[68] Husnik R, Gaschen F. Gastric Motility Disorders in Dogs and Cats. Vet Clin North Am Small Anim Pract 2021;51(1):43–59.

[69] Torres-Henderson C, Summers S, Suchodolski J, et al. Effect of Enterococcus Faecium Strain SF68 on Gastrointestinal Signs and Fecal Microbiome in Cats Administered Amoxicillin-Clavulanate. Top Companion Anim Med 2017;32(3):104–8.

[70] Whittemore JC, Mooney AP, Price JM, et al. Clinical, clinicopathologic, and gastrointestinal changes from administration of clopidogrel, prednisone, or combination in healthy dogs: A double-blind randomized trial. J Vet Intern Med 2019;33(6):2618–27.

[71] Garcia-Mazcorro JF, Suchodolski JS, Jones KR, et al. Effect of the proton pump inhibitor omeprazole on the gastrointestinal bacterial microbiota of healthy dogs. FEMS Microbiol Ecol 2012;80(3):624–36.

[72] Stavroulaki EM, Suchodolski JS, Pilla R, et al. Short- and long-term effects of amoxicillin/clavulanic acid or doxycycline on the gastrointestinal microbiome of growing cats. PLoS One 2021;16(12):e0253031.

[73] Robert A, Asano T. Resistance of germfree rats to indomethacin-induced intestinal lesions. Prostaglandins 1977;14(2):333–41.

[74] Werner M, Suchodolski JS, Straubinger RK, et al. Effect of amoxicillin-clavulanic acid on clinical scores, intestinal microbiome, and amoxicillin-resistant Escherichia coli in dogs with uncomplicated acute diarrhea. J Vet Intern Med 2020;34(3):1166–76.

[75] Espinosa-Gongora C, Jessen LR, Kieler IN, et al. Impact of oral amoxicillin and amoxicillin/clavulanic acid treatment on bacterial diversity and β-lactam resistance in the canine faecal microbiome. J Antimicrob Chemother 2020;75(2):351–61.

[76] Schmidt M, Unterer S, Suchodolski JS, et al. The fecal microbiome and metabolome differs between dogs fed Bones and Raw Food (BARF) diets and dogs fed commercial diets. PLoS One 2018;13(8):e0201279.

[77] Miyasaka EA, Feng Y, Poroyko V, et al. Total parenteral nutrition-associated lamina propria inflammation in mice is mediated by a MyD88-dependent mechanism. J Immunol 2013;190(12):6607–15.

[78] Dahlgren AF, Pan A, Lam V, et al. Longitudinal changes in the gut microbiome of infants on total parenteral nutrition. Pediatr Res 2019;86(1):107–14.

[79] Zaborin A, Smith DP, Garfield K, et al. Membership and Behavior of Ultra-Low-Diversity Pathogen Communities Present in the Gut of Humans during Prolonged Critical Illness. mBio 2014;5(5):e01361.

[80] Zaborina O, Lepine F, Xiao G, et al. Dynorphin activates quorum sensing quinolone signaling in Pseudomonas aeruginosa. PLoS Pathog 2007;3(3):e35.

[81] Winston JA, Theriot CM. Impact of microbial derived secondary bile acids on colonization resistance against Clostridium difficile in the gastrointestinal tract. Anaerobe 2016;41:44–50.

[82] Zaborin A, Gerdes S, Holbrook C, et al. Pseudomonas aeruginosa overrides the virulence inducing effect of opioids when it senses an abundance of phosphate. PLoS One 2012;7(4):e34883.

[83] Krezalek M, Yeh A, Alverdy J, et al. Influence of nutrition therapy on the intestinal microbiome. Curr Opin Clin Nutr Metab Care 2016;20:131–7.

[84] Babrowski T, Holbrook C, Moss J, et al. Pseudomonas aeruginosa virulence expression is directly activated by morphine and is capable of causing lethal gut-derived sepsis in mice during chronic morphine administration. Ann Surg 2012;255(2):386–93.

[85] Kullberg RFJ, Wiersinga WJ, Haak BW. Gut microbiota and sepsis: from pathogenesis to novel treatments. Curr Opin Gastroenterol 2021;37(6):578–85.

[86] Haak B, Wiersinga W. The role of the gut microbiota in sepsis. Lancet Gastroenterol Hepatol 2017;2 2:135–43.

[87] Wan Y, Zhu RX, Wu Z, et al. Gut Microbiota Disruption in Septic Shock Patients: A Pilot Study. Med Sci Monit 2018;24:8639–46.

[88] Klingensmith NJ, Coopersmith C. The Gut as the Motor of Multiple Organ Dysfunction in Critical Illness. Crit Care Clin 2016;32(2):203–12.

[89] Clarke TB, Davis KM, Lysenko ES, et al. Recognition of peptidoglycan from the microbiota by Nod1 enhances systemic innate immunity. Nat Med 2010;16(2): 228–31.

[90] Schuijt TJ, Lankelma JM, Scicluna BP, et al. The gut microbiota plays a protective role in the host defence against pneumococcal pneumonia. Gut 2016;65(4): 575–83.

[91] Gibson GR, Scott KP, Rastall RA, et al. Dietary prebiotics: current status and new definition. Food Sci Technol Bull Funct Foods 2010;7(1):1–19.

[92] Schneider SM, Girard-Pipau F, Anty R, et al. Effects of total enteral nutrition supplemented with a multifibre mix on faecal short-chain fatty acids and microbiota. Clin Nutr 2006;25(1):82–90.

[93] O'Keefe SJ, Ou J, DeLany JP, et al. Effect of fiber supplementation on the microbiota in critically ill patients. World J Gastrointest Pathophysiol 2011;2(6):138–45.

[94] Yang G, Wu XT, Zhou Y, et al. Application of dietary fiber in clinical enteral nutrition: a meta-analysis of randomized controlled trials. World J Gastroenterol 2005; 11(25):3935–8.

[95] Majid HA, Cole J, Emery PW, et al. Additional oligofructose/inulin does not increase faecal bifidobacteria in critically ill patients receiving enteral nutrition: a randomised controlled trial. Clin Nutr 2014;33(6):966–72.

[96] Rudinsky AJ, Parker VJ, Winston J, et al. Randomized controlled trial demonstrates nutritional management is superior to metronidazole for treatment of acute colitis in dogs. J Am Vet Med Assoc 2022;260(S3):S23–32.

[97] Batra P, Soni KD, Mathur P. Efficacy of probiotics in the prevention of VAP in critically ill ICU patients: an updated systematic review and meta-analysis of randomized control trials. J Intensive Care 2020;8:81.

[98] Johnstone J, Meade M, Lauzier F, et al. Effect of Probiotics on Incident Ventilator-Associated Pneumonia in Critically Ill Patients: A Randomized Clinical Trial. JAMA 2021;326(11):1024–33.

[99] Shimizu K, Yamada T, Ogura H, et al. Synbiotics modulate gut microbiota and reduce enteritis and ventilator-associated pneumonia in patients with sepsis: a randomized controlled trial. Crit Care 2018;22(1):239.

[100] Ziese AL, Suchodolski J, Hartmann K, et al. Effect of probiotic treatment on the clinical course, intestinal microbiome, and toxigenic Clostridium perfringens in dogs with acute hemorrhagic diarrhea. PLoS One 2018;13(9):e0204691.

[101] Arslan H, Aksu DS, Terzi G, et al. Therapeutic effects of probiotic bacteria in parvoviral enteritis in dogs. Rev Med Vet 2012;163(2):55–9.

[102] Hocquart M, Lagier JC, Cassir N, et al. Early Fecal Microbiota Transplantation Improves Survival in Severe Clostridium difficile Infections. Clin Infect Dis 2018;66(5): 645–50.

[103] Li Q, Wang C, Tang C, et al. Successful treatment of severe sepsis and diarrhea after vagotomy utilizing fecal microbiota transplantation: a case report. Crit Care 2015;19(1):37.

[104] Wei Y, Yang J, Wang J, et al. Successful treatment with fecal microbiota transplantation in patients with multiple organ dysfunction syndrome and diarrhea following severe sepsis. Crit Care 2016;20(1):332.

[105] Pereira GQ, Gomes LA, Santos IS, et al. Fecal microbiota transplantation in puppies with canine parvovirus infection. J Vet Intern Med 2018;32(2):707–11.

[106] Gal A, Barko PC, Biggs PJ, et al. One dog's waste is another dog's wealth: A pilot study of fecal microbiota transplantation in dogs with acute hemorrhagic diarrhea syndrome. PLoS One 2021;16(4):e0250344.

[107] Keskey R, Cone JT, DeFazio JR, et al. The use of fecal microbiota transplant in sepsis. Transl Res 2020;226: 12–25.

SECTION III: VETERINARIAN WELLNESS

Advances in Small Animal Care 4 (2023) 113–122

ADVANCES IN SMALL ANIMAL CARE

Early Career Veterinary Well-being and Solutions to Help Young Veterinarians Thrive

Addie R. Reinhard, DVM, MS[a,b,*]

[a]MentorVet, Lexington, KY, USA; [b]Lincoln Memorial University College of Veterinary Medicine, Harrogate, TN, USA

KEYWORDS
• Mentorship • Veterinary well-being • Burnout • Transition to practice • Veterinary graduates
• Professional skills

KEY POINTS
• Young veterinary professionals seem to be at the highest risk for mental health challenges within the profession, with approximately 75% of all young veterinarians experiencing moderate-to-severe burnout.
• A multifaceted approach is required to make an impact on mental health of young professionals, and workplaces, veterinary schools, organizations, and individuals must all take action.
• Quality mentorship and adequate training in professional skills are vital aspects for early-career success.
• Young veterinarians can support themselves by creating a stress management plan, setting healthy boundaries, seeking support from others, and obtaining training in professional skills.

INTRODUCTION

Well-being and mental health of veterinary professionals has recently become a topic of growing interest within the veterinary industry. There are growing concerns of poor mental health within the profession. Research dating back to the 1980s suggests that the mental health challenges facing the veterinary profession are not new but within the past 20 years, a growing body of literature is contextualizing this complex issue [1–4].

The risk of burnout and stress for veterinary professionals is significantly higher than the general population, and the Merck Animal Health Veterinary Wellbeing Study III revealed that young veterinarians seem to be at the highest risk for burnout and serious psychological distress [5,6]. It is estimated that around 75% of veterinarians under the age of 35 are experiencing moderate-to-high levels of burnout (Fig. 1) [7].

In addition, around 1 in 6 young veterinarians reported experiencing serious psychological distress (Fig. 2) [7].

One of the main contributing factors for high rates of burnout in the profession is the inherently stressful job, and the transition to practice seems to be one of the most stressful periods of the veterinary career [8]. Some of the key stressors for early-career veterinarians included the following:
• An expectation of self-sufficiency coupled with a sense of self-doubt
• Fear of making mistakes
• Ethical dilemmas
• The changing clientele from an academic institution to general practice
• Assuming a leadership role
• Conflict with clients and support staff
• Experiencing discrimination
• Inadequate mentorship [8].

*4045 Clearwater Way, Lexington, KY 40515. E-mail address: Addie@mentorvet.net

https://doi.org/10.1016/j.yasa.2023.05.005
2666-450X/23/

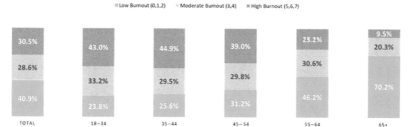

FIG. 1 Burnout levels from the Merck Animal Health Veterinary Wellbeing Study III. (*From* Volk JO, Schimmack U, Strand EB, et al. Veterinary Mental Health and Wellbeing and How to Improve Them. Learnings from the Merck Animal Health Veterinarian Wellbeing Study III. 2022. Page 19. https://www.merck-animal-health-usa. com/wp-content/uploads/sites/54/2022/02/2021-PSV-Veterinary-Wellbeing-Presentation_V2.pdf.)

Although it is important to understand the causal factors that contribute to burnout and stress in the profession, the majority of this article will be focused on solutions to this problem. To address this complex issue, we must have multifaceted solutions including workplace strategies, veterinary school strategies, organizational strategies, and individual strategies. By taking a multifaceted approach, we have the potential to help young veterinarians thrive in their careers.

SOLUTIONS TO HELP YOUNG VETERINARIANS THRIVE

When considering potential solutions to improve well-being of young veterinarians, we must approach this issue at various levels. Veterinary schools play an important role in preparing young professionals for the challenges and stressors they will be experiencing in their career. In addition, workplaces play a vital role in on-the-job training and mentorship for early-career veterinarians. Organizations can also take steps to promote well-being among young professionals, and finally, the young veterinarians themselves have the ability to support themselves through challenges they may be facing.

Veterinary school strategies

It is likely that no amount of education or training can fully prepare a young veterinarian to enter the workforce completely competent and confident. In most careers, there are substantial learning curves in the first few years of the career that require significant on-the-job training. That being said, there are many strategies we can take at the veterinary school level to begin to prepare our students for the challenges that they may face during the transition to practice.

Provide training in professional skills

One of the most important aspects for preparing veterinary students to be able to successfully navigate challenges and stressors in the career is to provide ample training in professional skills in veterinary school. It was found that professional skills such as communication and teamwork were ranked just as important for veterinarians as medical and surgical skills by veterinary students and veterinarians [9]. With this in mind, it is likely that more training in these skills will better prepare veterinary students for their transition to practice.

Early-career professionals reported experiencing challenges when navigating conflict with teammates

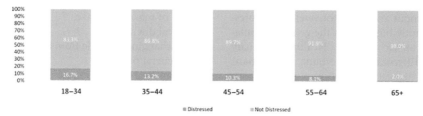

FIG. 2 Serious psychological distress rates from the Merck Animal Health Veterinary Wellbeing Study III. (*Adapted from* Volk JO, Schimmack U, Strand EB, et al. Veterinary Mental Health and Wellbeing and How to Improve Them. Learnings from the Merck Animal Health Veterinarian Wellbeing Study III. 2022. Page 15. Retrieved from https://www.merck-animal-health-usa.com/wp-content/uploads/sites/54/2022/02/2021-PSV-Veterinary-Wellbeing-Presentation_V2.pdf.)

and clients [8]. When stepping into clinical practice, young veterinarians are often asked to assume a role in which they are delegating tasks to their team and assuming the role of a leader even though they are often not in a managerial role when starting their careers. This poses unique challenges for young veterinarians who may not have much training in conflict management or leadership. Thus, it is recommended that a heavy focus be placed on these skills within the veterinary school curriculum.

Provide education in spectrum of care

Another key stressor for early-career veterinarians is working with clients given the context of limited client finances [8]. Many new graduates feel comfortable with offering gold-standard care to clients but many are unsure of how to navigate complex cases when client finances are limited. Previous research has revealed that client financial barriers to accessing pet care are very common, and this is one of the most frequent ethical dilemmas that veterinarians face in practice [10,11]. Experiencing frequent ethical dilemmas in practice can lead to moral stress, and this stress is exacerbated if a veterinary professional also has high levels of perfectionism [12]. Moral stress can contribute to burnout in the early career, so steps should be taken to provide training in understanding and coping with moral stress.

Given that veterinary students feel the lack of confidence in having challenging financial discussions with clients [13], and early-career veterinarians experienced stress when navigating these cases, it is recommended to provide training in communication of the cost of care with clients. In addition, training in providing care across a spectrum may result in more confidence working in the gray areas of veterinary medicine. For example, when discussing how to treat parvovirus in dogs, consider teaching students both the gold-standard treatment options as well as additional treatment options. Challenge students to consider how they might navigate the case with only a US$200 budget or a US$500 budget. In the context of limited client resources, have students consider each test they would like to perform and how those tests might alter the outcome of their treatment plan. If the test will not change the outcome of treatment, this might not be a diagnostic tool that they should prioritize when helping a client determine how to allocate their resources. Exposing students to this type of critical thinking will improve clinical decision-making and help young veterinarians feel more confident navigating these types of cases.

Keeping in mind some of the previously mentioned stressors for recent graduates as well as the skills veterinary professionals thought were most important, it is suggested that veterinary schools should place a high emphasis on teaching the skills and knowledge listed in Box 1.

Workplace strategies

There are many actions that can be taken within workplaces to promote the mental health and well-being of early-career veterinarians. Empowering leaders to participate in leadership training, creating a psychologically safe work environment, providing access to quality mentorship, and providing ample employee benefits are all ways in which we can empower young professionals to thrive within the workplace.

Leadership training

Research suggests that the quality of leadership provided is directly related to overall well-being of employees, so all mentors and leaders within the workplace should be given adequate opportunities for participation in leadership training [14]. Many veterinary professionals do not receive much leadership training throughout the veterinary school curriculum. Leadership competencies may come naturally to some but most individuals need training on how to be effective leaders. Providing opportunities for advanced leadership training for individuals who will be working directly with the young veterinarians will not only help the leaders feel more confident but will also help

> **BOX 1**
> **Skills and knowledge vital for early-career success**
>
> Communication with clients and coworkers
> Leadership
> Professional and personal identity development
> Conflict management
> Recognizing and responding to burnout
> Stress management
> Responding to discrimination
> Disclosing medical errors and coping with making a mistake
> Ethical decision-making
> Coping with moral stress
> Seeking quality mentorship
> Building trust and rapport
> Communicating the cost of care
> Spectrum of care

the rest of the veterinary team including young professionals.

Create an environment of psychological safety

Fear of making mistakes is a significant stressor for young veterinarians. One study found that around 75% of young veterinarians within their first 18 months of practice committed a mistake, and often, mistake-making had a significant impact on veterinarians, including feelings of guilt, sleepless nights, or even thoughts of leaving the profession [15]. Because of this, practices should create an environment of psychological safety where mistakes are not viewed on as failures but rather as opportunities for learning and growth. Psychological safety "leads employees to engage in open communication, voice their concerns, and seek greater feedback." [16].

Imagine an early-career veterinarian who just made a mistake. How likely are they to consult with a more experienced veterinarian about the mistake they made if they know that they will get reprimanded? However, how likely are they to disclose the error if they know that the experienced veterinarian will quickly help them mitigate the error then discuss with them how they will prevent the error from occurring in the future? To improve patient safety and help early-career veterinarians feel more comfortable within the practice, it is important to create an environment where mistakes will be viewed as a learning experience. Often when leaders can also demonstrate vulnerability and admit when they have made a mistake, this can further improve psychological safety in the workplace.

Provide quality mentorship

When veterinarians enter the workforce, there are many different challenges and stressors but a key contributor to positive experiences in the transition to practice was access to quality mentorship [8]. Traditionally, mentorship in the veterinary profession has been viewed as receiving advice and support from a more experienced veterinarian within a practice. This individual usually supports the growth of a new graduate by placing a heavy focus on mentorship of clinical knowledge and acumen. New graduates reported that a good mentor was someone who is

- Trusting and supportive of new graduate's medical knowledge
- Willing and available to answer questions
- Able to empathize with challenges faced in the early career [8].

Although supporting a mentee through clinical case support is important, mentors must also be able to support mentees through other challenges they may be facing such as navigating conflict and ethical dilemmas. This requires effective communication and listening skills as well as how to properly deliver feedback. After asking the mentee for permission to deliver feedback, mentors can use a feedback model such as the Pendleton Model (Table 1) to deliver feedback [17].

Mentors should encourage and model healthy self-care habits. When a mentee sees their mentor not setting healthy boundaries or not taking care of themselves, it can encourage the mentee to model this behavior as well. Alternatively, if mentors prioritize their own mental health and well-being and model healthy stress management, mentees may feel more comfortable practicing regular self-care. In addition, mentors should regularly encourage their mentees to care for themselves as well as set healthy boundaries for themselves. A good mentor will respect boundaries that a mentee sets for themselves.

A quality mentor will create safety and inclusivity within their mentoring practices by pursing advanced training and education in diversity, equity, inclusion, and belonging. Learning how to create inclusive environments within mentorship is a lifelong learning process that requires continual self-reflection of one's own biases and beliefs and doing self-guided study to learn more about other's cultures. Advanced training in diversity, equity, inclusion, and belonging can be obtained from the following:

- American Veterinary Medical Association (AVMA) Brave Space Certificate Program
- AVMA Journey for Teams
- Purdue Certificate Programs for Diversity and Inclusion in Veterinary Medicine

Mentors should also seek advanced training in suicide prevention to be able to recognize and respond to signs of mental health challenges because veterinary professionals are 1.6 to 2.4 times likely to die by suicide than the general population [18]. At the time of writing, any veterinary professional can participate in free suicide prevention training through the AVMA [19]. If you notice potential signs of a mental health condition such as behavior changes, mood disturbances, or social withdrawal, it is important to be a good listener, ask how you can help, and provide referral to appropriate mental health resources [20].

Although the traditional form of one-on-one mentorship within the practices are important for success in the early career, additional mentorship structures outside of the practice environment contribute to holistic support of the young professional. Ensure that additional support opportunities are provided for external mentorship outside of the practice by encouraging

TABLE 1
Pendleton model for effective feedback

Feedback Model Steps	Sample Question or Statement
1. Ask the veterinarian what they thought they did well	"What did you do well in this situation?"
2. Reflect back the successes that you heard then tell the veterinarian other things you think they did well	"I agree that you handled that angry client calmly and what I also thought you did well was asking for help from your practice manager when you needed extra support."
3. Ask the veterinarian what could be improved for next time, if anything	"What could make this go even better next time you experience a similar situation?"
4. Reflect back those ideas then add any additional feedback for what could be improved in the future	"It sounds like you think you could have done a better job of communicating all the treatment options for the case, and I think one way you could make it go even better next time is adding in some empathetic statements to your communication."

Adapted from Pendleton D, Schofield T, Tate P, Havelock P. The consultation: an approach to learning and teaching. Oxford: Oxford University Press; 1984.

young veterinarians to participate in external mentorship programming. In addition, young veterinarians should be encouraged by their mentors to seek out professional development opportunities and training to help them better cope with the challenges and stressors of practice.

Provide benefits and resources

In addition to providing mentorship, employers should consider offering an Employee Assistance Program (EAP), a voluntary, work-based program that typically includes free access to short-term counseling, assessment, and referrals designed to help employees with personal issues that they may be facing. Employers should also consider adequate time off, flexible scheduling options, paid maternity and paternity leave, and insurance coverage for mental health support. These additional resources and benefits can make individuals think that their workplace and employers care about their mental health and well-being. Ensure that benefits and resources are well communicated with employees so that they are well utilized. Often, young professionals may be unaware of resources available to them if they are not regularly communicated.

Organizational strategies

Organizations such as local, state, and national veterinary medical associations play a vital role in providing external structures outside of the practice environment to support young veterinary professionals. There are also an increasing number of organizations that have been established to support individuals from underrepresented groups within veterinary medicine. These organizations often provide early-career professionals with important

community and resources including mentorship and leadership programming.

Power of 10

Many veterinary medical associations have implemented Power of 10 programming. This program is a leadership development program for veterinarians in their early career designed to provide training in topics such as leadership, business, and communication [21]. These programs often leverage small peer group learning and professional skills training to support young veterinarians in leadership development. To the author's knowledge, there has been no published research to date showing the efficacy of these programs but a large body of positive testimonials exists revealing the impact that the Power of 10 programs have on early-career professionals.

Mentorship programs

Mentorship programming has been implemented within associations with varying success. Some mentorship programs fail due to the lack of intentional program development as well as barriers in funding, time, and personnel. Intentional program development requires understanding the challenges and stressors of a population and then creating a structured program to support that population. Particularly in paired mentorship programs, both the mentor and the mentee must be given training and structure to make the relationship successful. In addition, ongoing evaluation should be conducted to ensure the program is having the desired outcome.

Organizations attempting to develop mentorship programming should also research existing programming that might fit the needs of the organization because this could save the organization significant time and resources. There is an increasing number of existing mentorship programs that might fit the needs of an organization without having to create an entirely new program internally.

Leadership opportunities

Veterinary medical associations should give adequate opportunities for young professionals to participate in the leadership team of the organization. Early-career professionals can provide a unique perspective to some of the challenges faced within the profession, and when given a voice, these individuals may feel more engaged and involved within their organizations. Organizations should consider encouraging young professionals within the organization to get more involved including participating on the board of directors and getting engaged with committees. When young professionals feel a broader sense of connection to the veterinary industry, this may promote well-being in the early career.

Individual strategies

Even in the most supportive environments, it is possible that young veterinarians could still experience challenges and stressors in the transition to practice. Early-career veterinarians can take many actions to support themselves (Table 2). The Merck Animal Health Veterinary Wellbeing Study found that having a healthy way to manage stress was one of the most important predictors for good mental health and well-being within the veterinary profession [6]. Early-career professionals should consider the following strategies when creating an individualized stress management plan.

Self-care and stress management

The veterinary profession is inherently stressful. Early-career professionals must prioritize self-care and stress management to be successful in the transition to practice. There are common misconceptions that self-care is indulging on delicious food or binge-watching Netflix, yet self-care can be defined as the "the process of purposeful engagement in practices that promote effective and appropriate use of the self in the professional role within the context of sustaining holistic health and well-being." [22] Essentially, self-care is the intentional practice of regularly taking actions to support one's overall health. Self-care is extremely important to individuals within the veterinary profession as having a healthy method for dealing with stress was one

TABLE 2 Individual strategies to promote early-career well-being	
Strategy	**Example**
1. Self-care and stress management	Develop an individualized stress management plan including intentional and regular self-care activities
2. Set healthy boundaries	Establish a consistent 10–20 min daily lunch break
3. Create a strong support network	Establish and foster healthy relationships with others outside of the veterinary profession
4. Seek training in professional skills	Attend a leadership conference or pursue continuing education in conflict management
5. Establish mentoring relationships	Identify 3 individuals within the profession to serve as mentors—someone within the workplace, a peer, and someone outside of the workplace
6. Seek mental health support	Research options for mental health support
7. Obtain financial advice	Seek advice from a financial advisor to discuss strategies for debt repayment and budgeting
8. Find community	Join your state veterinary medical association and get involved with programming offered
9. Understand personal and professional values	Self-reflect about what you value both personally and professionally

of the most important predictors for good mental health and well-being in the veterinary profession [7].

Self-care and stress management are often individualized, so young professionals must find what is most effective for them. Often basic self-care includes adequate sleep, regular exercise, and good nutrition. In addition, young professionals should consider incorporating recreation and hobbies outside of the profession, quality time with loved ones, time in nature, volunteering, gratitude exercises, and/or mindfulness into their self-care plans because these strategies have all been shown to create positive impacts on mental health and well-being [23]. These self-care activities can help veterinary professionals develop a sense of personal identity outside of their career, which is important for promoting overall life satisfaction.

Self-care does not have to be laborious to be effective. As busy professionals, self-care can be challenging to fit into the schedule but taking small actions toward caring for yourself such as taking a 10-minute break to mindfully eat lunch, taking the dog for a walk after work every day, or actually leveraging vacation time can make large impacts on overall health and well-being. If veterinarians take small steps over time to improve their overall health and well-being, this can lead to big improvements.

Set healthy boundaries

Individuals will not have the time or ability to practice stress management and self-care without setting healthy boundaries. Boundary setting is not an easy task but it often requires speaking up about your own needs so that others know your emotional, mental, and physical limits. It requires first defining what your boundaries are then clearly and compassionately communicating these boundaries with others.

It is acceptable to say "no" if you are feeling overwhelmed, and only when you are able to prioritize yourself, will you be able to have the energy to help others and their pet. After you state your boundary, you may need to remind individuals of that boundary and uphold it. Remember that it likely that no one will advocate for you more than yourself. Setting boundaries can be incredibly challenging but are vital at promoting overall mental health.

Create a strong support network

Social support, which can be defined as being able to receive assistance and support from friends, family members, neighbors, and others appears to be important in contributing to overall life satisfaction [24]. Although having support from others is vital, feeling a lack of support has the potential to have negative impacts on mental health and well-being. One study found that around one-third of veterinarians felt bothered by a lack of social support [25].

To promote well-being in the transition to practice, it is recommended to foster healthy relationships with others. Creating a support network of friends and loved ones to support you is important when you are experiencing a major life transition—such as starting a new career. Try to set aside regular and intentional time for fostering healthy relationships with friends or loved ones. This could be as simple as reaching out to call a friend once a week on the way home from work or planning a weekly dinner with a loved one.

Seek training in professional skills

Many of the stressors in the transition to practice are related to communication, navigating conflict, and ethical decision-making. Although some stressors can be mitigated by feeling confident in medical skills, many of the stressors young veterinarians experience are unrelated to medical and surgical skills. To improve confidence in the transition to practice, new and recent graduates should consider seeking as much training in professional skills as possible. For example, learning strategies for conflict management can help early-career veterinarians feel more prepared for navigating conflict among colleagues and clients. In addition, learning strategies for navigating ethical dilemmas can make early-career veterinarians feel more confident practicing along a spectrum. Early-career veterinarians can seek this type of training from veterinary conferences, mentorship programming, workshops, and leadership programming.

Establish mentoring relationships

It is recommended that veterinarians have at least 3 mentors. The first mentor should be someone more experienced within the workplace. As previously discussed, the traditional form of mentorship sought in veterinary medicine is support from a more experienced veterinarian within a practice. Receiving this form of mentorship can provide a great starting point for early-career support but it may not be enough to meet the needs of young veterinarians.

Early-career veterinarians should consider seeking peer support from other young professionals in the transition to practice, so the second mentor should be a fellow new or recent veterinary graduate. Peer mentorship seems to be an extremely effective form of mentorship. In a facilitated monthly peer group meeting of veterinary interns, many professionals had positive experiences [26]. In addition, a pilot peer mentorship and professional development program showed significant influences on burnout among young veterinary professionals, and participants reported that the peer support received in the program made them think as if they were not alone in their challenges [27].

The final mentor should be someone external to the practice environment. External mentorship can provide a third-party safe space to talk about challenges faced within the workplace. Many veterinarians have a desire to provide mentorship to early-career veterinarians, so young professionals should take time to search for a mentor outside of the practice environment. Mentors can be found through organizations, networking events at conferences, social media, as well as staying engaged with veterinary schools.

Seek mental health support

Seeking support from a mental health professional in the transition to practice can be extremely helpful. Mental health professionals are trained to be able to identify and diagnose mental health conditions and provide treatment but they can also be helpful for providing individualized recommendations for coping with stress experienced in major life transitions. A mental health professional can provide additional tools and resources for navigating stress and burnout.

Young professionals should contact their medical insurance provider to determine if mental health coverage is included. In addition, early-career professionals should determine if their workplace has an EAP, and search for therapists in the area that may fit individual needs. Veterinary social workers often are a great resource because these are mental health professionals who also have knowledge and expertise working within the veterinary industry.

Obtain financial advice

The Merck Animal Health Veterinary Wellbeing Study III found that high levels of student debt and financial pressures can influence overall mental health, and thus recommended that veterinary professionals seek support from a financial advisor [7]. Financial advisors can help young professionals determine the best way to pay off student debt as well as provide resources and advice for budgeting, saving, and retirement planning. Many resources exist for veterinarians wanting support in addressing finances including the Veterinary Information Network Foundation Student Debt Center and the American Veterinary Medical Association's financial resources [28,29]. Early-career professionals should seek support from these resources in the transition to practice to further improve overall well-being.

Find community

Often early-career veterinarians are going from an environment where they have a large amount of support and resources in veterinary school to an environment with fewer resources and support in their first jobs. Early-career professionals should try to find a community within the veterinary profession to engage with. Many communities exist from within local to national

organizations. Getting involved with organized veterinary medicine such as the local, state, and national veterinary medical associations can provide young professionals with additional resources in the transition to practice. Other organizations listed below can also provide access to resources and community for early-career professionals.

- Multicultural Veterinary Medical Association
- Pride Veterinary Medical Community
- Women's Veterinary Leadership Development Initiative
- BlackDVM Network
- Association of Asian Veterinary Medical Professionals
- MentorVet
- Pawsibilites Vet Med
- Jewish Association of Veterinarians
- Latinx Veterinary Medical Association
- American Association of Veterinarians of Indian Origin
- National Association of Black Veterinarians
- Native American Veterinary Association
- Veterinarians as One Inclusive Community for Empowerment

Understand personal and professional values

Often young veterinarians have been so busy during veterinary school that they have little time to reflect on what they value both personally and professionally. In the early career, young professionals should set aside time to discover what is important to them within their careers. By identifying these professional values, they will be able to find workplaces that have values that closely align with their own values. In addition, exploring personal values will help young professionals develop a sense of identity outside of their career in veterinary medicine.

Young professionals can start by reading through a list of common values and narrowing the list down to their top 3 to 5 values. After the list is established, young professionals should write a few sentences describing why this value is so important to them. By uncovering these values, veterinarians will then be able to take actions that align with their personal and professional values, which has the potential to improve their overall mental health and well-being.

AREAS OF FUTURE RESEARCH

Although there has been a large amount of research done within the veterinary profession to conceptualize the issue of mental health and well-being, greatly lacking within the research are evidence-based interventions. A future area of focus for veterinary well-being researchers should be placed on evaluating interventions to support the mental health and well-being of the profession. We should also continue to track trends of mental health and well-being at a national scale so that we can continue to provide an ongoing assessment of the issue.

Particular areas of further research could include the intersection of mental health and well-being and diversity, equity, inclusion, and belonging within the veterinary profession. There is scant literature on the mental and emotional impact of discrimination within the workplace, so this could be a potential area of exploration. This is particularly important among young veterinary professionals who reported one of the challenges in the transition to practice was experiencing discrimination [8].

SUMMARY

The early career and particularly the transition to practice is a stressful time for veterinarians. Research shows that this period is associated with some of the highest rates of burnout and stress within the career. Although there are challenges faced during this period including discrimination, conflict with clients and support staff, challenges assuming a leadership role, and navigating ethical dilemmas, there is much that can be done to support early-career professionals. Taking a multifaced approach that includes workplace and organizational support, veterinary school strategies, and individual strategies will lead to a pathway of success for young veterinarians. Given the right tools, education, resources, and community, any veterinary professional in this industry has the potential to thrive within the career.

CLINICS CARE POINTS

- Young veterinarians should seek support from at least 3 mentors in their early career—a more experienced professional within the workplace (workplace mentor), a fellow early-career professional (peer mentor), and a veterinarian outside of the workplace to provide third party support (external mentor).
- Workplace mentors should seek additional training in diversity, equity, inclusion, and belonging, as well as how to support the mental health and well-being of mentees through emotional support training and suicide prevention training.

- A strong focus should be placed on education in professional skills for early-career veterinarians and veterinary students as challenges with conflict, leadership, and ethics seem to be common in the transition to practice.
- Organizations such as veterinary medical associations play a vital role at providing additional external support to the young professional and should consider offering leadership and mentorship programming.

DISCLOSURE

The author is CEO of MentorVet, LLC who receives sponsorship and funding from Merck, United States Animal Health and other corporate entities.

REFERENCES

[1] Kinlen LJ. Mortality among British veterinary surgeons. Br Med J 1983;287:1017–9.

[2] Bartram DJ, Yadegarfar G, Baldwin DS. A cross-sectional study of mental health and well-being and their associations in the UK veterinary profession. Soc Psychiatry Psychiatr Epidemiol 2009;44(12):1075–85. https://doi.org/10.1007/s00127-009-0030-8.

[3] Gardner DH, Hini D. Work-related stress in the veterinary profession in New Zealand. N Z Vet J 2006;54(3):119–24. https://doi.org/10.1080/00480169.2006.36623.

[4] Volk JO, Schimmack U, Strand EB, et al. Executive summary of the Merck Animal Health Veterinary Wellbeing Study. J Am Vet Med Assoc 2018;252(10):1231–8. https://doi.org/10.2460/javma.252.10.1231.

[5] Hatch PH, Winefield HR, Christie BA, et al. Workplace stress, mental health, and burnout of veterinarians in Australia. Aust Vet J 2011;89(11):460–8. https://doi.org/10.1111/j.1751-0813.2011.00833.x.

[6] Volk JO, Schimmack U, Strand EB, et al. Executive summary of the Merck Animal Health Veterinarian Wellbeing Study III and Veterinary Support Staff Study. J Am Vet Med Assoc 2022;260(12):1547–53. https://doi.org/10.2460/javma.22.03.0134.

[7] Volk JO, Schimmack U, Strand EB, et al. Veterinary Mental Health and Wellbeing and How to Improve Them. Learnings from the Merck Animal Health Veterinarian Wellbeing Study III. 2022. Retrieved from https://www.merck-animal-health-usa.com/wp-content/uploads/sites/54/2022/02/2021-PSV-Veterinary-Wellbeing-Presentation_V2.pdf. Accessed January 15, 2023.

[8] Reinhard AR, Hains KD, Hains BJ, et al. Are They Ready? Trials, Tribulations, and Professional Skills Vital for New Veterinary Graduate Success. Front Vet Sci 2021;8:785844. https://doi.org/10.3389/fvets.2021.785844.

[9] Haldane S, Hinchcliff K, Mansell P, et al. Expectations of graduate communication skills in professional veterinary

practice. J Vet Med Educ 2017;44:268–79. https://doi.org/10.3138/jvme.1215-193R.

[10] Wiltzius AJ, Blackwell MJ, Krebsbach SB, et al. Access to veterinary care: barriers, current practices, public Policy, Faculty Publications Other Works – Small Animal Clinical Sciences, 2018. Tennessee Research and Creative Exchange. https://trace.tennessee.edu/utk_smalpubs/17/.

[11] Batchelor CE, McKeegan DE. Survey of the frequency and perceived stressfulness of ethical dilemmas encountered in UK veterinary practice. Vet Rec 2012;170:19. https://doi.org/10.1136/vr.100262.

[12] Crane MF, Phillips JK, Karin E. Trait perfectionism strengthens the negative effects of moral stressors occurring in veterinary practice. Aust Vet J 2015;93:354–60. https://doi.org/10.1111/avj.12366.

[13] Meehan MP, Menniti MF. Final-year veterinary students' perceptions of their communication competencies and a communication skills training program delivered in a primary care setting and based on Kolb's Experiential Learning Theory. J Vet Med Educ 2014;41:371–83. https://doi.org/10.3138/jvme.1213-162R1.

[14] Shanafelt TD, Noseworthy JH. Executive Leadership and Physician Well-being: Nine Organizational Strategies to Promote Engagement and Reduce Burnout. Mayo Clin Proc 2017;92(1):129–46. https://doi.org/10.1016/j.mayocp.2016.10.004.

[15] Mellanby RJ, Herrtage ME. Survey of mistakes made by recent veterinary graduates. Vet Rec 2004;155(24):761–5.

[16] Newman A, Donohue R, Eva N. Psychological safety: A systematic review of the literature. Hum Resour Manag Rev 2017;27(3):521–35.

[17] Pendleton D, Schofield T, Tate P, et al. The consultation: an approach to learning and teaching. Oxford: Oxford University Press; 1984.

[18] Witte TK, Spitzer EG, Edwards N, et al. Suicides and deaths of undetermined intent among veterinary professionals from 2003 through 2014. J Am Vet Med Assoc 2019;255(5):595–608. https://doi.org/10.2460/javma.255.5.595.

[19] QPR suicide prevention training. AVMA. Retrieved from https://www.avma.org/resources-tools/wellbeing/qpr-suicide-prevention-training. Accessed January 15, 2023.

[20] Brister, T. Navigating a mental health crises: A NAMI resource guide for those experiencing a mental health emergency. 2018. Retrieved from https://www.nami.org/Support-Education/Publications-Reports/Guides/Navigating-a-Mental-Health-Crisis/Navigating-A-Mental-Health-Crisis?utm_source=website&utm_medium=''' cta&utm_campaign=crisisguide. Accessed January 15, 2023.

[21] Maine Veterinary Medical Association. Power of 10 Program. Retrieved from https://www.mainevetmed.org/power-of-10-program. Accessed January 15, 2023.

[22] Lee JJ, Miller SE. A self-care framework for social workers: Building a strong foundation for practice. Fam Soc: The Journal of Contemporary Social Services 2013;94(2):96–103.

[23] Walsh R. Lifestyle and mental health. Am Psychol 2011;66(7):579–92.

[24] Siedlecki KL, Salthouse TA, Oishi S, et al. The Relationship Between Social Support and Subjective Well-Being Across Age. Soc Indic Res 2014;117(2):561–76. https://doi.org/10.1007/s11205-013-0361-4.

[25] Rivera AC, Geronimo-Hara TR, LeardMann CA, et al. Behavioral health and sleep problems among US Army veterinarians and veterinary technicians participating in the Millennium Cohort Study. J Am Vet Med Assoc 2021;258(7):767–75. https://doi.org/10.2460/javma.258.7.767.

[26] Blum NR. Professional development groups help physicians; why not veterinarians? J Am Vet Med Assoc 2018;253(6):704–8. https://doi.org/10.2460/javma.253.6.704.

[27] Reinhard AR. Stress, Burnout, and Well-Being in New Veterinary Graduates: Evaluating a Pilot Online Professional Development Program. 2021. Theses and Dissertations—Community & Leadership Development. 54. https://uknowledge.uky.edu/cld_etds/54 Accessed January 15, 2023.

[28] VIN Foundation. Student Debt Center. Retrieved from https://vinfoundation.org/resources/student-debt-center/. Accessed January 15, 2023.

[29] American Veterinary Medical Association. Managing personal finances. Retrieved from https://www.avma.org/resources-tools/personal-finance. Accessed January 15, 2023.

Advances in Small Animal Care 4 (2023) 123–131

ADVANCES IN SMALL ANIMAL CARE

Veterinarians' Personality, Job Satisfaction, and Wellbeing

John Volk, BS[a,*], Ulrich Schimmack, PhD[b], Elizabeth Strand, PhD, LCSW[c]

[a]Brakke Consulting, 806 Green Valley Road, Suite 200, Greensboro, NC 27408, USA; [b]Department of Psychology, University of Toronto, Mississauga, ON, Canada; [c]College of Social Work and the College of Veterinary Medicine, University of Tennessee, Knoxville, TN, USA

KEYWORDS
• Veterinarians • Personality • Neuroticism • Mental health • Wellbeing • Job satisfaction

KEY POINTS
• The personality trait Neuroticism is the main personality predictor of veterinarians wellbeing.
• One important mediator is job satisfaction.
• Out of 13 job dimensions, work-life balance is the most important predictor of veterinarians' wellbeing.
• The results suggest that negative effects of Neuroticism on wellbeing can be managed by increasing work-life balance.

The wellbeing and mental health of veterinarians has been a longstanding concern in the profession. Recent studies have documented reports of compassion fatigue, burnout and other forms of job stress [1], as well as a suicide rate higher than in the general population [2].

A series of biennial studies beginning in 2017 documented that stress and suicide were among the most critical issues facing the profession [3–5]. These studies, the Merck Animal Health Veterinarian Wellbeing Studies, were conducted by Brakke Consulting in collaboration with the American Veterinary Medical Association (AVMA) and sponsored by Merck Animal Health, a supplier of vaccines, pharmaceuticals, and digital tools to the veterinary profession.

The Veterinarian Wellbeing Studies measured the wellbeing and mental health of veterinarians, and examined factors that contributed to higher levels of wellbeing and better mental health. Prominent predictors of lower wellbeing were high student debt and working more hours per week than desired. Consistent with the broader wellbeing literature, having a higher income was related to higher wellbeing [5–7].

However, wellbeing is not only influenced by environmental stressors. It is also influenced by personality traits; that is, internal dispositions that influence how individuals experience their lives. Personality traits explain why individuals with similar lives can have different levels of wellbeing. In this monograph, we review the literature on personality and wellbeing and present new results from the Merck Animal Health Veterinarian Wellbeing Studies, a national representative sample of veterinarians.

LITERATURE REVIEW
Definition of wellbeing

The concept of wellbeing measured in the Veterinarian Wellbeing Studies, sometimes called subjective wellbeing, assumes that individuals create their own conceptions of their ideal lives and are capable of evaluating their actual lives in comparison to their subjective ideals [8]. These evaluations are commonly called life satisfaction judgments. A widely used life

---

*Corresponding author, *E-mail address:* john@volkonline.com

https://doi.org/10.1016/j.yasa.2023.05.006
2666-450X/23/

satisfaction measure is Cantril's ladder that is used to measure wellbeing around the world [9]. Respondents are asked to think about a ladder that ranges from the worst possible life to the best possible life and then place their actual life on a ladder with 11 steps ranging from 0 to 10. A score of 10 out of 10 would imply that an individual's actual life perfectly matches their ideal life. Other life satisfaction measures ask similar questions and elicit similar responses. Our research on veterinarians' wellbeing is based on subjective theories of wellbeing and uses the average of 3 life satisfaction ratings to create a well-being index [3].

Top-down and bottom-up effects on wellbeing

Diener distinguished top-down effects and bottom-up effects on wellbeing [10]. Bottom-up effects are effects of objective life-circumstances (debt, long work hours) on wellbeing. Top-down effects are effects of personality on wellbeing. For example, the same number of work hours can have opposite effects on wellbeing, depending on individuals' preferences and personality. Modern theories of wellbeing recognize that wellbeing is influenced by bottom-up and top-down processes [11,12]. For example, financial satisfaction is influenced by actual income (bottom-up) and by materialism (top-down) [13].

A major challenge for wellbeing researchers is that human lives are complex and that wellbeing is influenced by hundreds of bottom-up and top-down processes. Moreover, the specific factors that contribute to wellbeing can vary from person to person. To study subjective wellbeing empirically, it is therefore necessary to focus on factors that influence most people's wellbeing. Wellbeing researchers have identified a number of life-domains that shape individuals' conceptions of the ideal life. The core life domains are health, material wellbeing, close relationships (partner, family), and work. An additional factor is affect; that is, individuals do care about the amount of pleasure versus displeasure in their life experiences [14]. Integrated top-down/bottom-up models assume that personality influences the evaluations of these life aspects and that these life-aspects mediate the effects of personality on life satisfaction judgments [11,12]. The more individuals focus on a domain, the more satisfaction in this domain contributes to wellbeing. For veterinarians, who are highly invested in their work, it is possible that most personality effects on wellbeing are mediated by personality effects on job satisfaction. Thus, we also review the literature on personality and job satisfaction.

Personality

Many veterinarians may be familiar with personality because they took the popular Myers-Briggs Types Indicator (MBTI) [15]. While this test provides meaningful information about personality, it has 2 main limitations. One problem is that there is little evidence for Jung's theory of personality that motivated the creation of the test. Second, the creation of types is problematic because personality differences are gradual rather than categorical. For example, there are no introverts or extraverts. Rather, individuals are introverted or extraverted to varying degrees.

Personality researchers have conducted many studies using factor analysis of personality ratings to develop an empirically grounded model of personality. In the 1980s, a consensus emerged that specific personality traits such as being helpful, sociable, orderly, moody, or creative reflect 5 broad and largely independent factors. These factors are called the Big Five because they capture variation in many specific personality traits. The names for these 5 broad dimensions of personality are Neuroticism, Extraversion, Openness, Agreeableness, and Conscientiousness [16]. Each Big Five dimension is characterized by distinct, but related specific personality traits (Fig. 1). The specific traits capture unique aspects of personality, but most specific traits are related to one or more of the Big Five [17].

Neuroticism

Neuroticism is a salient dimension of individual difference that has been studied since the beginning of empirical psychology. The core feature of neuroticism is a disposition to have negative thoughts and experiences. It is related to greater vulnerability to stress, more experiences of anxiety, anger, sadness, and self-conscious emotions such as shame and guilt. Individuals higher in neuroticism also tend to have lower self-esteem. While neuroticism itself is not a mental illness, high levels of neuroticism are a risk factor for mood disorders, especially during times of high stress [5,18]. It is not surprising that Neuroticism is the strongest Big Five predictor of wellbeing [19].

Looking at specific predictors of wellbeing, however, shows that the main reason for this strong relationship are experiences of sadness and low self-esteem [19,20]. A salient concern among veterinarians is burnout [4,5]. Burnout symptoms overlap considerably with depressive symptoms, but burnout is linked to work experiences, whereas depression can also be triggered by other life stressors as well. We are particularly interested in the effects of neuroticism on work-related aspects of

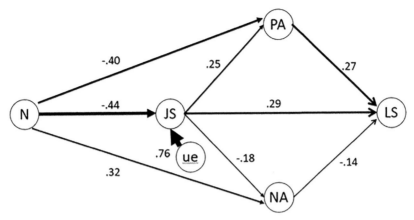

FIG. 1 Path diagram of neuroticism, job satisfaction, and life satisfaction. Note. JS, job satisfaction; LS, life satisfaction; N, neuroticism; NA, negative effect; PA, positive effect; ue, unexplained factors, numbers are standardized regression coefficients.

wellbeing (ie, burnout). According to the integrative top-down/bottom-up model, neuroticism is predicted to have a negative influence on job satisfaction and this effect may partially contribute to lower well-being [21].

Extraversion

Extraversion is the second oldest personality trait to be studied. Unfortunately, the terms extraversion and introversion have become everyday terms and are also used in the MBPT, but they have different meanings in different contexts. Even personality researchers do not agree about the core feature of this dimension. Some researchers assume that the core feature is sociability, which is consistent with the everyday meaning of the term. However, in the Big Five model Extraversion is a broad factor that is related to sociability, assertiveness, excitement seeking, and cheerful affect. Out of these specific personality traits, cheerfulness appears to be the main predictor of life satisfaction [19,20]. Thus, the correlation between sociability and life satisfaction may be spurious. More cheerful individuals are more likely to socialize and are more satisfied with their lives, but being more sociable is not a cause of higher wellbeing.

The influence of extraversion on job-satisfaction is more complex. Population studies suggest that extraverted workers tend to have higher wellbeing. However, this finding may be limited to work environments with many social interactions [22]. While veterinary medicine does involve social interactions, these interactions do not require a high level of sociability. Thus, extraversion may be a relatively weak predictor of veterinarians' job satisfaction and wellbeing.

Openness to experience

Openness to Experiences is a relatively new dimension of personality that only received attention after the Big Five model gained acceptance. Individuals high in this dimension are thinkers. They enjoy daydreaming and fantasizing, cognitively stimulating arts such as poetry, and reading thought-provoking literature. Less central aspects of openness are curiosity and novelty seeking, more intense emotional experiences, and more progressive attitudes. This dimension of the Big Five consistently shows very weak relationships with wellbeing [19].

Agreeableness

The core aspect of agreeableness is the extent to which individuals are competitive (low agreeableness) or cooperative (high agreeableness). Low agreeableness can manifest in different ways, including immoral actions, but low agreeableness itself may have benefits and costs. The main benefit is that self-interested individuals are more likely to maximize their wellbeing. The cost is that low agreeableness can undermine social relationships and create a hostile work environment. In general, agreeableness tends to show a small positive relationship with wellbeing [19], job satisfaction [23], and a small negative relationship with burnout [24]. However, most of these results rely on self-ratings of personality and outcomes and may be distorted by rating biases. Studies that control for response styles show mixed results [20,25–27].

It is unclear how agreeableness influences job satisfaction and well-being of veterinarians. On the one hand, agreeableness may help with social relationships at work and with finding meaning in helping patients and their owners. On the other hand, agreeableness may also undermine work-life balance and be a risk factor for burnout.

Conscientiousness

Conscientiousness is a personality trait that distinguishes individuals with a short-term (low conscientiousness) and a long-term (high-conscientiousness) focus. Conscientious is a key predictor of working hard towards long-term goals. As a result, it predicts higher grades in high school and in university, and better job performance in work settings [28]. The better performance of conscientious workers is reflected in the correlation between conscientiousness and income [29].

Conscientiousness is also a weak predictor of wellbeing [19]. One possible explanation for this relationship is a top-down effect of conscientiousness on income and a bottom-up effect of income on financial satisfaction and wellbeing. Conscientiousness also has a small positive relationship with job satisfaction, but the relationship is not as strong as one might expect, given the relationship with job performance [23] One possible explanation is that conscientious people have higher performance goals, which makes it more difficult for them to be satisfied with their performance. Conscientious people may also be at higher risk of burnout if they overexert themselves.

Veterinarian wellbeing and personality

Our first study in 2017 provided the first, extensive examination of personality influences on veterinarians' wellbeing. For the survey, a random sample of 20,000 email addresses was obtained from the American Veterinary Medical Association's (AVMA's) database of working US veterinarians. An email signed by AVMA then-president Dr Michael Topper and executive vice president and CEO Dr Janet Donlin was sent by the AVMA to alert recipients to the upcoming survey and encourage them to participate. An email and 2 reminder emails were sent to these emails by Kynetec, a market research firm. Nearly 3,600 veterinarians responded to the survey invitation, with a net of 3,540 usable survey responses, representing a response rate of 17.7%.

Personality was measured with a brief, 15-item questionnaire of the Big Five that was also used in a national representative sample of US Americans, namely the wellbeing module of the University of Michigan Panel Study of Income Dynamics (PSID) [30]. This allowed us to compare the personality profile of veterinarians to the personality profile of working US Americans. To correct for the unreliability of the short scales and

response biases, a latent variable model was used [31]. The model also controlled for age and gender differences between the 2 populations. The most notable difference was that veterinarians are, on average, less extraverted/more introverted than the average American. The difference was d = 0.3 to 0.5, depending on different model specifications. This effect size is considered a moderate effect size by conventional standards [32]. An effect size of d = 0.5 implies that a veterinarian has a 37.5% probability to be above the US average of extraversion or a 62.5% probability to be below the US average of extraversion. There was also a small difference for Neuroticism, with effect sizes in the range from 0.1 to 0.2 depending on different model specifications. A single item "worry a lot" accounted for most of the variation in effect size estimates. Thus, veterinarians might worry more, but the difference in neuroticism to the general population may be negligible (full results at https://osf.io/uypz6/). Thus, the key finding is that veterinarians tend to be more introverted than the general population.

We now turn to the more important findings of the relationship between personality and life satisfaction in the veterinarian sample. The data were analyzed using structural equation modeling to control for measurement error in the measures of personality and wellbeing (see https://osf.io/uypz6/for the complete results). We found no notable relationships between openness, agreeableness, conscientiousness, and extraversion with veterinarians' wellbeing or job satisfaction. This finding suggests that the veterinary profession allows individuals with different personality traits to have high levels of wellbeing. However, consistent with the broader literature, neuroticism was a notable, negative predictor of wellbeing. We found 3 mediators of this relationship. Consistent with other studies, the influence of neuroticism on wellbeing (life satisfaction, LS) was mediated by positive effect (PA) and negative affect (NA) [12,27]. More important, job satisfaction was an additional mediator. That is, Neuroticism lowered job satisfaction (b = - .44) and job satisfaction was a unique predictor of life satisfaction, b = 0.29 (see Fig. 1).

These results suggest that neuroticism has a top-down effect on work-related experiences that contribute to overall wellbeing. Neuroticism also influenced other life aspects, but the effect on job satisfaction was by far the strongest. Thus, work-related experiences are important to understanding how neuroticism lowers veterinarians' wellbeing.

This finding shows that the effects of neuroticism on wellbeing are also influenced by factors that are unrelated to being a veterinarian. For individuals, it can be difficult to distinguish between work-related and other aspects of their lives, and some veterinarians may falsely attribute lower wellbeing to their work. A systematic evaluation of life domains may help to avoid this attribution mistake. Moreover, a personality assessment may help to recognize that a negative bias may contribute to dissatisfaction with work.

The third finding is that neuroticism is only one of the many factors that influence job satisfaction. Fig. 1 makes it salient that neuroticism is not the only predictor of job satisfaction. Unexplained factors (ue) also make a substantial contribution to job satisfaction, $b = 0.76$, which in turn also influence life satisfaction, $b = 0.76 * 0.38 = 0.29$. These factors are likely to be environmental factors. A better understanding of these factors can help veterinarians to improve their wellbeing by changing work conditions that are under their control. Yet, it is important to keep the influence of personality in mind. People often overestimate the influence of situational factors on their wellbeing because they are more salient than stable, internal factors. Recognizing the influence of personality is important to avoid futile attempts to improve wellbeing with coping strategies that do not work (eg, changing jobs).

A key limitation of the first study was that work-related experiences were measured with a single, global item. To address this limitation, the second study included 14 specific items about job experiences [4]. This made it possible to compare 2 different top-down models of personality. One model assumes that neuroticism produces a global bias that colors all experiences negatively. The alternative model assumes that people are generally able to regulate their emotions, but that this ability fails under specific circumstances (eg, stressful situations, situations not under control). Accordingly, neuroticism might be negatively related to some work aspects, but not to all of them. Consistent with the later model, we already found in the first wave that neuroticism was more strongly related to work experiences than to other life aspects such as marriage and friendships. Thus, it seemed plausible that neuroticism would also show different relationships to different job aspects.

The data collection for the second wave was similar to the first wave. The main difference in the survey was that we included only neuroticism and extraversion items to measure personality and added 14 questions about specific job aspects. Respondents were asked to rate their agreement or disagreement with each of these dimensions as follows using a 6-point Likert scale,

where 6 represented strongly agree and 1 represented strongly disagree.

1. Absorption: I am often intensely focused on my work and time goes by quickly.
2. Autonomy: I decide how I structure my work and how the work gets done.
3. Contribution: My work makes a positive contribution to other people's lives.
4. Coworkers: I have a warm, friendly, and supportive relationship with my coworkers.
5. Enjoyment: I am enjoying the work that I do.
6. Flexibility: I have flexible work hours and can determine the amount of work I do.
7. Fair pay: I think that I am paid fairly and adequately for my work.
8. Invested: I am invested in my work and take pride in doing a good job.
9. Invigorated: I feel invigorated after working with clients.
10. Learning: I often learn something new at work.
11. Negative climate: A coworker or supervisor is creating a negative work environment.
12. Position/promotion: I am satisfied with my position and promotion opportunities.
13. Supervisor: My supervisor treats me with respect and values my work.
14. Work-life balance: I have a good balance between my work life and my personal life.

Preliminary analysis suggested that one of the 14 items measured global job satisfaction rather than a specific job aspect ("I am enjoying the work that I do"). For statistical reasons this item was excluded from the model to examine the unique contribution of specific aspects to overall job satisfaction. The remaining 13 aspects all made unique contributions to overall job satisfaction and combined accounted for 60% of the variance in job satisfaction. This is close to the reliability of the single-item measure of job satisfaction, suggesting that the job aspects provided a comprehensive assessment of job satisfaction. The 13 aspects also fully mediated the effect of neuroticism on job satisfaction, with an effect size similar to Study 1, ($r = -0.38$ in Study 2 vs. $r = -0.44$ in Study 1). Thus, our list of job aspects seems to capture most of the relevant aspects that contribute to job satisfaction.

We discuss the results for the 13 job aspects in decreasing order of their relationship with neuroticism. By far the strongest relationship was found for the aspect "I have a good balance between my work life and my personal life," $r = -0.73$. One possible explanation for this finding is that neuroticism makes it more difficult for individuals to cope with the stress of a demanding job and other stressors. While the present results do not provide insights into specific problems of neurotic individuals to balance work and non-work related tasks, they do point towards stress as a key factor that lowers job satisfaction and wellbeing.

The aspect with the second strongest relationship to neuroticism was "I have flexible work hours and can determine the amount of work I do," r = −0.46. Although the effect size is still strong, it is notably smaller than the relationship with work-life balance. It seems unlikely that this relationship is due to objective differences in the work conditions of veterinarians high and low in neuroticism. A more likely explanation is that neurotic individuals would prefer to have more control over their work conditions because their actual work conditions have a negative effect on their job satisfaction. Measuring objective and ideal work conditions could help to clarify this relationship.

The next aspect was "I think that I am paid fairly and adequately for my work," r = −0.38. One explanation for this finding could be that pay or compensation is perceived as a compensation for the negative aspects (what economists call disutility) of work. Individuals high in neuroticism are experiencing more disutility and might therefore believe that there are not compensated enough. Alternatively, they might think that higher pay would help them to manage their stress better (eg, paying for services, paying down debt faster). Another possibility is that neuroticism may be related to financial worries, especially for young veterinarians with high student debt, but we did not find a particularly strong effect of neuroticism on financial satisfaction to support this hypothesis.

The fourth aspect was "I decide how I structure my work and how the work gets done," r = −0.35. This finding suggests that neuroticism affects perceptions of autonomy. One explanation is that neurotic individuals may require more autonomy because they may have episodes of negative affect and low energy that make it hard for them to be productive on a fixed schedule. Future research could examine how individuals manage their emotions at work and pinpoint the specific struggles of neurotic individuals to do so. Veterinarians have a reputation for being reluctant to delegate; for example, they would rather pull a blood sample themselves than have a technician draw it. Neuroticism likely contributes to the tendency to do the work themselves rather than trust others do to it perfectly.

The fifth aspect was "I am satisfied with my position and promotion opportunities," r = −0.34. There are various explanations for this finding. First, individuals

high in neuroticism may not be as productive at work as individuals low on neuroticism [28]. These differences may be independent of effort and neurotic individuals may feel unfairly treated, if they work as hard as others without getting similar recognition. Once more, objective indicators would help to disentangle the effects of neuroticism on objective work conditions and perceptions of these conditions.

The sixth aspect was "I feel invigorated after working with clients," r = −0.31. This finding is consistent with evidence that neuroticism is related to higher negative affect and lower positive affect [12,19]. Neurotic individuals may receive fewer emotional benefits from work for a number of reasons. Future research could examine how personality influences responses to positive and negative events at work.

The next 3 aspects are related to social relationships at work: (a) "I have a warm, friendly, and supportive relationship with my co-workers," r = −0.29, .(b) "My supervisor treats me with respect and values my work," r = −0.27, and (c) A coworker or supervisor is creating a negative work environment, r = −0.21. These results are consistent with other evidence that neuroticism can have negative effects on social relationships [21]. This may be particularly true when people work together in a stressful work environment. Indeed, neuroticism was a weak predictor of satisfaction with friendships in Study 1 and Study 2, r = −0.07. The present results suggest that neurotic individuals may benefit from working alone or in smaller clinics rather than in big organizations, but this hypothesis needs to be tested with objective measures of the size of clinic.

The final 4 aspects had relatively weak relationships with neuroticism, r < 0.20. Aspect 10, "My work makes a positive contribution to other people's lives," r = −0.19, shows that neuroticism is only weakly related to perceptions of meaning. Nevertheless, neurotic individuals show a negative bias in their perceptions of meaning. This bias might reflect a tendency to focus on negative events when it was not possible to help a client or an animal had to be euthanized. However, the more important finding is that the effect size of personality is low and that neurotic individuals may especially benefit from doing meaningful work, which contributes to higher job satisfaction. Neuroticism had a very small relationship with "I learn something new at work," r = −0.11. However, this aspect also had a negligible unique relationship with job satisfaction. The 2 items with the weakest relationships reflected intrinsic aspects, namely "I am often intensely focused on my work, and time goes by quickly,"

−0.09, and "I am invested in my work and take pride in doing a good job," r = −0.06. These results are interesting because they show that neuroticism is not a dark cloud that colors all aspects of work. According to our results, even veterinarians high in neuroticism have a favorable attitude towards the work they do. Overall, these results do not support the hypothesis that neuroticism is a general negative bias that influences all aspects of work. The results are more consistent with the hypothesis that neuroticism affects some aspects of work, but not all of them. The biggest effects were observed for aspects related to the external aspects of work with work-balance ranking number 1.

DISCUSSION

Negative effects of neuroticism on mental health and wellbeing have been documented in many populations. Our results provide evidence of the same relationships among veterinarians. Our results also provide evidence for the top-down model of wellbeing [11,12,21]. Most important, we found that top-down effects of neuroticism on job satisfaction contribute to the negative effect of neuroticism on wellbeing. Thus, personality effects on veterinarians' wellbeing are related to their work, pointing to the importance of understanding personality effects on work experiences of veterinarians.

Our investigation of 13 specific job aspects uncovered that neuroticism influences vary across job aspects. The strongest relationship was found for work-life balance. This finding suggests that veterinarians high in neuroticism may benefit especially from life style changes that can improve work-life balance. In contrast, we found only negligible relationships between neuroticism and work aspects that reflect the enjoyment of the work itself (eg, being focused on work, proud of work, time goes by quickly). This suggests that neuroticism has small effects on finding meaning in veterinarian medicine. Rather the problem may be that neuroticism makes it harder for individuals to work long hours and to manage the stress associated with working in veterinarian medicine. Alternatively, it might be possible that they use all of their energy at work and then have little energy left for chores and other demands outside of work. Overall, our results suggest that work-related stress and neuroticism are risk factors that can lead to lower wellbeing and burnout among veterinarians. A closer investigation of these factors may help to develop advice to improve the wellbeing of veterinarians with low wellbeing. We discuss 3 possible strategies to do so.

Reduce neuroticism

nWhile personality psychologists generally consider variation in personality traits to be normal and healthy, it has been difficult to find an upside to Neuroticism. Maybe being sensitive to threats and stressors was more adaptive in the past when life was filled with risks and negative events threatened survival. In modern Western societies, Neuroticism has yet to show some positive effects. Not surprisingly, lowering neuroticism is the most common answer when individuals are asked what aspect of their personality they would like to change [33].

A few intervention studies have examined whether voluntary personality change is possible [33–35] While these studies reported some success in lowering neuroticism at least temporarily, the effect sizes are relatively small. Moreover, longitudinal studies show that adult personality is highly stable [36]. Personality is more stable than weight. Thus, wanting to be considerably less neurotic may be as difficult as losing weight; not impossible, but difficult. On a positive note, however, studies suggest that neuroticism decreases somewhat with age. Similarly, we also observed a negative correlation between age and neuroticism in our study of veterinarians [31]. However, it is unknown what causes this relationship. Thus, it does not help younger veterinarians to increase their well-being.

At the very high end of neuroticism, individuals are at risk of meeting diagnostic criteria of mood disorders, especially during times of prolonged stress [5,18]. Evidence shows that individuals who are suffering from a mood disorder benefit from pharmacological interventions as well as psychotherapy. However, it may also require life-style changes to reduce stress. Our results do suggest that neuroticism in combination with chronic work-related stress is a risk factor for burnout–a state of physical or mental exhaustion accompanied by a sense of reduced personal accomplishment.

In sum, there are currently no proven interventions to reduce neuroticism. Thus, neurotic individuals have to find other ways to avoid burnout and to improve their wellbeing.

Reduce work stressors

An obvious strategy to improve work-life balance is to reduce work or work stressors. However, an equally obvious problem is that workers do not have control over their work condition. Especially young veterinarians with high student debt may feel the need to work long hours to pay down their debt. However, work hours and work conditions of veterinarians vary. Owners, in contrast, may be able to reduce work by hiring more staff or outsourcing some tasks. A closer look at veterinarians with good work-life balance might help to shed light on strategies that can benefit all veterinarians.

Reduce stress outside of work

Psychologists distinguish between big life events and everyday events that can produce stress. Some big stressors may be unavoidable, but daily hassles may be something that individuals can control and manage. How veterinarians spend their time out of work may be just as important for their work-life balance than the time at work. However, we found that satisfaction with hobbies and friendships was a very weak predictor of wellbeing. A much bigger factor was satisfaction with family relationships, including marriage for married veterinarians. This finding suggests that close social relationships are important for wellbeing. While social relationships can produce some challenges to maintain work-life balance, they also provide emotional and instrumental support. This does not mean that we recommend marriage to all single veterinarians, but our results suggest that close social relationships are an important factor that contributes to wellbeing. Our results also suggest that neurotic individuals may benefit especially from these relationships because neuroticism had relatively weak effects on satisfaction with social relationships.

SUMMARY

Our results showed that veterinarians' personality profiles are not very different from the profiles of average Americans. Thus, there does not appear to be a specific personality profile for veterinarians. Veterinarians can have different personalities, and most of this variation is unrelated to their wellbeing. The main exception is neuroticism. Like other neurotic individuals, neurotic veterinarians experience more negative affect, less positive affect, and lower life satisfaction. We found that work experiences contributed to this relationship and that the key factor was low work-life balance. Future research needs to uncover the specific obstacles to work-life balance for neurotic veterinarians to develop strategies that can improve the wellbeing of neurotic individuals. We also found that neuroticism has little influence on the enjoyment of the actual work. This suggests that the neurotic veterinarians could be happy veterinarians if they can find a way to manage the stressors in their lives better.

CLINICS CARE POINTS

- Understanding your personality profile can help you manage your approach to work and stress. For an assessment on the Big Five Personality Traits, go to https://www.merck-animal-health-usa.com/offload-downloads/big-five-mah.

- Understanding personality type can help individuals identify tendencies that can contribute to burnout and lower wellbeing.

- Veterinarians as a group score higher in neuroticism than the general population. Individuals with this characteristic benefit by paying close attention to achieving a good work-life balance.

- Individuals with personalities high in neuroticism tend to be more vulnerable to stress. Veterinary medicine, such as other medical professions, is an inherently stressful profession. Consequently, developing an effective stress management technique is especially valuable and contributes to higher wellbeing.

- How veterinarians spend time outside of work is as important to work-life balance as time at work. Research suggests that fostering close social relationships with family and friends contributes significantly to wellbeing.

REFERENCES

[1] Dicks M, Bain B. Chipping away at the soul: new data on compassion fatigue—and compassion satisfaction—in veterinary medicine. DVM360 Magazine 2016;1–5.
[2] Nett RJ, Witte TK, Holzbauer SM, et al. Risk factors for suicide, attitudes toward mental illness, and practice-related stressors among US veterinarians. J Am Vet Med Assoc 2015;247:945–55.
[3] Volk JO, Schimmack U, Strand EB, et al. Executive summary of the merck animal health veterinary wellbeing study. J Am Vet Med Assoc 2018;252(10):1231–8.
[4] Volk JO, Schimmack U, Strand EB, et al. Executive summary of the merck animal health veterinarian wellbeing Study II. J Am Vet Med Assoc 2020;256(11):1237–44.
[5] Volk JO, Schimmack U, Strand EB, et al. Executive summary of the merck animal health veterinarian wellbeing study III and veterinary support staff study. J Am Vet Med Assoc 2022;260(12):1547–53.
[6] Killingsworth MA, Kahneman D, Mellers B. Income and emotional well-being: a conflict resolved. Proc Natl Acad Sci U S A 2023;120(10):e2208661120.
[7] Lucas RE, Schimmack U. Income and well-being: How big is the gap between the rich and the poor? J Res Pers 2009;43(1):75–8.
[8] Diener E, Helliwell J, Lucas R, et al. Well-being for public policy. New York, NY: Oxford University Press; 2009.

[9] Helliwell JF, Layard R, Sachs JD, et al, editors. World happiness report 2022. New York: Sustainable Development Solutions Network; 2022.

[10] Diener E. Subjective well-being. Psychol Bull 1984;95(3): 542–75.

[11] Brief AP, Butcher AH, George JM, et al. Integrating bottom-up and top-down theories of subjective well-being: the case of health. J Pers Soc Psychol 1993; 64(4):646–53.

[12] Schimmack U, Diener E, Oishi S. Life-satisfaction is a momentary judgment and a stable personality characteristic: the use of chronically accessible and stable sources. J Pers 2002;70(3):345–84.

[13] Yu GB, Lee DJ, Sirgy MJ, et al. Household income, satisfaction with standard of living, and subjective well-being. The moderating role of happiness materialism. J Happiness Stud: An Interdisciplinary Forum on Subjective Well-Being 2020;21(8):2851–72.

[14] Suh E, Diener E, Oishi S, et al. The shifting basis of life satisfaction judgments across cultures: emotions versus norms. J Pers Soc Psychol 1998;74(2):482–93.

[15] Myers IB. The Myers-Briggs type indicator manual. Princeton, NJ: Educational Testing Service. Published online; 1962. https://doi.org/10.1037/14404-000.

[16] Digman JM. Personality structure: emergence of the five-factor model. Annu Rev Psychol 1990;41:417–40.

[17] Paunonen SV, Jackson DN. What is beyond the big five? Plenty! Journal of Personality 2000;68(5):821–35.

[18] Kendler KS, Kuhn J, Prescott CA. The interrelationship of neuroticism, sex, and stressful life events in the prediction of episodes of major depression. Am J Psychiatry 2004;161(4):631–6.

[19] Anglim J, Horwood S, Smillie LD, et al. Predicting psychological and subjective well-being from personality: A meta-analysis. Psychol Bull 2020;146(4):279–323.

[20] Schimmack U, Oishi S, Furr RM, et al. Personality and life satisfaction: a facet-level analysis. Pers Soc Psychol Bull 2004;30(8):1062–75.

[21] Heller D, Watson D, Ilies R. The role of person versus situation in life satisfaction: a critical examination. Psychol Bull 2004;130(4):574–600.

[22] Huang JL, Bramble RJ, Liu M, et al. Rethinking the association between extraversion and job satisfaction: the role of interpersonal job context. J Occup Organ Psychol 2015;89(3):683–91.

[23] Bruk-Lee V, Khoury HA, Nixon AE, et al. Replicating and extending past personality/job satisfaction meta-analyses. Hum Perform 2009;22(2):156–89.

[24] Swider BW, Zimmerman RD. Born to burnout: a meta-analytic path model of personality, job burnout, and work outcomes. J Vocat Behav 2010;76(3):487–506.

[25] Schimmack U, Schupp J, Wagner GG. The influence of environment and personality on the affective and cognitive component of subjective well-being. Soc Indic Res 2000;89:41–60.

[26] Kim H, Schimmack U, Oishi S. Cultural differences in self- and other-evaluations and well-being: a study of European and Asian Canadians. J Pers Soc Psychol 2012; 102(4):856–73.

[27] Schimmack U, Kim H. An integrated model of social psychological and personality psychological perspectives on personality and wellbeing. J Res Pers 2020;84. https://doi.org/10.1016/j.jrp.2019.103888:Article 103888.

[28] Zell E, Lesick TL. Big five personality traits and performance: a quantitative synthesis of 50+ meta-analyses. J Pers 2022;90(4):559–73.

[29] Alderotti G, Chiara R, Silvio T. The Big Five personality traits and earnings: a meta-analysis. J Econ Psychol 2023;94. https://doi.org/10.1016/j.joep.2022.102570.

[30] Freedman Vicki A. The Panel study of income Dynamics' well being and daily life supplement (PSID-WB); user guide, final release 1. Ann Arbor, MI: University of Michigan; 2017 Institute for Social Research Available at: https://psidonline.isr.umich.edu/WB/WBUserGuide.pdf.

[31] Schimmack U, Strand EB, Volk JO. A top-down, bottom-up model of personality effects on veterinarians' well-being. Manuscript in Preparation. 2023

[32] Cohen J. Statistical power analysis for the behavioral sciences. 2nd edition. New York, NY: Lawrence Erlbaum Associates, Publishers; 1988.

[33] Hudson NW, Briley DA, Chopik WJ, et al. You have to follow through: attaining behavioral change goals predicts volitional personality change. J Pers Soc Psychol 2019;117(4):839–57.

[34] Stieger M, Flückiger C, Rüegger D, et al. Changing personality traits with the help of a digital personality change intervention. Proc Natl Acad Sci U S A 2021; 118(8):2017548118.

[35] Olaru G, Stieger M, Rüegger D, et al. Personality change through a digital-coaching intervention: Using measurement invariance testing to distinguish between trait domain, facet, and nuance change. Eur J Pers 2022; 0(0). https://doi.org/10.1177/08902070221145088.

[36] Anusic I, Schimmack U. Stability and change of personality traits, self-esteem, and well-being: Introducing the meta-analytic stability and change model of retest correlations. J Pers Soc Psychol 2016;110(5):766–81.

Advances in Small Animal Care 4 (2023) 133–144

ADVANCES IN SMALL ANIMAL CARE

Practice Culture

The Golden Ticket to Increasing Well-Being in Practice

Josh Vaisman, MAPPCP (PgD)

Flourish Veterinary Consulting, 10279 Dover Street, Firestone, CO 80504, USA

KEYWORDS
• Culture • Well-being • Leadership • Retention • Turnover

KEY POINTS
- Recent research suggests many veterinarians and veterinary support staff struggle with burnout, psychological distress, and low well-being.
- Workplace climate can impact veterinary professionals' experience of burnout, psychological distress, and well-being.
- Specifically, veterinary professionals who work in environments with a high sense of belonging, high degree of organizational trust, candid and open communication, and ample time to provide high-quality care, report significantly lower burnout and psychological distress and higher well-being.
- Veterinary leaders can develop and employ specific behaviors to encourage and enable the four workplace climate qualities that appear to support veterinary well-being.

INTRODUCTION

In many ways, veterinary professionals are like a seed from a large tree, full of potential and possibility. As with actual seeds, when planted in an environment that provides crucial nutrients, they sprout and grow. So long as the new plant is continually nurtured, it will thrive. Absent these nutrients, wilting is inevitable. If we are to think of veterinarians, technicians, and other members of a veterinary team as seeds, it can be helpful to think of the environment they practice in—the workplace culture—as the soil in which they will thrive or wilt.

Veterinary professionals are as much a result of the environment they work in as they are contributing members to it. To wit, their well-being is influenced by that environment. Tim Lomas, Kate Hefferon, and Itai Ivtzan, pioneers in third-wave positive psychology, argue for a systems-thinking approach to well-being. They make the case that while we are all individuals with unique lived experiences, we are also, "…inextricably embedded in sociocultural networks that sustain [or inhibit]," well-being [1].

Recent research seems to confirm this, suggesting that veterinarians and support staff employed in positive work climates are more likely to report high levels of well-being [2]. This article will explore the four key elements of a healthy veterinary workplace environment and the role they play in supporting veterinary well-being. Furthermore, this article will discuss the role leaders play in crafting healthy veterinary workplace environments that support team members' well-being.

SIGNIFICANCE

In a lecture attended by this article's author in 2017, Dr Martin Seligman, Director of the University of Pennsylvania Positive Psychology Center, shared his belief that the absence of illness is not necessarily wellness. Seligman argues that well-being is not simply the absence of suffering, but the presence of *at least* five essential psychological elements: positive emotions, engagement, positive relationships, meaning, and achievement (PERMA) [3].

E-mail address: josh@flourish.vet

https://doi.org/10.1016/j.yasa.2023.04.002
2666-450X/23/

Seligman's PERMA model has spurred, among many things, a call for culture change in medical schools [4].

It seems clear that employees are influenced and impacted by the workplace environment to which they are routinely exposed. To that end, Julie Butler and Margaret L. Kern developed a tool to measure PERMA, called the PERMA-Profiler [5]. A workplace version of the tool has also been developed and used to identify, among other things, relationships between PERMA and individual work outcomes [6]. As Seligman's influence on well-being and happiness studies has permeated the literature for the last 20 years, workplace well-being seems to have become a common concern as a result.

Citing "growing concern … about mental distress and suicide among veterinarians," the first Merck Animal Health Veterinary Wellbeing Study was launched to assess general mental health and well-being among current veterinarians. The results of the study were published in the *Journal of the American Veterinary Medical Association* in 2018 [7]. The study has been repeated biennially since, with the most recent executive summary published in 2022.

The initial study found that veterinarians report slightly lower well-being than the general US population (Fig. 1). However, while male veterinarians reported better well-being than the general male US population, female veterinarians reported worse well-being than the general US female population. This may be of importance as the American Veterinary Medical Association suggests the percentage of female veterinarians is growing [8].

The 2021 Merck Animal Healthy Veterinary Wellbeing Study (the third edition of this biennial study) was unique compared to the prior two studies in at least two distinct ways:

1. It included responses from veterinary support staff (prior studies were exclusive to veterinarians).

2. It sought to measure the relationship between workplace climate and team members' mental health and well-being.

Nearly 2500 veterinarians participated in the third study alongside 448 veterinary support staff. Overall, well-being among veterinarians has not significantly changed across the three studies (Fig. 2). However, the third study discovered a large difference in well-being between veterinarians and support staff, with support staff reporting significantly lower overall well-being (Fig. 3).

The study identified several correlates to veterinary well-being and mental health. For example, the personality trait of neuroticism was the strongest predictor of low well-being, serious psychological distress, and high levels of burnout among veterinarians. This correlation closely matched findings from the prior two veterinary well-being studies. Furthermore, "having a healthy coping method was the strongest predictor of high well-being, low burnout," and the absence of serious psychological distress among participants.

Certainly, individual characteristics influence the presence or absence of workplace well-being and mental health. However, as mentioned above, one of the unique aspects of the third edition of the Merck Veterinary Wellbeing Study was the measurement of participant perception of workplace climate. The study sought to measure 15 factors thought to relate to workplace climate. Multiple regression analysis found that of these 15 factors, four defined a healthy practice culture. Those four factors are

1. A strong sense of belonging to a team.
2. A high degree of trust in the organization.
3. Candid, open communication within the team.
4. Sufficient time for each appointment to provide high-quality care.

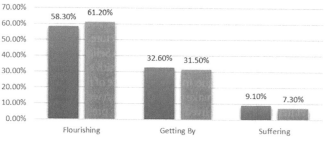

FIG. 1 Veterinarian well-being compared to US general population. (*Data from* Volk JO, Schimmack U, Strand EB, Lord LK, Siren CW. Executive summary of the Merck Animal Health Veterinary Wellbeing Study. J Am Vet Med Assoc. 2018;252(10):1231-1238.)

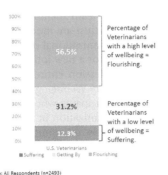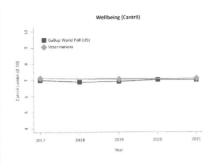

Base: All Respondents (n=2493)

FIG. 2 Veterinarian well-being over time. (*From* Veterinary Mental Health and Wellbeing and How to Improve Them. Learnings from the Merck Animal Health Veterinarian Wellbeing Study III. January 2022. https://www.merck-animal-health-usa.com/wp-content/uploads/sites/54/2022/02/2021-PSV-Veterinary-Wellbeing-Presentation_V2.pdf.)

In the executive summary, the study authors note, "The impact [of a healthy practice culture] was significant. Having a healthy practice culture was second only to a healthy coping mechanism in predicting high well-being, low burnout, and a lack of serious psychological distress." They go on to recommend veterinary employers' work to develop workplace climates that mirror these four factors of healthy practice culture.

A Strong Sense of Belonging

A need to connect with other people in meaningful ways is as essential to human psychology as breathing is to our biology. One critical way this need manifests in the human psyche is in our drive to experience belongingness. In fact, some research suggests the need to belong may be a hardwired feature of the human brain. The human brain at rest appears to default

to neural activity that matches activity when we engage in social connection. Gao and colleagues found this default neural network active in infants as young as 2 weeks old [9].

Psychologists have long argued that the need to belong is a fundamental human drive, a necessary condition for psychological well-being. According to Baumeister and Leary, the drive to belong is satisfied when people have frequent, enduring, positive interactions with other people who appear to share a mutual concern for each other's welfare [10].

The benefits of experiencing belongingness are myriad, including better social connection, improved personal and professional performance, and stronger mental and physical health [11]. In one study, a social belonging intervention led to improvements in academic and health outcomes among young minority

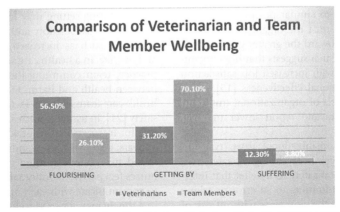

FIG. 3 Comparison of veterinarian and staff well-being. (*Data from* Volk JO, Schimmack U, Strand EB, et al. Executive summary of the Merck Animal Health Veterinarian Wellbeing Study III and Veterinary Support Staff Study. J Am Vet Med Assoc. 2022;260(12):1547-1553. Published 2022 Jul 1.)

students [12]. In the 2021 Merck Wellbeing Study work team belongingness was highly predictive of higher levels of well-being, lower burnout, and lower risk of serious psychological distress. In fact, participants who were not psychologically distressed were more than twice as likely to report belongingness in their team.

Trust in the Organization

In an organizational context, trust can be defined as the willingness to behave and accept vulnerability, "based upon positive expectations of the intentions or behavior of another." [13] In other words, team members who believe the intentions of other team members are positive tend to trust those fellow team members. Team members who believe the organization's intentions are positive (eg, as represented by the behaviors of a hospital manager, practice leadership, an entity's ownership, etc.) tend to have a high level of trust in the organization.

In relationships, trust tends to contribute to a higher-quality connection between individuals. Relationships high in trust are more collaborative and cooperative, and individuals will perceive each other as members of the same unit, sometimes referred to as "in-grouping" [14]. The psychological attachment of in-grouping can be a powerful connective force resulting in a high level of interpersonal commitment and prosocial behavior. Of note, trust appears to be reciprocal. When another individual places their trust in us, we tend to reciprocate with trustworthy behavior. This applies in both directions and, as such, trust seems to beget trust, building connection.

The social contract between employee and employer is, in many ways, like the psychological agreements within interpersonal relationships. As such, organizational trust likely leads to similar positive outcomes. Presumably, those who trust the organization will be more willing to "work toward the greater good" of the relationship. In fact, research suggests that high organizational trust is linked with increased job satisfaction and perceived organizational effectiveness [15]. Team members with high levels of organizational trust tend to be higher performers and report lower turnover intention [16].

A unique form of organizational trust, typically localized at the team level, is psychological safety. We can think of psychological safety as a belief that interpersonal risks, such as admitting to an error or asking for help, can be taken in the workplace without risk of punishment or retribution [17]. In other words, team members trust that they will not be unduly punished for speaking up. A survey conducted in 2022 found

that veterinary team members who have this kind of organizational trust are more likely to report job satisfaction and organizational commitment, and less likely to be looking for a new job or considering leaving the veterinary profession entirely (Fig. 4) [18]. The 2021 Merck Veterinary Wellbeing Study echoed this, finding that study participants who reported a high degree of trust in the organization in which they were employed were more likely to report high well-being and less likely to report psychological distress or burnout.

Candid, Open Communication Within the Team

Effective communication is an essential element of a high-performing team. Defined as the exchange of information, high-quality communication within teams can benefit interpersonal relationships, individual and team learning, error avoidance, and overall team performance [19]. In some research, the quality and valence of inter-team communication are highly predictive of a team's perceived performance, as judged by the organization in which they work [20]. Specifically, team communication was measured along three metrics: positive (supportive, encouraging, or appreciate) v. negative (disapproving, sarcastic, or critical) language, inquisitive (curiosity, asking questions) v. self-advocacy (explaining, defending a position) style, and "other" focused v. self-focused approaches. Teams that were more positive than negative, more inquisitive than self-advocating, and more other-focused than self-focused were significantly more likely to be deemed high-performing by organization leadership.

In a health care setting, the quality of team communication may be of exceptional importance. The outcomes of effective communication in, say, a manufacturing setting may lead to personal outcomes such as job satisfaction and engagement or business outcomes such as increased production of "widgets" and the like. In a health care setting, such as a veterinary practice, team communication may be the difference between health and harm. Effective communication in health care teams may, in fact, directly influence patient safety [21]. In teams of nurses, the belief that the team is safe for interpersonal risk-taking (psychological safety) appears to predict the candid, open communication found in effective learning environments [22]. When nurses feel psychologically safe, they appear more likely to communicate with each other candidly, openly, and in a timely manner so as to limit mistakes, improve co-learning, and provide better medicine. As a result, medical errors are significantly less common in these environments.

	POSITIVE LEADERSHIP PRACTICES HAPPENING	POSITIVE LEADERSHIP PRACTICES NOT HAPPENING
Consider quitting job	Rarely	Often
Consider leaving profession	Rarely	Sometime
Happy with job	Agree	Disagree
Perceived Wellbeing	Doing well	Getting by
Psychological Safety	High	Low

FIG. 4 The positive leadership difference in veterinary workplaces.

Furthermore, psychological safety allows for a style of candid, open communication that fosters improved interpersonal relationships and connections. Nurses who feel psychologically safe tend to report their work relationships as supportive and trusting [23]. In this way, candid communication may contribute to a great sense of belonging and improve the quality of workplace relationships, a strong predictor of overall job satisfaction [24].

The 2021 Merck Veterinary Wellbeing Study found that for veterinarians and support staff, candid and open communication was predictive of higher levels of well-being, lower prevalence of burnout, and a decreased likelihood of experiencing psychological distress. The 2022 Flourish Leadership & Workplace Experience study found a strong positive relationship between team psychological safety and team member job satisfaction and organizational commitment as well as a negative relationship to turnover intention.

Sufficient time to provide high-quality care
Veterinary professionals come to the work of veterinary medicine in large part to fulfill a desire to serve the health and well-being of animals [25]. Some form of quality clinical outcomes is among the most cited sources of job satisfaction among surveyed veterinarians. Early career veterinarians cite the ability to effectively communicate with clients among the most important skills, even beyond technical skills [26]. This may be in part to their desire to provide sufficient and effective care for both the patient and client.

The 2021 Merck Veterinary Wellbeing Study found that a participant's agreement that they had sufficient time to provide high-quality care correlated positively with well-being and negatively with burnout and serious psychological distress.

The Role Leaders Play in Crafting Positive Veterinary Work Climates

A full-time team member working approximately 40 hours per week spends almost one-quarter of their entire week in the workplace. With veterinary professionals often citing an imbalance in work–life balance, marked by working hours beyond the norm, it is likely the typical veterinarian or technician is spending significantly more than 25% of their time at work.

Clearly, workplace experiences carry weight and influence over all areas of life. In fact, one large-scale survey suggests that 25% of the variance in life satisfaction scores are explained by job satisfaction [24]. The same survey found that almost 40% of job satisfaction ratings are explained by the quality of relationships at work, of which nearly 90% of them explained by how team members rate the quality of the relationship they have with their direct leader. When it comes to workplace experience, leadership matters.

Veterinarians in the United States take an oath to, "... use my scientific knowledge and skills for the benefit of society," and prevent and alleviate suffering. This author argues that those of us in leadership positions within veterinary organizations hold a moral obligation to mirror the veterinary oath by preventing and alleviating workplace suffering for veterinary professionals and using our knowledge and skill to benefit them so they might best benefit society. Recognizing not every leader is compelled by a moral imperative, leaders may be further be implored with a business case. One meta-analysis found that, across a variety of business types (including health care units), team member job satisfaction correlated positively with a variety of business outcomes, including productivity, profit, customer satisfaction, and employee retention [27]. Considering the impact leaders appear to have on team member job satisfaction, it behooves leaders to develop and implement behaviors, actions, policies, and programs that improve or enhance the workplace climate.

Where is a leader to begin? Below are suggestions to improve the four factors found to correlate with a positive work climate in veterinary organizations.

Improving belonging within a team

An attempt to understand the experience of belonging at work might solicit discomfort in a leader attempting to cultivate and amplify it in their organization. On the one hand, there is simplicity in the concept. Most team members, when queried with a simple binary question, "Do you feel as if you belong here?", will respond quickly with confidence. Many "know" the answer almost instinctually.

Complexity arises in the "why" behind the response. The experience itself is highly subjective, driven by both an individual's lived experience and their interpretation of that experience. For a veterinary leader trying to cultivate belonging within their team, this reality may make the effort feel daunting. Of course, given the positive impact belonging seems to have in veterinary workplaces, the effort is a worthy one.

Although the antecedents to workplace belongingness can be highly subjective, there may exist some common threads linking lived experience with the result of belonging. A veterinary leader could leverage these threads to cultivate a workplace environment in which belonging is more likely to emerge among the team. Three of these threads are

1. Belonging as being accepted and valued in a social environment [28].
2. Belonging as being a part of something [29].
3. Belonging as performing together [29].

Of note, this is where we might make the important, if subtle, distinction between "belonging" and "inclusion". In the context of this article, think of inclusion as the efforts and actions leaders take to include team members in the work environment. For example, when a leader asks a team member for their opinion or invites that team member to contribute to a project they have chosen to include them. Belonging is the subjective feeling within a team member based on inclusive efforts. Put another way, inclusion is the nutritious diet that, when balanced and offered in

the right amounts, enables the vitalizing experience of belongingness.

Based on experience in veterinary hospital leadership, positive psychology practice, and veterinary workplace culture consulting, the following are offered as opportunities for current veterinary leaders to cultivate more belonging within their teams.

CULTIVATING ACCEPTANCE AND VALUE

Onboarding is a critical time in a team member's journey with an organization. The onboarding experience can impact integration into the team and organizational culture. Some surveys have found that team members who rate their onboarding experience as excellent may be nearly 70% more likely to remain with the organization 3 years later [30].

Research has found that in organizations where a formalized new-employee support program is in place, outcomes like organizational commitment are significantly higher, likely contributing to better retention, job satisfaction, and an improved sense of belonging by increasing prosocial behavior and experience [31]. Of interest, the support programs not only appear to benefit the incoming new team member but also the "supporter". Team members who provide support in welcoming new employees also show an increased sense of organizational commitment (and likely belonging).

The keyword here is "support". These programs were not about training and skill development (eg, integrating the new team member into their job role). Rather, the goal of the program is to provide the new team member with a ready-made "work buddy" whose role is to welcome them into the team, get to know their strengths and values, introduce them throughout the organization, and help them integrate into the social fabric of the workplace. In doing so, they are likely to cultivate a sense of acceptance and value early on in the onboarding process.

Veterinary leaders can leverage this approach in at least two ways; during the onboarding process and throughout the employment journey. By implementing a "work buddy" program hospital leaders are in essence delegating belongingness interventions across the entire team, both increasing the opportunity to instill a sense of acceptance and value early in a new team member's tenure and empowering the entire team to develop high-quality connections. Then, leaders can continue the effort in ongoing interactions with team members, well beyond the onboarding phase. For example, managers can use motivational interviewing in one-on-one sessions to explore each team member's strengths and contributions, thus reinvigorating the sense of value.

BEING A PART OF SOMETHING

One veterinary practice utilizes a unique culture assimilation program. The interview process for all positions is a group effort. Multiple members of the team are included in all interviews and are prompted to identify the "must-have" qualities in all potential new hires. When a decision is made to add someone to the team, each interviewer is asked by management to share their answer to this question: "What is the one thing about this person that made you feel they absolutely had to be a part of our team?" They are coached to seek out qualities that will add to or amplify the current culture and goals of the hospital.

Shortly after their start date, new team members sit in on a "culture talk" with one of the hospital owners or core leaders. They learn about the practice's history, aspirations and values, cultural norms and expectations, and how they came to be. Each new team member is also told, often in front of multiple other new hires, what interviewers said were the "must-have" qualities they bring to the team and organization. It is framed in this way: "This is who we hope to be and the impact we strive to have. This is why we needed you on the team to help us get there." In this way, they instill early on that new team members are not just filling an empty seat, they are on the team because they bring valuable qualities that make the whole team better. They are a part of something.

Another practice implemented a community volunteer program that is likely to enhance belonging in at least two important ways. The program includes community service conducted on a rotational basis (eg, quarterly). For each community service event, team members are recruited from various departments across the large organization. Alongside key hospital leaders, they participate in meaningful volunteer activities in the community. This shared effort making a meaningful impact in the community writ large instills a sense of being a part of something that matters within the participants. It also builds bridges and breaks down barriers between inter-hospital silos. In these ways, a sense of belonging grows.

PERFORMING TOGETHER

Achieving things together in meaningful ways may be helpful in instilling a sense of belonging among teams. This path to belonging can manifest in a variety of ways from shared activities both inside and outside the workplace to accomplishing meaningful goals together. It can also come from a team member's belief that they are involved in important workplace decisions.

Team building through shared activities outside of work may be a valuable endeavor for building a sense of collective performance and belonging. For example, the community service program discussed above may enable both a sense of "being a part of something" and mutual performance among participating team members. One veterinary hospital has a longstanding annual tradition of inviting the entire team to participate in a pseudo-competitive event such as a Tough Mudder. These events involve timed obstacle courses in which a sense of competition and camaraderie is found by timing the event, creating a community environment, and limiting the competitive aspects to "self-competition". That is, participants do not win an award for finishing ahead of others. Rather, they are competing against their own time and the personal capacity to complete the course. Competitors find these events invigorating, uplifting, and empowering, and tend to find a sense of belonging within the Tough Mudder community.

This practice further enhances these benefits by inviting the entire team to participate either as a competitor or a cheering observer. Participation is fully funded by the hospital and matching shirts are made and distributed. Team members have a voice in designing the shirts and team photos are captured and shared internally and externally during the event. In this way, the team comes together and bonds over a challenging and fun experience.

Within the hospital, leaders can enable the benefits of co-performance by

- Actively including team members in tasks, activities, and events.
- Inviting the team's perspective in decision-making both in group contexts such as team meetings.
- Encouraging "cross-pollination" by exposing team members to work outside their normal role or department.
- Establish a goal-setting structure in which individual and workgroup goals are clearly tied to the greater goals of the organization.
- Celebrating (and rewarding) collective accomplishments in addition to or above individual performance.

Building Organizational Trust and Cultivating Open Communication

Trust and communication may be inextricably linked in the workplace and so both are included together here.

As discussed above, in the context of work, trust can be defined as a team member's positive expectations regarding the intentions and expected behaviors of the people and structures within and throughout the organization. When trust is present, team members are more likely to adopt a willingness to be vulnerable [32]. Willingness to be vulnerable is a driver of a type of psychological safety that encourages open communication within teams likely, at least in part, due to the minimized risk of retribution or humiliation for speaking candidly.

Vis a vis when a team member uses their voice and experiences what feels to them like punishment or humiliation, trust erodes likely mediated by a loss in psychological safety. If that experience involves hospital leadership (either directly or indirectly), trust in the organization may erode globally. As trust erodes, team members are likely to at best measure their candor or, worse, withhold perspectives or opinions. This contributes to a decrease in open, candid communication.

Some research suggests a close relationship between psychological safety and both organizational trust and navigating group conflict (one element of open, candid communication) [33]. This is important because trust and effective communication drive goal achievement, learning and development, innovation, and effective teaming. Psychological safety appears to be an antecedent to organizational trust and candid communication. All this is to argue that to cultivate organizational trust and open candid communication within their teams, veterinary leaders should focus first on developing psychologically safe workplaces (Fig. 5).

A culture of psychological safety is cultivated through an interpersonal action and response loop. In nearly every interpersonal interaction in a workplace environment, some sort of response occurs (even a non-response is deemed to be a form of response). In essence, each response is categorized as either "supportive" or "harmful". Supportive responses tend to build trust and encourage further communication. Harmful responses tend to erode trust and encourage interpersonal withholding. Either way, future interactions are influenced by the lived experience of prior interactions. In this way, communication is a dynamic, ever-changing aspect of the workplace environment.

In a veterinary setting, a variety of team members in a variety of roles are routinely interacting. As such, psychological safety is constantly evolving within and throughout the team and every team member is influencing its evolution. However, those team members who are formal (by title or role) or informal (by influence or tenure, for example) leaders have the greatest influence over the norms that enhance or deplete team psychological safety [34].

Leaders can cultivate a greater sense of psychological safety among their team and encourage trust-building and candid communication in a variety of ways. Three examples include
1. Behavioral Modeling
2. Inviting Voice
3. Productive Response

BEHAVIORAL MODELING

Veterinary team members tend to look to their leads, supervisors, managers, directors, and other leadership roles for examples of behaviors that are encouraged or accepted. That is to say, leaders are tone-setters for cultural norms. In the case of organizational trust and open communication, it behooves leaders to define these terms for themselves, consider the observable outcomes of a culture in which those definitions are being lived out, and to adopt intentional behaviors likely to nurture such a culture. In the book, "Lead to Thrive: The Science of Crafting a Positive Veterinary Culture", Vaisman (2023) describes culture as a set of behaviors

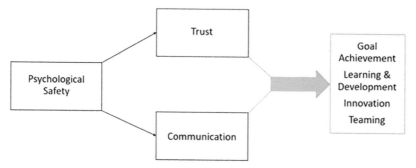

FIG. 5 Psychological safety drives trust and communication.

that occur consistently enough to become a habit which, in turn, drive norms and expectations of "how we do things here" [35]. For leaders, this begins with modeling.

For example, a leader may envision a psychologically safe culture in which team members view mistakes or shortcomings as collective learning opportunities. An observable outcome of such a culture may include trusting, open conversations in which team members explore procedural improvements to avoid future mistakes. To model this outcome, leaders could take note of their own mistakes or shortcomings and find the opportunity to share them candidly and vulnerably with their team. They could further model the learning environment they wish to nurture by either describing what they have learned (and how they plan to improve) or inviting problem-solving interaction with the team (eg, "What do you think I should do differently?").

The "Error Audit" program is a tool to systematically embed psychological safety enhancing behavioral modeling in a workplace environment. Typically applied during structured meeting time, such as team or all-staff meetings, this can begin with an individual in a leadership position sharing a recent error, stumble, or shortcoming *in front of the team* and describing what they have learned through the challenge. Once normalized, the program can shift to a rotation in which both leaders and team members are included.

INVITING VOICE

It can be suggested that veterinary team members desire a workplace with high trust and candid communication because they value a healthy, productive form of dissent called "intellectual tension". That is, veterinary team members are likely driven to learn and develop skills and practices so that they may deliver high-quality medical care. However, when trust is low, communication manifests in unhealthy ways. Low trust in a candid environment tends to appear as rumination, complaining, bickering, or worse. These are the workplace environments many refer to as "toxic". Low trust in the absence of candid communication may, at first glance, appear calm, peaceful, and even inviting. This deceptive façade is indicative of a complete absence of healthy intellectual tension. In the former, silos form and interpersonal relationships suffer. In the latter, apathy sets in as individual and team growth and development stagnate (Fig. 6).

To prevent or counteract these environments, leaders can invite intellectual tension. To begin, veterinary leaders can seek opportunities to utilize curiosity. For example, when discussing policies, procedures, new

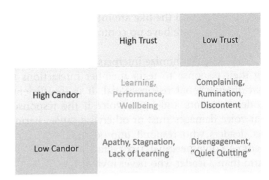

FIG. 6 Outcomes of trust and candor in a work environment.

ideas, and the like, leaders can build a habit of asking questions such as

- "What do you think?"
- "Thanks for sharing your perspective. That's one possible view, what's another?"
- "What am I missing?"
- "What would make this better?"

As with behavioral modeling, an opportunity exists here to both formalize and normalize intellectual tension in team meetings. Leaders can assign a "voice of dissent" for each team meeting to be sure that at least some form of intellectual tension exists. Some suggestions for successful implementation of an assigned dissenter include

- Establish a clear purpose. We are not assigning someone to dissent simply for the sake of dissent. Their counter perspective should have a purpose. For example, to help us improve our policies and procedures by finding their flaws.
- Assign one individual.
- Provide clear guidelines. When will this person speak up? For how long?
- Rotate the assignment. Do not assign the same person at every meeting.

Leaders can then invite healthy dissension for a specific, learning-focused purpose. They can also guide the conversation in a healthy way, providing coaching when necessary.

PRODUCTIVE RESPONSE

In teams seeking to develop a culture of trust and candid communication, psychological safety is a necessary condition. Psychological safety is cultivated through interpersonal interaction and is heavily influenced by how individuals feel during and after these interactions. In a work environment, speaking up, productively challenging, admitting mistakes or shortcomings, and the like are interpersonally risking actions because we have no control over the response of others.

Leaders can minimize interpersonal risk by managing their response to team member interactions that have interpersonal risk potential. It is insufficient to model behaviors and invite voice if the response to that voice damages trust or otherwise causes harm. In fact, leaders who respond unproductively to a team member's interpersonal risk-taking may cause more harm than a leader who never invited voice in the first place. Put another way, it is in the response that psychological safety is built or demolished.

Some actions supportive of productive response might include

- Hit the pause button. Leaders should develop a habit of noticing when they are becoming defensive and pause before responding. This pause can be brief or may even include a request to reconvene the conversation at a later time.
- Consider possible alternatives. All brains are built to tell stories. Often the stories in our minds are inaccurate. When a team member shares something interpersonally risky, especially when the information they share makes us upset, one way to manage our response could be to challenge ourselves to imagine an explanation that gives that person the benefit of the doubt.
- Practice gratitude. Always thank team members for using their voice, even when what they say upsets us or goes against our perception. Remember, there is power in the word, "and". For example, if a team member shares a failure with us, we can practice gratitude and hold them accountable *at the same time* with a response like, "I'm disappointed in this mistake and I'm grateful you've brought it to me so we can work through it together."

Leaders that model psychologically safe behaviors, invite voice and perspective, and respond productively to the interpersonal risk of speaking up, nurture a loop that builds trust and encourages productive communication.

Providing Sufficient Time for High-Quality Patient Care

This author does not feign expertise in operational efficiencies nor intends to offer suggestions for providing team members with sufficient time for each appointment. In truth, how team members define "sufficient time" and "high-quality care" likely differs from practice to practice. Recommendations for improvement here may be highly contextual.

That said, leaders play a critical role in improving this metric for their team. First and foremost, hospital leaders typically hold purview over the variable that impact a team's perception of patient care. Leadership tends to dictate appointment duration, frequency, and types on the hospital schedule. It is often hospital leaders who assess role needs, facilitate recruitment and hiring, and set the staff schedules. Furthermore, leadership establishes, communicates, and manages hospital goals which likely impact where and how a team's efforts are directed. Finally, leaders are directly responsible for the training and development of their teams and individual team members.

From appointment duration to service efficiency, as with psychological safety, leaders have the most influence. Of course, leaders are often not providing patient care or may only be privy to their unique experience. Understanding the day-to-day experience of the team, how that experience matches or deviates from their values, and exploring actionable steps to improving both efficiency and quality of care should be a primary goal for veterinary practice leaders. Who best to make that picture clear than the team members living it each day?

Proactive, positive leaders can leverage the lessons above (building belonging and psychological safety) to cultivate practice efficiency and patient care and ensure team members find the time they have to provide the said care feels sufficient and effective. Proactive, positive leaders can leverage the above lessons (building belonging and psychological safety) to ensure team members have the time they need to deliver high-quality care. Then, explore where things are already efficient and high-quality as well as areas for improvement. Invite collective exploration of possible adjustments, changes, and solutions to bridge the gap between the current state and your team's ideal. As a group, select an intervention to experiment with, establishing the details necessary to implement, play with, and assess its success. Apply the intervention and, after a predetermined time, analyze its efficacy with the team. Adjust accordingly.

In this way, leaders are not only facilitating improvements in practice efficiency and patient care, they are engendering a greater sense of belonging and psychological safety.

DISCUSSION AND FUTURE INVESTIGATION

Workplace well-being and employee outcomes such as burnout, psychological distress, and turnover intention, appear to be influenced both by individual variables and the workplace climate. Recent studies support this assertion in the veterinary profession, suggesting that a veterinary professional's experience in the practice environment may be a primary driver of these outcomes for them. Throughout the literature, we find that workplace leadership is highly influential when it comes to workplace climate and experience. Therefore, veterinary leaders who envision a workplace in which team members stay, perform at their best and thrive in and through their work should consider practices, policies, and behaviors likely to enhance those outcomes. For example, leaders who enable belongingness and psychological safety among their teams, and facilitate sufficient time for their teams to provide high-quality care are more likely to develop thriving teams.

This article has leveraged literature and experience to suggest methods leaders can apply to that end. However, the literature is limited in scope and veracity. Although recent studies have uncovered several antecedents to these desired workplace experiences, little experimental research exists offering specific approaches. Although evidence-based, the suggestions in this article are not borne of a controlled study. In the future, this area of study would benefit from research focused on testing interventions meant to enhance belongingness, organizational trust, candid communication, and the like in the veterinary setting.

CLINICS CARE POINTS

- Leadership practices influence workplace climate and employee experience in veterinary settings.
- To enable belongingness in their workplaces, leaders can cultivate acceptance, build up employee self-worth, instill cultural norms, and craft opportunities for collaborative and inclusive work.
- To build trust and encourage candid, open communication, leaders can build a culture of psychological safety with behavioral modeling, inviting employee voice, and productive interpersonal response.
- Leaders can work to enhance workplace efficiency by inviting the team to share their day-to-day experience, exploring efficiency improvement together, experimenting with initiatives, and collectively analyzing their efficacy.

DISCLOSURE

The author is the founder and Lead Positive Change Agent at Flourish Veterinary Consulting, a for-profit organization focused on positive leadership and culture development in veterinary practices.

REFERENCES

[1] Lomas T, Hefferon K, Ivtzan I. The LIFE Model: A Meta-Theoretical Conceptual Map for Applied Positive Psychology. J Happiness Stud 2015;16(5):1347–64.

[2] Volk JO, Schimmack U, Strand EB, et al. Executive summary of the Merck Animal Health Veterinarian Wellbeing Study III and Veterinary Support Staff Study. J Am Vet Med Assoc 2022;260(12):1547–53.

[3] Seligman M. PERMA and the building blocks of well-being. J Posit Psychol 2018;13(4):333–5.

[4] Slavin SJ, Schindler D, Chibnall JT, et al. PERMA: A Model for Institutional Leadership and Culture Change. Acad Med 2012;87(11):1481.

[5] Butler J, Kern ML. The PERMA-Profiler: A brief multidimensional measure of flourishing. International Journal of Wellbeing 2016;6(3):1–48.

[6] Yang CC, Wantanabe K, Kawakami N. The Associations Between Job Strain, Workplace PERMA Profiler, and Work Engagement. J Occup Environ Med 2022;64(5):409–15.

[7] Volk JO, Schimmack U, Strand EB, et al. Executive summary of the Merck Animal Health Veterinary Wellbeing Study. J Am Vet Med Assoc 2018;252(10):1231–8.

[8] Nolen R S. Women practice owners projected to overtake men within a decade. In: AVMA website. 2020. Available at: https://www.avma.org/javma-news/2020-12-15/women-practice-owners-projected-overtake-men-within-decade. Accessed March 2, 2023.

[9] Gao W, Zhu H, Giovanello KS, et al. Evidence on the emergence of the brain's default network from 2-week-old to 2-year-old healthy pediatric subjects. Proc Natl Acad Sci U S A 2009;106(16):6790–5.

[10] Baumeister RF, Leary MR. The Need to Belong: Desire for Interpersonal Attachments as a Fundamental Human Motivation. Psychol Bull 1995;117(3):497–529.

[11] Allen KA, Kern ML, Rozek CS, et al. A Review of Conceptual Issues, an Integrative Framework, and Directions for Future Research. Aust J Psychol 2020;73(1):87–102.

[12] Walton GW, Cohen GL. A brief social-belonging intervention improves academic and health outcomes of minority students. Science 2011;331(6023):1447–51.

[13] Rousseau DM, Burt RS, Camerer C. Not so different after all: a cross-discipline view of trust. Acad Manag Rev 1998;23:393–404.

[14] Borum 4. The Science of Interpersonal Trust. Mental Health Law & Policy Faculty Publications 2010. In: University of South Florida Digital Commons. Available at: https://digitalcommons.usf.edu/cgi/viewcontent.cgi?article=1573&context=mhlp_facpub. Accessed March 2, 2023.

[15] Schockley-Zalabak PE, Ellis K, Winograd G. Organizational trust: What it means, why it matters. Organ Dev J 2000;18(4):35–48.

[16] Kath ML, Magley VJ, Marmet M. The role of organizational trust in safety climate's influence on organizational outcomes. Accid Anal Prev 2010;42:1488–97.

[17] Vaisman J, Davison A. Leadership & Workplace Experience Study: The Impact of Positive Leadership on Veterinary Teams. 2022. Available at: https://www.flourish.vet/positive-workplace-study-results. Accessed March 2, 2023.

[18] Edmondson A, Zhike L. Psychological Safety: The History, Renaissance, and Future of an Interpersonal Construct. Annual Review of Organizational Psychology and Organizational Behavior 2014;1(1):23–43.

[19] Marlow SL, Lacerenza CN, Paoletti J, et al. Does team communication represent a one-size-fits-all approach?: A meta-analysis of team communication and performance. Organ Behav Hum Decis Process 2018;144:145–70.

[20] Losada M, Heaphy E. The Role of Positivity and Connectivity in the Performance of Business Teams: A Nonlinear Dynamics Model. Am Behav Sci 2004;47(6):740–65.

[21] Lee CT, Doran DM. The Role of Interpersonal Relations in Healthcare Team Communication and Patient Safety. Can J Nurs Res 2017;49(2):75–93.

[22] Edmondson A. Psychological Safety and Learning Behavior in Work Teams. Adm Sci Q 1999;44(2):350–83.

[23] Pfeifer L, Vessey J. Psychological safety on the healthcare team. Nurs Manag 2019;50(8):32–8.

[24] Alas T, Schaninger B. The Boss Factor: Making the world a better place through workplace relationships. McKinsey Quarterly 2020. Available at: https://www.mckinsey.com/capabilities/people-and-organizational-performance/our-insights/the-boss-factor-making-the-world-a-better-place-through-workplace-relationships. Accessed March 2, 2023.

[25] Cake MA, Bell MA, Bickley N, Bartram DJ. The life of meaning: A model of the positive contributions to well-being from veterinary work. J Vet Med Educ 2015;42(3):184–93.

[26] A.R. Renhard, K.D. Hains, B.J. Hains, E.B. Strand, Are They Ready? Trials, Tribulations, and Professional Skills Vital for New Veterinary Graduate Success. Frontiers in Veterinary Science 2021, 8. Available at: https://www.frontiersin.org/articles/10.3389/fvets.2021.785844/full. Accessed March 2, 2023.

[27] Harter JK, Schmidt FL, Hayes TL. Business-Unit-Level Relationship Between Employee Satisfaction, Employee Engagement, and Business Outcomes: A Meta-Analysis. J Appl Psychol 2002;87(2):268–79.

[28] Hagerty BM, Lynch-Sauer J, Patusky KL, et al. Sense of belonging: a vital mental health concept. Arch Psychiatr Nurs 1992;6(3):172–7.

[29] Filstad C, Traavik LEM, Gorli M. Belonging at work: the experiences, representations and meanings of belonging. J Workplace Learn 2019;31(2):116–42.

[30] Hirsch AS. Don't Underestimate the Importance of Good Onboarding. Society for Human Resource Management 2017. Available at: https://www.shrm.org/resourcesandtools/hr-topics/talent-acquisition/pages/dont-underestimate-the-importance-of-effective-onboarding.aspx. Accessed March 2, 2023.

[31] Grant AM, Dutton JE, Rosso BD. Giving Commitment: Employee Support Programs and the Prosocial Sensemaking Process. Acad Manag J 2008;51(5):898–918.

[32] Schoorman FD, Mayer RC, Davis JH. An Integrative Model of Organizational Trust: Past, Present, and Future. Acad Manag Rev 2007;32(2):344–54.

[33] Joo BK, Yoon SK, Galbraith D. The effects of organizational trust and empowering leadership on group conflict: psychological safety as mediator. Org Manag J 2023;20(1):4–16.

[34] Frazier ML, Fainshmidt S, Klinger RL, et al. Psychological Safety: A Meta-Analytic Review and Extension. Person Psychol 2017;70:113–65.

[35] Vaisman J. Lead to thrive: the science of crafting a positive veterinary culture. Lakewood, CO: AAHA Press; 2023.

SECTION IV: ACCESS TO VETERINARY CARE

Advances in Small Animal Care 4 (2023) 145–157

ADVANCES IN SMALL ANIMAL CARE

Access to Veterinary Care–A National Family Crisis and Case for One Health

Check for updates

Michael J. Blackwell, DVM, MPH*, Augusta O'Reilly, MSSW, LCSW, VSW

College of Social Work, Center for Behavioral Health Research, University of Tennessee, 600 Henley Street Suite 221, Knoxville, TN 37996, USA

KEYWORDS

- Access to veterinary care • One health • AlignCare • Interprofessional collaboration • Health care
- Mental health • Veterinary social work

KEY POINTS

- Due to the significance of the human–animal bond in our society, the lack of veterinary care negatively influences both human and nonhuman members of communities.
- More than 1 out of 4 families struggle to access veterinary care in the United States.
- Barriers to veterinary care are human-related, requiring a One Health solution.
- Access to veterinary care is the social justice call to action of veterinarians.

INTRODUCTION

Bob lost his best friend and constant companion, Chief, a Shepherd mix, because he could not pay for veterinary care after Chief sustained a treatable injury (Table 1 [a]). As a Vietnam veteran, Bob lived with health issues, most recently recovering from a stroke. His health prohibited him from working, so he lived on a limited budget from assistance. It was Chief's companionship, support, and unconditional love that Bob says most helped him to survive. Due to their circumstances, Chief's untimely and preventable death was via euthanasia.

Stories such as this occur daily because of the lack of a system that helps ensure access to veterinary care, regardless of socioeconomic status. Most who are struggling to access veterinary care contribute (or have contributed) to our society, including public servants, wage earners, many in service industries, senior retirees, and others. This article will discuss the nature of the issue of access to veterinary care, the human costs, possible ways to begin to address the issue through a One Health system (eg, AlignCare), and patient management through an incremental care approach.

A National Crisis

Pets have coexisted with humans in societies around the globe for ages. Approximately 70% of US households have pets [1]. The Harris Poll found that 95% of people living with pets consider them members of the family [2]. The Program for Pet Health Equity coined "bonded family" to describe families with human and nonhuman members in a human–animal bond relationship. Bonded families exist across the whole socioeconomic spectrum. Due to income inequality, it is important to understand how many face barriers. The Access to Veterinary Care Coalition's (AVCC) national study found that more than 1 out of 4 (28%) US families did not receive

*Corresponding author, E-mail address: mblackw1@utk.edu

[a]Definition of owned pets: Animals kept primarily for a person's or family's companionship, protection, and/or pleasure. They typically live in the home or on the property of their owner, and the owner is responsible for the animal's overall health care and well-being.

https://doi.org/10.1016/j.yasa.2023.05.003

TABLE 1
Benefits of the Human–Animal Bond

Physical	• Increased physical activity • Decreased physical isolation • Hypertension management and prevention • Cardiovascular risk reduction
Emotional	• Joy • Emotional comfort • Security • Companionship • Decreased social isolation

Data from Wein H, ed. The Power of Pets. News in Health (NIH). March 6, 2018. Accessed January 10, 2023. https://newsinhealth.nih.gov/2018/02/power-pets.

veterinary care during the previous 2 years, primarily because they could not afford it [3].

In the fiscal year 2022, the United States Department of Agriculture (USDA) indicated that 21,612,065 households participated in the Supplemental Nutrition Assistance Program (SNAP) [4]. There are no census data on the number of pets in these households. However, using the national average of 2 pets per household, it is estimated that there are 30,256,891 dogs and cats living in SNAP households.

The lack of access to veterinary care is the greatest threat to the health and well-being of pets with loving families. The AVCC made 5 recommendations to address access to veterinary care.

1. Improve veterinary care delivery systems to serve all socioeconomic groups.
2. Provide incremental veterinary care (IVC) to avoid nontreatment.
3. Improve the availability of valid and reliable information to educate pet owners.
4. Develop public policies that improve access to veterinary care and pet retention.
5. More research is needed.

Families in Crisis

Some suggest that a pet is a luxury, and those who cannot afford veterinary care should not have one. However, when families talk about their pets, they use terms of endearment like "my best friend," "my fur baby," "my babies," and "my kids"; the word "luxury" is not used. When someone cannot pay for veterinary care, generally it is not because of the human–animal bond (relationship); instead, it is the lack of a system that better ensures accessible veterinary care. The costs

of veterinary services are beyond what most low-income families can pay out of pocket. Their lack of available funds is exacerbated by their difficulty acquiring a loan, including using a credit card. Furthermore, many middle class families struggle to access veterinary care. In the US, only 48% of middle-income adults report having enough savings to support them for a period of least 3 months [5]. With limited emergency funds, not many people can pay out-of-pocket for their health care. Most of us depend on assistance, that is, private or public insurance and other financial assistance programs. As the costs of providing veterinary care continue to increase, the need for financial assistance becomes more critical. Consequently, improving access to veterinary care for all families requires new public policies resulting in One Health systems that
• Address the primary barriers families face, that is, financial,
• Reduce the frequency of nontreatment with patient management strategies that control costs, and
• Strategically connect human health care and veterinary medicine by adjusting financial resources and strengthening interprofessional collaborations.

The US Centers for Disease Control and Prevention (CDC) defines One Health as a collaborative, multisectoral, and transdisciplinary approach—working at the local, regional, national, and global levels—to achieve optimal health outcomes by recognizing the interconnection between people, animals, plants, and their shared environment [6].

A Case for One Health

Access to veterinary care is a broad complex topic affecting multiple animal species. However, this article will limit the focus to One Health systems specific to bonded families. Improving access to veterinary care requires a One Health approach, where resources and activities are aligned to serve bonded families better. In the One Health system, veterinary medicine is integrated into family health care, providing care to nonhuman family members.

The Program for Pet Health Equity, with its 3-fold mission of service, research, and education, was established to address all 5 AVCC recommendations. AlignCare, a One Health system developed by the Program for Pet Health Equity in collaboration with many others, is an example of how communities can improve access to veterinary care.

. . . for the benefit of society. . .
AN ETHICAL DILEMMA

All US veterinarians take the Veterinarian's Oath [7], pledging to use their "…scientific knowledge and skills for the benefit of society…" The veterinary oaths of other countries contain similar pledges. Yet currently, not all of society is being served. Negative impacts include the following.

- Injured or ill pets (nonhuman family members) experience prolonged recovery or premature death, including euthanasia or being relinquished, thus losing their family.
- Families, especially vulnerable individuals, experience emotional distress and trauma, affecting their health and well-being.
- Veterinary care teams experience ethical dilemmas and moral distress when wanting to help but are unable.
- Communities are at risk of zoonotic diseases, threatening overall health and well-being.

Many consider access to veterinary care a fundamental right, as with human access to health care. Access to veterinary care means an individual can obtain services and treatments and pay for them when needed. Access includes economic, physical, and geographical access and availability of Veterinary Service Providers (VSPs) and facilities. Yet, millions of families have limited or no access to veterinary care due to poverty, geographic isolation, and systemic barriers.

Compassion is an excellent reason to ensure underserved families gain access to veterinary care. Equal or more compelling reasons other than compassion include the following.

- Safeguarding public health through the prevention and control of zoonotic diseases.
  - Changes in the climate may lead to the growth and migration of microbial and vector populations.
- Supporting human health and well-being through the benefits of the human–animal bond.

Intentionality requires that we see underserved families; that is, meaning they are no longer marginalized, and we endeavor to understand their needs without judgment. In the United States, most of the underserved are not indigent, although this is an important subgroup. Most underserved families are ALICE, that is, Asset Limited, Income Constrained, Employed [8]. They are members of the essential workforce, including cashiers, servers, teachers, sanitation workers, childcare providers, and others (Fig. 1). They are essential, working, struggling, earning just above the Federal Poverty Level but less than what it costs to make ends meet. ALICE workers are the backbone of our economy. They deserve companionship with a pet and access to veterinary care. Households of color are disproportionately ALICE, a compelling reason for veterinarians to commit to

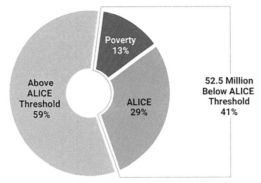

* In the U.S., out of 127 million households, there were 16.2 million (12.8%) in poverty plus 36.3 million (28.6%) that were ALICE, which totals to 52.5 million (41.4%) below the ALICE Threshold and rounds to 41% in this Report.

FIG. 1 Percentage of US Households who are Asset Limited, Income Constrained, Employed (ALICE). (United For ALICE. (2023). "ALICE in the Crosscurrents: COVID and Financial Hardship in the United States." UnitedForALICE. org/National-Overview.)

diversity, equity, and inclusion as critical to improving access to veterinary care.

Middle-income families also struggle to access veterinary care. Recent studies show that more than 3 out of 4 Americans working full-time live paycheck-to-paycheck [3], including 10% of those earning more than US$100,000 annually. Having the disposable income necessary to provide veterinary care can be a struggle for these families, mainly when an unforeseen expensive problem occurs. Proportionately, the US middle class has been shrinking in recent decades. According to the Pew Research Center [9], the percentage of American adults living in middle-income households declined from 61% in 1971 to 50% in 2021, with most shifting into a lower income bracket (Fig. 2). The main reason for this decline includes stagnating wage, increasing income inequality, and the increasing cost of living. This widening income gap and shrinkage of the middle class have led to a steady decrease in the proportion of US aggregate income held by middle-class households. In 1970, adults in middle-income households accounted for 62% of aggregate income, a proportion that fell to 42% in 2020 [8]. These socioeconomic trends inform the delivery of veterinary services during the next few decades. The current veterinary practice business models may not be aligned with these trends.

ACCESS TO VETERINARY CARE—THE HUMAN COSTS

Historically, programs facilitating access to veterinary care have primarily focused on the pets' needs, that is, not a

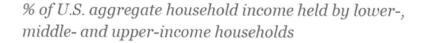

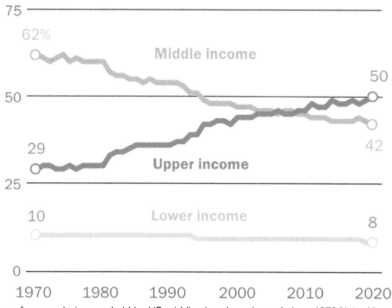

FIG. 2 Share of aggregate income held by US middle class has plunged since 1970. Note: Households are assigned to income tiers based on their size-adjusted income in the calendar year before the survey year. Their unadjusted incomes are then totaled to compute the share of US aggregate household income held by each income tier. Shares may not add to 100% due to rounding. (*From* Kochhar R, Sechopoulos S. How the American middle class has changed in the past five decades. Pew Research Center. April 20, 2022. Accessed January 5, 2023. https://www.pewresearch.org/fact-tank/2022/04/20/how-the-american-middle-class-has-changed-in-the-past-five-decades/. Source: Pew Research Center analysis of the current population survey, annual social and economic supplement (IPUMS).)

One Health approach. However, barriers to veterinary care are associated with human realities, not pets. Undeniably, a pet is negatively affected without access to veterinary care, but so are humans, including the pet's family, the veterinary care teams wishing to help, communities, and society.

Costs to Families

The entire household is affected when a family member has fallen ill or sustained an injury. If that member is a young child or a pet, the family's distress may be heightened because of their limited ability to communicate what is wrong. The illness or injury of one family member, especially a dependent, can threaten the physical and mental health of the household. Families that lack a network of emotional and practical support when these incidents arise are especially vulnerable members of society.

Looking at the extensive list of benefits the human–animal bond provides, vulnerable individuals may be seen as at significant risk of harm when denied these benefits. Studies show how interacting with animals can decrease cortisol levels, lower blood pressure, reduce loneliness, increase feelings of social support, and boost mood [10]. When pets are surrendered or euthanized due to the family's inability to overcome human-related barriers, the family loses these health benefits. In a 2019 US national study conducted by the Program for Pet Health Equity with 1781 people who live with pets, 31% of those who experienced barriers to needed care stated that having a pet always caused them stress. However, only 2% of those without a barrier to veterinary care experienced this same stress level. The people who had experienced at least one type of barrier to veterinary care also reported a higher number of days in the past 30 days that their mental health was not good: 5.7 days compared with

2.8 days reported by those who did not experience a barrier. If an individual is already enduring physical or emotional health-related hardships within a bonded family unit, one may infer the potentially catastrophic aftermath of not providing needed veterinary care. It can be understood how losing a pet this way could especially devastate vulnerable individuals who rely on their nonhuman family member(s) for enhanced emotional or physical well-being.

Being confronted with barriers to veterinary care contributes to the crisis that vulnerable families are experiencing. When pet owners cannot provide their nonhuman family members proper care, they can lose self-assurance. Rather than attributing their lack of resources to more significant socioeconomic factors, some may see themselves as unfit pet parents.

In many societies, value tends to be placed on the ability to afford care for loved ones rather than the person's capacity for affection—especially regarding dependents. People often feel accountable for their loved ones' well-being, and when they cannot provide needed care, they question their integrity.

Costs to Veterinary Service Providers

The level of bondedness is similar across the socioeconomic spectrum [11]. Therefore, systems to improve access to veterinary care should reflect this. Low-income families' limited means should not be confused with not caring about their pets. A One Health system facilitating access to veterinary care for bonded families with limited means will incentivize and enable VSPs to help. Without such a system, the financial burden is disproportionately carried by VSPs, who cannot address the barriers.

Historically, veterinarians have taken steps to make veterinary care accessible. These actions help many, but on a societal level, many are still not served. There are limits to the kind and amount of assistance VSPs can offer without negatively affecting the financial health of their business. Veterinarians participating in the AVCC US national study reported various efforts to serve families with limited means [3]. See Fig. 3 for the most common steps taken.

Moral distress is the psychological and emotional anguish the veterinary care team experiences when they cannot act according to their ethical and moral beliefs [12]. It typically develops when put in situations where they cannot provide the care or treatment they think is best for their patients or when they feel compelled to act in ways that conflict with their values or professional standards. Examples of situations that may cause moral distress include decisions about end-of-life care, conflicts over treatment options, or

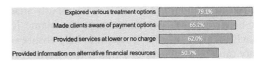

FIG. 3 US veterinarians reported having employed a variety of strategies to address needs of underserved pets (n = 470). (*Adapted from* Wiltzius AJ, Blackwell MJ, Krebsbach SB, et al. Access to Veterinary Care: Barriers, Current Practices, and Public Policy. Published December 17, 2018. Accessed January 5, 2023. https://trace.tennessee.edu/cgi/viewcontent.cgi?article=1016&context=utk_smalpubs.)

allocation of limited resources. Veterinary care teams risk experiencing moral distress when they turn away a family without helping or euthanize the pet while having the desire and ability to help. From literature reviews and personal anecdotal experiences, the experience of moral distress can lead to a range of adverse outcomes, including burnout, depression, and decreased job satisfaction. VSP organizations must recognize and address moral distress among their members and provide support and resources to help them navigate these difficult situations.

Veterinarians in the United States and abroad have a higher proportionate mortality ratio for suicide than the general public. For example [13].

- In comparison to the general US population, male veterinarians are more than 2.1 times as likely to die by suicide, and female veterinarians are 3.5 times as likely to die by suicide.
- Those in small animal practice experience a higher rate of suicide than veterinarians in other types of practice.

There is much to learn about the factors contributing to the rates of suicide among veterinarians.

Researchers continue to try and better understand the determinants of veterinarians' declining mental health. Contributing factors include the following [14].

- Student debt
- Profound grief that accompanies the loss of a pet
- The "caring-killing paradox," which occurs when performing or exposed to euthanasia of pets under your care

Sometimes when people cannot access veterinary care, their crisis leads them to blame the VSPs. They can express their dismay that people who claim to love animals will not help. The age of social media enables accusatory stories to be broadly shared, negatively influencing the veterinary care team.

When bonded families need out-of-reach veterinary care, they are likely in crisis, and emotions can run high. The veterinary care team may be unfairly attacked for not helping. However, most of the blame legitimately lies in not having a system to help ensure veterinary care across the socioeconomic spectrum. Human health care provides numerous examples of systems to help ensure access. Just about everyone who receives human health care depends on financial assistance, generally from insurance (private or public). Those with limited means achieve equity by accessing health care through programs designed to reach them. The driving principle leading to assistance across the socioeconomic spectrum is that all deserve access to health care. Without that belief being broadly held, many would not have health care. Believing all pets deserve access to veterinary care will help drive the creation of systems to achieve this outcome. When we see them as the family members they are, we will also see that their needs mirror those of the human members of the family. Similarly, they need a system that sees them regardless of socioeconomic status.

Costs to Animal Welfare Organizations

Because of a lack of standardized reporting, the number of pets in the United States who are relinquished to animal shelters/rescues due to treatable medical conditions is unknown. Most of these organizations are underresourced, given the job they are tasked to perform for the community. A system that improves access to veterinary care will benefit these organizations by reducing the number of pets they take in due to needing veterinary care. Individuals engaged in animal shelter/rescue-related work are at a disproportionately high risk of:

- Secondary trauma occurs from knowing about an animal's traumatizing event and the stress resulting from helping or wanting to help that animal [15].
- Posttraumatic stress disorder is at a 5 times greater risk of developing it than the national average [15].
- The "caring-killing paradox" [14].

Access to veterinary care is a family rights issue. It is also veterinarians' social justice issue as primary providers of such care. Social justice in this context means that everyone, regardless of socioeconomic status, race, ethnicity, or gender, has an equitable opportunity to receive quality, affordable services. Receiving care includes physical access to veterinary care facilities, providers, treatments, and financial access to care. Within this definition, access to veterinary care is a social justice call to action.

In a socially just veterinary care system, the distribution of services is equitable. Everyone has access to the care they need to maintain and improve their family's overall health and well-being. Such a system would help to reduce health disparities and improve the health outcomes of marginalized communities. Pursuing social justice in veterinary care involves addressing broader social determinants of health, such as poverty, education, housing, and employment, which can significantly affect an individual's health and access to care. Veterinarians cannot alone achieve the objectives of a socially just veterinary care system. It takes collaborations with others in a One Health system that factors in the realities of the humans in the pet's life and their shared environment or ecosystem.

PROVIDERS OF FAMILY HEALTH CARE—A TWENTY-FIRST CENTURY SOCIETY PARADIGM

Veterinarians who provide medical care to pets are providers of family health care. They attend to the medical needs of nonhuman family members just as pediatricians attend to the medical needs of the minors in a family. The "provider of family health care" paradigm is strategic to improving access to veterinary care. Otherwise, there is the risk of using twentieth-century thinking and approaches to solving twenty-first-century societal problems, for example, access to veterinary care.

Family health care refers to the medical care and treatment of individuals and their families, focusing on preventive and primary care. This type of health care involves a team-based approach that includes physicians, nurses, and other health-care professionals working together to provide comprehensive and personalized care to families. Family health care is concerned with the physical, emotional, and social well-being of individuals and their families throughout their lifetimes. It involves regular check-ups, immunizations, health screenings, and managing chronic conditions such as diabetes, asthma, and high blood pressure. Veterinary care teams who provide care to pets should be better integrated with human health-care professionals. This integration is One Health, and a structured system will better ensure these collaborations that are critical to overall family health and well-being.

A One Health Health-care System

- Integrates an interdisciplinary/interprofessional approach to health care, recognizing the interconnectedness of humans, animals, and their shared environment (Fig. 4).

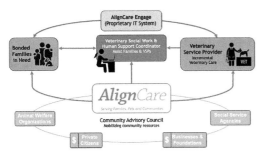

FIG. 4 The AlignCare system.

- Involves collaborations and coordination among health-care providers, veterinarians, public health officials, social service professionals, and others to address the full range of health threats facing families and communities.
- Health-care providers consider the environmental and social factors that contribute to health and well-being, including the presence and influence of nonhuman family members and work with other health-care professionals and organizations to address these factors holistically.
- Veterinarians are essential to achieving a holistic approach to improving bonded family and community health and well-being. Human health care and veterinary medicine are not adequately connected; thus, the health-care system is fragmented.

AlignCare—A One Health Solution

With generous funding from Maddie's Fund [16], the University of Tennessee Program for Pet Health Equity researched, developed, and tested AlignCare [17,18], a One Health system to improve access to veterinary care (see Fig. 4). The system aligns resources and activities with a community's funding to assist qualified families with veterinary care. Data about bonded families with limited means captured through the AlignCare Engage software include the following.

- Reason(s) veterinary care is needed at the time of enrollment.
- The severity of the problem(s) needing a veterinarian.
- Average costs and expenditures.
- Family health and well-being.

A One Health Health-care System

- Integrates an interdisciplinary/interprofessional approach to health care, recognizing the interconnectedness of humans, animals, and their shared environment (see Fig. 4).
- Involves collaborations and coordination among health-care providers, veterinarians, public health

officials, social service professionals, and others to address the full range of health threats facing families and communities.

- Health-care providers consider the environmental and social factors that contribute to health and well-being, including the presence and influence of nonhuman family members and work with other health-care professionals and organizations to address these factors holistically.
- Veterinarians are essential to achieving a holistic approach to improving bonded family and community health and well-being. Human health care and veterinary medicine are not adequately connected; thus, the health-care system is fragmented.

The AlignCare System makes serving bonded families with limited means easier by spreading and controlling costs and facilitating the VSP–family relationship.

- Family eligibility is established by confirming demonstrated need, for example, participation in a means-tested public assistance program. This confirmation ensures all who are contributing support that their help is reaching the intended families.
- Spreading costs among 3 or more entities:
  - Families pay the VSP 20% of the charges when services are received.
  - AlignCare pays the VSP 60% of the charges after invoicing.
  - For-profit VSPs offer a 20% discount (or other negotiated amount) for their services. Nonprofit VSPs are not required to discount their services.
  - Others may help by paying:
    - The family's 20% copayment, especially when they cannot, or make up the difference when a family does not have the whole amount.
    - Some of the total amount due, which then lowers the family's 20% copayment net amount.
- Controlling costs by utilizing IVC as a patient management strategy to ensure some level of care available, thus avoiding nontreatment.

As observed with the families enrolled in AlignCare, the veterinary care needs are not that different from what is reported nationally (Table 2). A common question is how much it costs to provide veterinary care to underserved families. No one can provide a valid answer, partly because these are marginalized families, meaning their needs have not been adequately characterized and understood. There is a need for more community assessments to gain an understanding of these families and their needs. This information will enable better estimates of the cost.

TABLE 2
Most Common Conditions Among Pets Enrolled in AlignCare

Internal Medicine—49.6% • Benign prostatic hyperplasia • Cancer • Cystitis/urinary tract disease • Diarrhea • Hepatopathy • Pyometra • Neurologic	Dental Conditions—17.0% • Fractured teeth • Periodontitis	Musculoskeletal——15.8% • Dysplasia • Luxating patella • Osteoarthritis • Spondylosis
Skin conditions—15.0% • Alopecia • Fleas • Mass • Mast cell tumor • Pyoderma	Chronic illness—14.0% • Diabetes • Heart murmur • Obesity • Pancreatitis	Ear/eye condition—10.9% • Cherry eye • Otitis Allergies—6.5%

AlignCare offers a wide range of benefits to VSPs and communities wanting to help bonded families with limited means by reducing complexity, including.

• Reducing the number of bonded families VSPs turn away due to their inability to pay for services.
• Eliminating the need to renegotiate fees for every case; that is, VSPs receive payment for services based on their fee schedule discounted by 20% (for-profits).
• Having transparent processes with minimal impact, integrating well into current practice operations. For example, the VSP follows routine procedures with client appointments and treatment decisions.
• Permitting predictable implications for practice profitability and cash flow. The structured system enables decisions about how many families can be served given the discounts.
• Promoting greater workplace satisfaction and well-being of the veterinary care team by enabling them to reach families they otherwise would not have been able to help.
• Enabling VSPs to help their community.
• Reducing the likelihood of surrender to animal shelters and economic euthanasia rates.

AlignCare includes interprofessional collaborations with Veterinary Social Work (VSW) [19]. Veterinary Social Workers (VSWs) support the human side of the human–animal bond, that is, the pet's human family member(s). In addition, VSWs support the veterinary care team because they tend to the pet's needs in the bond.

Support from VSWs includes the following.
• Connecting families to local resources, such as

  ○ Human food and pet food pantries,
  ○ Therapy referrals,
  ○ Housing needs, and others
• Mediation between families and veterinarians.
• Pet loss support groups for families.
• Guidance and support with end-of-life decision-making with the attending veterinarian.

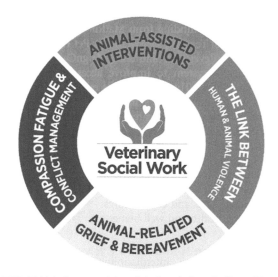

FIG. 5 Veterinary social work is founded on 4 pillars. (*From* Attending to human needs at the intersection of veterinary and social work practice. Veterinary Social Work. Published 2015. Accessed January 7, 2023. https://vetsocialwork.utk. edu/.)

The issues at the intersection of humans and animals are often associated with one of the 4 pillars of VSW, as shown in Fig. 5.

The role of a VSW is vital because they advocate for policy changes within a more extensive system. They also identify community support, helping to ensure access to veterinary care because it plays a crucial role in the mental health of people bonded with pets and the veterinary care team. The ideal interdisciplinary team includes family support professionals, animal care professionals, physical and mental health professionals, and relevant government officials.

An example of how a VSW and veterinary care team worked together is the story of Paul and Stella, his service dog. Paul had to be hospitalized due to coronavirus disease 2019, so he contacted his veterinarian in crisis, hoping they could care for Stella in his absence. He had no natural support, and she required regular treatment after developing cancer. His veterinarian was not able to board Stella. Paul then remembered to contact the AlignCare VSW to see what could be done. The VSW contacted the local animal shelter, an AlignCare partner, and arranged for temporary boarding. The VSW also provided check-ins with Paul, updating him on Stella's care and providing emotional support from being separated.

As the years passed, Stella's cancer progressed, and the veterinary care team became concerned about her quality of life. They contacted the AlignCare VSW, who partnered with them, guiding Paul through treatment decision-making, quality-of-life discussions, and end-of-life options. The passing of Stella left a mark on all, and the AlignCare VSW was able to provide support for Paul and the veterinary care team, lessening the emotional burden of a loved one's passing.

This story is One Health, where the alignment of resources, people, and activities resulted in holistic health care for a bonded family with limited means. All communities can benefit from such a One Health system.

Incremental Veterinary Care and Spectrum of Care

When providing veterinary care to families with limited means, a veterinarian is often unable to do all that the patient needs. However, something can usually be done to safeguard the quality of life. The veterinarian uses scientific knowledge and professional judgment to decide what is most important in addressing the patient's needs within available resources. The Program for Pet Health Equity refers to this decision-making process of managing a patient's care as IVC. It is not a new concept because veterinarians have historically needed to alter desired treatment plans to fit a client's ability or willingness to pay. Using IVC to manage a patient's needs, by default, usually means not being able to do all that is medically recommended.

There are excellent discussions of the spectrum of care (SC), notably by Stull and colleagues [20] and Brown and colleagues [21], as well as others. It is noted that SC may refer to the range of services and interventions available for individuals with a particular health condition or need, from prevention and early detection to diagnosis, to treatment, and long-term management. As seen in Fig. 6, the AlignCare system uses SC and IVC regarding patient management and the range of

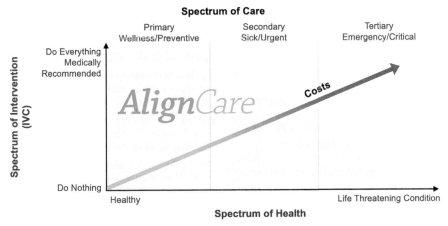

FIG. 6 Correlation of cost and the continuum of SC and IVC. The shaded area is intended to show that as the costs of care increase, fewer families receive care, even with AlignCare assistance.

services and interventions. In other words, a healthy individual's level or type of care needs is in the wellness and preventive end of the SC. Similarly, a critically ill individual's level or type of care needs is in the emergency critical care end of the spectrum. Although Fig. 6 shows 3 broad categories, SC and IVC occur on a continuum. Both clinical and nonclinical, including the following.

- Patient-centered experience-based medicine focused on a problem-solving approach to achieve the best possible outcomes for the family and human–animal bond in the context of limited resources.
- Experience-based medicine as a case management style, based on the practitioner's clinical experience and judgment relative to managing various clinical presentations.
- Utilizing the intuitive judgment of the veterinarian to develop a tiered diagnostic and dynamic therapeutic approach over time.
- Avoiding noncritical procedures to help control costs. IVC relies on the veterinarian's clinical judgment, active follow-up of case progression, and, when appropriate, in-home care that the client can provide.
- Relying on the veterinarian educating the client about the most pressing issues and guiding them with allocating their money toward what is most helpful for the pet.
- Focusing on prevention and early diagnosis and intervention.
- Emphasizing the need for the pet's primary caregiver and veterinary care team to closely monitor the patient's response, which requires a commitment of timely and accurate ongoing communication between the two. In developing a treatment plan, 2 prognostic indicators are as follows:
  - ○ The willingness of the pet's primary caregiver to actively participate in the pet's medical care. Active participation involves a commitment to collaborate and coordinate with the veterinary care team.
  - ○ The capability of the pet's primary caregiver to communicate with the veterinary care team, and carry out recommendations, need to be considered when developing a treatment plan.

More discussion is needed to achieve a shared understanding and use of terms and approaches to improving access to veterinary care.

As with any case management strategy, client dissatisfaction is always possible. There are potential liabilities when doing less for the patient than is recommended; that is, IVC. It is essential to create and guide reasonable client expectations and have documentation of informed consent to prevent or mitigate liability. Informed consent better protects the public by ensuring that veterinarians provide sufficient information so clients may reach appropriate decisions regarding the care of their pets. The American Veterinary Medical Association (AVMA) recommends that veterinarians, to the best of their ability, inform the client or authorized agent, in a manner that would be understood by a reasonable person, of the diagnostic and treatment options, risk assessment, and prognosis, and should provide the client or authorized agent with an estimate of the charges for veterinary services to be rendered [22]. The client or authorized agent should indicate that the information is understood and consent to the recommended treatment or procedure. In addition, the AVMA recommends that there is documentation of verbal or written informed consent and the client's understanding [22].

Education

Access to veterinary care raises numerous questions regarding the adequacy of the Doctor of Veterinary Medicine curricula in preparing veterinarians to serve bonded families with limited financial capability. US veterinary students get exposure to cutting-edge medical technologies and procedures taught by capable clinical specialists. However, some think these curricula do not adequately focus on general medical care, especially when working with limited resources. Because most veterinarians cannot do all that is medically recommended every time for many of their patients, it stands to reason that the DVM curricula would reflect this reality. It is a question of whether enough focus is on these issues. We are encouraged to see multiple organizations and individuals focusing on access to veterinary care. A notable example is the recent initiative on SC by the Association of American Veterinary Medical Colleges [23].

When resources are limited, more training is needed in the decision-making process and strategic procedures. Most of the medical problems occurring each day do not require a specialist, and when one is indicated, many bonded families may not be able to pay for that level of care. Yet, they are still in need of care, thus relying on general practitioners to do all they can. This reality should inform what is taught and emphasized by veterinary colleges and schools.

The Program for Pet Health Equity is collaborating with colleges/schools of veterinary medicine to share curricula ideas on incorporating access to veterinary care content. Ideally, veterinarians will enter clinical practice confident in developing individualized treatment plans based on the client's abilities/resources. Curricula addressing access to veterinary care should be broader than clinical procedures. They will include content about society, bonded families, One Health as a critical system, what it means to deliver family health care, in addition to patient management strategies. Continuing education courses will have a more immediate influence on veterinarians in practice.

Colleges and schools of social work also need to include access to veterinary care in their curricula, preparing social workers to serve a bonded family society. Assisting families without regard to the pets in the home may lead to suboptimal decisions when helping, for example, finding housing that does not accept pets because of underappreciation of the pet as family.

What can you do to help?

1. Embrace the new paradigm; veterinarians are providers of family health care.
   a. The public created this paradigm by integrating pets into their lives as family members. Do not overstate the "pets are private property" mantra. Although that is legally and technically correct, society has afforded pets a status above the living plants in the home. Society will hold someone accountable for what is done to or not done for a pet.
   b. Words matter. Attitude matters even more. Veterinary care teams may reflect an "animal" centric mindset in the words they use. They are reminded that the veterinarian (and team by extension) enters into a veterinarian–client–patient relationship. However, in the authors' experience, the patient is often called "the animal" in practice. Remember, the patient is someone's family member and ensure this is conveyed in the attitudes that are reflected and actions that occur in daily practice.
2. Be open to new interprofessional/interorganizational collaborations.
   a. A One Health system requires interprofessional collaborations that, up to now, have minimally existed. These collaborations should be driven by a belief that they are critical to a more effective health-care system.
   b. A family health-care attitude is essential to building new collaborations and realigning health care where veterinarians are in interprofessional collaborations. A good starting point is establishing a relationship with a social worker or social service agency that may facilitate client services. Partake and seek out trainings that increase skills and knowledge about supporting humans such as communication skills and trauma-informed care.
3. Be an advocate for the underserved. They can use the help.
   a. Veterinarians still have a significant influence on policy-makers and legislators. The new paradigm means broadening that advocacy to be about families.
4. Consider becoming a provider in the AlignCare (or similar One Health) system when it comes to your community. If you are not able to engage in a One Health system, consider other ways to support the bonded family system. These include the following:
   a. Practicing incremental care to meet the family where they are financially and otherwise.
   b. Connect with local animal welfare organizations as a referral source for families you cannot service.

Engage in trainings that support your staff's mental health when challenges arise from access to veterinary care [6]. Stay current of wellness resources available to practice personnel, recognizing access to care challenges place great stress on the veterinary care team.

Summary

Pets are an integral part of human societies. In the United States, 7 out of 10 households have one or more pets, and 95% of those households report that their pet is a family member. Unfortunately, millions of these bonded families struggle to access veterinary care primarily because they cannot pay the costs. There are other barriers, such as transportation and location, and what they all have in common is their association with the people in the pet's life. Pets themselves rarely present barriers to veterinary care. Socioeconomic trends suggest that access to veterinary care will continue to be a problem for some time and may worsen. Veterinarians know there is an access to veterinary care problem and play a vital role in making changes for access to care. Advocating for system changes, partnering with programs that follow the One Health model, and engaging with other disciplines working in the access to care field are just a few of the ways they can make a difference. Even with veterinarians taking steps to assist families, this societal crisis extends beyond the capacity of veterinary medicine alone to solve.

There are human costs that must be considered when discussing the veterinary access to care crisis, that is, negative human impacts when veterinary care is not accessible. The mental/emotional health of affected individuals needs additional attention from health-care professionals. Those most affected include the following.

- Families who may be experiencing distress and are at risk of losing a member due to relinquishment or premature death. This is of particular concern for vulnerable individuals who are significantly dependent on their pets for support.
- Veterinary care teams that want to help but never see the underserved, or when they do, are too often turning them away, not helping, or euthanizing a beloved pet whose medical problem can be addressed. These teams are at risk of compassion fatigue, moral distress, and other mental/emotional health problems. These scenarios create ethical and moral dilemmas for veterinary care team members, including the support people who do not provide the medical care but are knowledgeable of these situations.
- Communities cannot be healthy without healthy families, bonded or not. The public health consequences of a community having numerous individuals without access to health care, including veterinary, are real and should not be ignored.

A new paradigm that aligns all health care, that is, One Health, is needed. This paradigm's foundation is family health care for a bonded family society. In this paradigm, veterinarians treating nonhuman family members are providing family health care. Identifying with family health care creates a new context, meaning, and value for VSPs. Furthermore, aligning with family health-care facilitates the development of new approaches to assist with veterinary care.

AlignCare is a working example of a One Health system designed to reach families with limited means. It facilitates financial support for qualified families, addressing the primary barrier to veterinary care. The costs of veterinary care are spread among a few entities, and costs are controlled by veterinarians using an IVC (or similar) patient management strategy. AlignCare Veterinary Social Workers provide support for families and veterinary care teams. They facilitate communications with VSPs when a family needs such help. They also help families with other needs, as they often have, by aligning them with community resources such as food, housing, and human health-care services.

AlignCare changes lives by helping keep bonded families healthy and united. Kibou, described as a loving, nurturing, and happy dog, joined Dawn's family in February 2022. It did not take long for Kibou to endear himself to them, becoming best friends with Dawn's grandson. Life changed for this family when Dawn received a call that her mother, who resided on the other side of the country, was terminally ill. The family, now including Kibou, traveled to be with Dawn's mother during this time. Although the journey was long, Kibou is recounted as simply being happy to be with his new family.

Unfortunately, when they returned home, another tragedy struck the family. Kibou was hit by a car while chasing a rabbit, shattering his pelvis. Having spent most of their money taking care of her mother, Dawn's family had no resources remaining for emergency veterinary care—and in this case, surgery. Facing limited options, she reached out to Determined for Everyone to Gain Access (DEGA) Mobile Veterinary Care for guidance. DEGA Mobile Veterinary Care is a 501(c) (3) nonprofit located in the Triangle area of North Carolina that provides free basic veterinary care to low/no income and homeless bonded families all across the state.

Kibou's injuries needed emergency surgery beyond DEGA's scope of services, so DEGA recommended that Dawn reach out to AlignCare. Families are only asked to pay a 20% copay while AlignCare covers the rest. To this end, Dawn raised Kibou's 20% through donations and volunteering time with DEGA Mobile Veterinary Care. With the skilled help of XDS Inc., a partnering VSP, AlignCare was able to help Kibou gain access to the care he needed.

When asked about her experience, Dawn said, "AlignCare saved our family... I cannot even bear to think of what would have happened to Kibou if they had not helped us. He has a long recovery ahead of him, but he is home with us and is healing. We will never be able to express the amount of gratitude we have for both DEGA and AlignCare. They have given Kibou and our family a second chance."

CLINICS CARE POINTS

- When a client expresses they cannot afford the treatment plan presented, use an incremental care approach by identifying the most critical procedures within the means of the client's ability to pay, thus avoiding nontreatment.
- Deliver services within One Health by establishing a relationship with a social service agency or professional who can assist when certain barriers to care arise since barriers are usually associated with the client's realities.
- When presented with a patient who should have been seen sooner, resist prejudging the client, not understanding the barriers that needed to be overcome to get care.

DISCLOSURE

The authors have nothing to disclose.

REFERENCES

[1] American Pet Products Association. Pet Industry Market Size & Ownership Statistics. APPA. Available at: https://www.americanpetproducts.org/press_industrytrends.asp. Published 2021. Accessed January 17, 2023.

[2] The Harris Poll. More Than Ever, Pets are Members of the Family. Prnewswire.com. Available at: https://www.prnewswire.com/news-releases/more-than-ever-pets-are-members-of-the-family-300114501.html. Published July 16, 2015. Accessed January 10, 2023.

[3] Wiltzius AJ, Blackwell MJ, Krebsbach SB, et al. Access to Veterinary Care: Barriers, Current Practices, and Public Policy. Published December 17, 2018. Available at: https://trace.tennessee.edu/utk_smalpubs/17. Accessed January 5, 2023.

[4] U.S. Department of Agriculture. Supplemental Nutrition Assistance Program (SNAP). USA.gov. Available at: https://www.fns.usda.gov/pd/supplemental-nutrition-assistance-program-snap. Published 2019. Accessed February 8, 2023.

[5] Parker K, Menasce Horowitz J, Brown A. About Half of Lower-Income Americans Report Household Job or Wage Loss Due to COVID-19. Pew Research Center's Social & Demographic Trends Project. Published April 21, 2020. Available at: https://www.pewresearch.org/social-trends/2020/04/21/about-half-of-lower-income-americans-report-household-job-or-wage-loss-due-to-covid-19/. Accessed April 27, 2023.

[6] One Health Basics. Centers for Disease Control and Prevention. Available at: https://www.cdc.gov/one-health/basics/index.html. Published November 8, 2018. Accessed February 2, 2023.

[7] American Veterinary Medical Association. Veterinarian's Oath. AVMA. Available at: https://www.avma.org/resources-tools/avma-policies/veterinarians-oath. Accessed January 15, 2023.

[8] United For ALICE. (2023). ALICE in the Crosscurrents: COVID and Financial Hardship in the United States. Available at: UnitedForALICE.org/National-Overview. Accessed May 26, 2023.

[9] Kochhar R, Sechopoulos S. How the American middle class has changed in the past five decades. Pew Research Center. Published April 20, 2022. Available at: https://www.pewresearch.org/fact-tank/2022/04/20/how-the-american-middle-class-has-changed-in-the-past-five-decades/. Accessed January 5, 2023.

[10] Wein H, ed. The Power of Pets. News in Health (NIH). Available at: https://newsinhealth.nih.gov/2018/02/power-pets. Published March 6, 2018. Accessed January 10, 2023.

[11] Nugent WR, Daugherty L. A measurement equivalence study of the family bondedness scale: measurement equivalence between cat and dog owners. Front Vet Sci 2022;8. https://doi.org/10.3389/fvets.2021.812922.

[12] Jameton A. What moral distress in nursing history could suggest about the future of health care. AMA Journal of Ethics 2014;19(6):617–28.

[13] Tomasi SE, Fechter-Leggett ED, Edwards NT, et al. Suicide among veterinarians in the United States from 1979 through 2015. J Am Vet Med Assoc 2019;254(1):104–12.

[14] Lucchesi ELB. Researchers try to understand high suicide rate among veterinarians. Discover Magazine. Available at: https://www.discovermagazine.com/mind/researchers-try-to-understand-high-suicide-rate-among-veterinarians. Published May 12, 2022. Accessed January 17, 2023.

[15] Hoy-Gerlach J, Ojha M, Arkow P. Social workers in animal shelters: a strategy toward reducing occupational stress among animal shelter workers. Front Vet Sci 2021;8. https://doi.org/10.3389/fvets.2021.734396.

[16] AlignCare. Maddie's Fund. Available at: https://www.maddiesfund.org/aligncare.htm. Accessed January 20, 2023.

[17] About AlignCare. AlignCare Health. Available at: https://www.aligncarehealth.org/about. Accessed January 5, 2023.

[18] Veterinary Pet Insurance. Top 10 Most Common Medical Conditions for Dogs and Cats. Prnewswire.com. Available at: https://www.prnewswire.com/news-releases/top-10-most-common-medical-conditions-for-dogs-and-cats-300065935.html.Published April 15, 2015. Accessed January 10, 2023.

[19] Attending to human needs at the intersection of veterinary and social work practice. Veterinary Social Work. Available at: https://vetsocialwork.utk.edu/. Published 2015. Accessed January 7, 2023.

[20] Stull JW, Shelby JA, Bonnett BN, et al. Barriers and next steps to providing a spectrum of effective health care to companion animals. J Am Vet Med Assoc 2018; 253(11):1386–9.

[21] Brown CR, Garrett LD, Gilles WK, et al. Spectrum of care: more than treatment options. J Am Vet Med Assoc 2021; 259(7):712–7.

[22] American Veterinary Medical Association. Principles of veterinary medical ethics of the AVMA. AVMA. Available at: https://www.avma.org/resources-tools/avma-policies/principles-veterinary-medical-ethics-avma. Published 2019. Accessed January 16, 2023.

[23] American Association of Veterinary Medical Colleges. The Spectrum of Care Initiative. AAVMC. Available at: https://www.aavmc.org/the-spectrum-of-c. Accessed March 10, 2023.

Advances in Small Animal Care 4 (2023) 159–170

ADVANCES IN SMALL ANIMAL CARE

Competency and Controversies Along the Spectrum of Care

Gary Block, DVM, MS, DACVIM*

Ocean State Veterinary Specialists, 1480 South County Trail, East Greenwich, RI 02818, USA

KEYWORDS

- Standard of care • Spectrum of Care • Gold standard • Evidence-based medicine (EBM)
- Clinical practice guideline (CPG)

KEY POINTS

- Standard of care is a frequently misunderstood term in veterinary medicine and failure to understand this concept will hamper clinicians, regulatory bodies, and the legal system from assessing care provided by veterinarians
- Understanding and incorporating Spectrum of Care medicine into clinical practice will provide more pets with better veterinary care and will maintain and enhance the human–animal bond
- Gold standard care, while often the most expensive, has driven many improvements in veterinary care and occupies an important position on the Spectrum of Care
- Veterinarians are not adequately embracing or utilizing evidence-based medicine which is limiting their ability to create clinically valuable Spectrums of Care for pet owners
- Although not interchangeable with clinical practice guidelines, there are many resources (consensus statements, white papers, and disease monographs) that veterinarians need to become aware of to enhance their ability to appropriately utilize the concept of Spectrum of Care medicine.

As a progressively higher percentage of the pet-owning public finds veterinary care out of their financial reach, incorporating the concept of Spectrum of Care into practice has become an ethical and practical imperative. Understanding the terminology, limitations, and some of the unresolved controversies surrounding this concept will allow practitioners to provide the best quality care to the largest number of patients.

STANDARD OF CARE

The term "standard of care" has been part of the legal and medical lexicon for almost 200 years, with one of the oldest legal references to standard of care being found in *Vaughn v Menlove* where the court noted that

an individual with a duty of care must have "proceeded with such reasonable caution as a prudent man would have exercised under such circumstances" [1]. Although the term "standard of care" is firmly rooted in the law, there are no universally accepted definitions of standard of care in veterinary medicine. In veterinary tort law, the standard of care has been defined as "the standard of care required of and practiced by the average reasonably prudent, competent veterinarian in the community" [2]. Veterinarians should also remember that "a mere error of judgment, mistaken diagnosis, or the occurrence of an undesirable result" does not constitute a breach of the standard of care [3]. This is important to emphasize as the public (and some veterinarians) assume that an unexpected or untoward outcome

*Corresponding author. Ocean State Veterinary Specialists, 1480 South County Trail, East Greenwich, RI 02818. *E-mail address:* GBYLC@AOL.com

with one of their patients by definition, amounts to negligent care.

Although the standard of care in veterinary medicine essentially represents the minimum acceptable level of care, the standard of care is frequently mischaracterized as equivalent to "best practices". Part of this confusion is almost certainly related to the way standard of care is defined in human medicine, where the term is used very differently than in veterinary medicine. For example, the National Institute of Health defines the standard of care as "Treatment that is accepted by medical experts as a proper treatment of a certain type of disease and that is widely used by health care professionals. Also called best practice … and standard therapy" [4]. These conflicting definitions likely end up confusing many veterinarians, and explains why occasionally, veterinary publications use the human "gold standard" definition of standard of care. Examples of this include an article in which the authors contend that failure to submit uroliths for quantitative analysis constitutes negligent care and another that concludes CO_2 lasers have "become a standard of care in general practices and in specialty and referral practices" [5,6]. Regardless of these conflicting definitions of standard of care, even veterinarians well-versed in the concept of standard of care are hamstrung by the lack of practical, easily accessible, clinically relevant guideline to help direct the care they provide. Further complicating the issue is the fact that until recently, "SOC" was often used to represent "standard of care" in many scientific publications, and now, it is more frequently used as an acronym in veterinary medicine for "Spectrum of Care" [7].

SPECTRUM OF CARE

How one defines "Spectrum of Care" is an important part of understanding how embracing this concept can promote access to veterinary care. There have been numerous descriptions of Spectrum of Care, most of which refer to providing a continuum of diagnostic and treatment options that take into account the best available evidence, clients' financial means, client expectations and family circumstances, available resources, experience of the attending veterinarian, and proximity to tertiary care facilities when referral is warranted [8] (Fig. 1).

Veterinarians should take care not to define the Spectrum of Care as simply giving clients *a lot* of options. Spectrum of Care medicine is as much an effort to create as wide a palate of diagnostic and treatment options for the client to consider as it is to present *good* options,

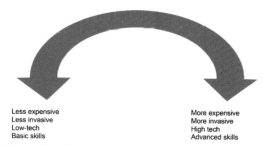

Less expensive
Less invasive
Low-tech
Basic skills

More expensive
More invasive
High tech
Advanced skills

FIG. 1 Simplified diagram of spectrum of veterinary care.

ideally grounded in evidence-based medicine (EBM), but at minimum, based on the most contemporary peer-reviewed resources available. Anecdote and personal experience may be important and sometimes all that is available, but these are considered to be near the bottom of the hierarchy of scientific evidence [9]. Recommending widely discredited, completely unvalidated, and physiologically dubious diagnostic or treatment options does a disservice to the entire concept of using the Spectrum of Care to increase access to veterinary care.

Notwithstanding the above caveats, if veterinarians are to take theory to practice, then the "widest spectrum" should always be the goal as it is most likely to allow clients to find a landing spot that synchs their financial preferences with their expectations and other factors noted above. Although this may be true for the typical general practitioner, the proliferation of for-profit and non-profit veterinary clinics that focus solely on preventive or wellness care have essentially carved out niches on the Spectrum of Care to focus on a subset of the pet-owning public. By not trying to be "everything to everyone" these models have proven successful by marketing to clients an intentionally more narrow spectrum of care [10,11].

Unfortunately, too many veterinarians have unknowingly adopted a practice philosophy of "your pet doesn't have what is has, it has what I know" —an indictment of their not having kept up with advances in veterinary medicine and likely to result in a more limited selection of legitimate options for the pet owner. Even when veterinarians *are* capable of presenting a wide Spectrum of Care, it appears that a significant number of them may be withholding this information from clients. Though the majority of surveyed veterinarians noted that they offer more than one treatment option to clients, a large-scale study of veterinarians in 2018 found that 21% of veterinarians said that they did not "explore various treatment options" as a strategy to address the needs of underserved pets [12]. A more recent study found that over 30% of veterinarians *disagreed* with the statement that "all treatment options should be presented to owners" [13]. This failure to provide legitimate options to pet owners may be a vestige of the paternalistic approach that was the historical communication style in both human and veterinary medicine. Another theory may be because there appears to be a difference of opinion as to whether veterinarians or pet owners are better able to assess a pet's quality of life [14]. Regardless, veterinarians should consciously strive to respect client's autonomy and take pains to avoid assuming what approach to care any particular client may be interested in pursuing. *How* veterinarians present information can be as important as what specific options are being presented, as veterinarians almost certainly can influence clients' decisions given the high regard and respect the public has for the profession. Sharing details regarding not only cost but likely outcomes, requirements for additional testing or follow-up, and what if any evidence exists supporting a particular course of action should all be included in these discussions [15]. A genuine dialogue with the client that promotes shared decision-making and presents diagnostic and treatment options in a non-judgmental fashion is an important component of how one increases access to care as well as how truly informed consent can be obtained [16]. This should also help both the client and veterinarian feel better about their ultimate decision on where along the spectrum they choose to place their pet.

Most veterinarians and pet owners assume that there is a linear relationship between the amount one spends on an ill or injured pet's veterinary care and the likelihood of a positive outcome. Although this is a commonsense generalization, the "you get what you pay for" assumption may not always be the case as has been disturbingly noted in human medicine [17]. The author is aware of numerous examples of more expensive treatment and diagnostic options not necessarily being more effective than their less expensive counterparts. A 1995 study on traumatic intervertebral disc extrusions found no difference in outcomes between dogs undergoing expensive spinal surgery and those managed medically [18]. Another study that evaluated the benefit of culturing acute, open, traumatic wounds found that routine bacterial culturing of such wounds is "not likely to predict subsequent wound infection, nor is likely to guide early selection of antimicrobials to treat wounds that become infected" [19]. Routine culturing of such wounds is a ubiquitous example of increasing the cost of care without a concomitant demonstrable benefit, and unfortunately is still common practice. Other examples include using significantly more expensive Telmisartan in lieu of benazepril for cats with pathologic proteinuria, and the unproven belief that dogs with immune-mediated hemolytic anemia always require second agent therapy such as cyclophosphamide or Azathioprine in addition to prednisone [20–22]. These examples make an important point because most charts and depictions of Spectrum of Care medicine create a straight-line graph where increasing costs are directly related to improved outcomes [23]. In fact, a more accurate depiction of the relationship between cost of care and outcome would likely look like this (Fig. 2).

Given the almost complete absence of research on outcome measures as a function of costs compared to human medicine, it is highly likely that veterinary care also routinely utilizes more expensive diagnostics and care without a concomitant improvement in patient outcomes [24].

"Gold STANDARD" CARE

Most descriptions of Spectrum of Care describe "gold standard" care as the most expensive, most invasive, most technologically advanced option, and often presupposing a medically successful outcome. We would be wise though to look to history when thinking about the "gold standard" when we are describing it as part of the Spectrum of Care and remembering that today's "gold standard" may be tomorrow's supplanted or abandoned diagnostic or treatment recommendation. The most dramatic example of this may be taken from human medicine where, in 1949, a Nobel Prize was bestowed upon Egas Moniz who pioneered the frontal lobotomy as a treatment of depression, schizophrenia, and other mental health disorders [25]. Now widely regarded as barbaric, tens of thousands of people

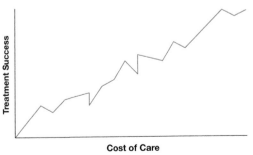

FIG. 2 The relationship between the cost of veterinary care and likelihood of treatment success.

including children as young as 4 years of age underwent this procedure, which rarely improved their signs. When the author was in veterinary school, high-dose injectable steroids were routinely administered to animals in shock or suffering acute spinal cord injuries. This was considered the gold standard at the time but is now actively discouraged because of their use being linked to increasing morbidity and mortality. Similarly, and under the banner of "less is more", the gold standard for a cutaneous histiocytoma on a young dog is to do nothing and let it go away on its own, whereas a more expensive and invasive option would be to recommend surgical removal of the tumor [26]. Gold standard specifically and Spectrum of Care generally, are thus an ever-evolving set of options to be considered and it should not always be assumed that gold standard care is synonymous with the most expensive or invasive care.

Some recent articles on increasing access to care have taken aim at "gold standard" care as one of the culprits increasing costs of veterinary care, often assuming that veterinary schools and other (private practice) tertiary care facilities are driving this runaway financial train [27,28]. Veterinarians would be well-served by remembering that the growth and success of tertiary care facilities have been driven by the dramatic change in the role companion animals play in people's lives. Over the last 50+ years, dogs and cats have, for many pet owners, become "part of the family" and these pet owners have demanded and been willing to pay for advanced veterinary care that often rivals what human medicine provides [29]. The number of veterinarians in the United States working in referral or specialty practice grew by almost 98% between 2008 and 2013 reflecting both the public's demand for ever-improving pet care and the economic willingness to pay for such care [30]. This has almost certainly expanded the Spectrum of Care "to the right" with procedures like brain surgery, dialysis, and interventional cardiology—once the exclusive purview of human medicine now routinely performed in veterinary hospitals. Many pet owners continue to present their pets to hospitals prepared to spend large sums of money including taking on debt in an effort to increase the quantity and quality of the animal's life and there is no reason a subset of veterinarians and veterinary practices should not be encouraged to practice gold standard care when financially feasible. Regardless, it is undeniable that *whatever* the standard of care for treating companion animals is, tertiary care facilities have—for better or worse—been raising the bar across the profession. The answer to increasing access to care is not to disparage "gold standard care" or discourage referral, but rather to understand that these options are just one end of what should be as wide a Spectrum of Care as possible.

MONEY AND THE SPECTRUM OF CARE; REDEFINING SUCCESS?

Greater attention being paid to increasing access to care and understanding the benefits of presenting clients with as wide a spectrum of diagnostic and treatment options is undeniably having a positive impact on our patients and clients by improving the health of pets not currently receiving adequate or in some cases, any veterinary care, decreasing pet-associated public health issues and increasing the likelihood of keeping pets in families. That said, one of the legitimate criticisms of all the research, educational initiatives, and attention being paid to the access to care issue is that it skirts an important detail that needs to be honestly acknowledged: having the ability to practice "farther to the right" on the spectrum more often than not, and notwithstanding the above admonitions, is going to result in decreased morbidity, decreased mortality, and improved medical outcomes. Crudely stated, there is likely a link between how much a pet owner can afford and the quality of the care their pet is going to receive. Pretending that money does not play the most important role ignores what we all observe in practice every day and ignores all the research that has studied barriers to veterinary care [31]. As noted previously, there may not be a direct linear relationship between cost and outcome, but no sane veterinarian would argue that treating a sick ketoacidotic cat or dog with a comminuted femoral fracture is going to go better for the client with only $400 to spend compared to the client willing to spend $4000. This financial truth is, in fact, one of the main selling points of pet insurance. A recent article in *Today's Veterinary Business* suggested it would cost over 20 billion dollars annually just to provide *basic* veterinary care to all the pets in the country not currently receiving it, so it should not be at all surprising that providing emergent care would be even more restricted by financial limitations [32].

When viewed within the context of Spectrum of Care, how then do we balance the trade-off between treatment success and cost of care? For example, is a 70% lower vet bill worth a 20% higher risk of treatment failure? Is a 20% lower bill worth risking a 70% higher risk of treatment failure? Holding up the success of pinning—instead of plating—a simple femoral fracture or simply "putting the broken cat in a box and waiting for it to heal" is absolutely appropriate for financially limited clients, but pretending that these are legitimate options for a hit-by-car cat with a crushed pelvis, broken jaw, and bilateral femoral fractures is divorced from reality. Unlike human medicine, where at least in theory, the quality of care provided is not related to one's ability to pay, veterinarians cannot avoid the reality that pet owners often make medical decisions based on their financial means [33]. Trumpeting the benefits of increasing access to care by broadening the Spectrum of Care cannot act as a "fig leaf" for veterinarians or be a mechanism to create a patina of equivalence for options that by most objective standards are going to be considered less likely to succeed. And redefining success by focusing on the client's expectations, improving one's empathy, or spending less of the client's money cannot be surrogates for actually improving an animal's quantity and quality of life. In one recent trade publication, the writer noted that "lesser options often provide optimal, affordable outcomes," seemingly redefining the word "optimal" to validate their practice along the Spectrum of Care [28]. Admittedly, how one defines medical "success" can be multifactorial and vary between individuals, but most veterinarians and pet owners would agree that lower morbidity, improved quality of life, and higher survival rates would rank high on that list. Until we create a society that views animal health care as a right (admittedly unlikely given the fact that this is not yet the case for people in the United States), honestly acknowledging the link between having money and more successful outcomes and accepting that we are attempting to balance sometimes competing goals and interests is an important component of those interested in increasing access to care.

With appropriate deference to the fact that Spectrum of Care should not only be viewed through a financial prism, the goal for veterinarians should be to find the "biggest bang for the buck". Even vets well-versed in the concept of Spectrum of Care and able to present the widest range of treatment options must, at some point, recognize that the "lowest" end of the spectrum becomes an exercise in futility when the likelihood of treatment success is so small that the veterinarian must direct the client to other options or, when warranted, humane euthanasia. Unsurprisingly, agreement about what constitutes futile care may not be universal between veterinarians and clients [34]. Regardless, veterinarians should familiarize themselves with and provide resources designed to help clients grappling with whether to forego or discontinue treatment of their pet and whether palliative or hospice care is warranted [35,36].

Understanding and embracing all the facets of the concept of Spectrum of Care do not automatically give veterinarians the knowledge that makes the Spectrum of Care clinically valuable to clients and their pets. As noted previously, almost all definitions of Spectrum of Care include taking account of "best available evidence" as a prerequisite to veterinarians counseling clients about the Spectrum of Care. A recent article on Spectrum of Care notes that "all *evidence-supported* [emphasis added] diagnostic testing and treatment options are filtered through the lens of the specific circumstances of the pet and owner ...," further emphasizing the importance of EBM along the Spectrum of Care [15]. It is thus logically impossible to make wise decisions—financial or otherwise—that respect and support clients' needs if veterinarians are not adequately versed in the breadth and depth of these diagnostic and treatment options.

CLINICAL PRACTICE GUIDELINES
In human medicine, recognition that the public was not receiving sufficient value for the resources that were being expended on health care was one of the main drivers for creating clinical practice guidelines (CPGs). CPGs have been defined by the Institute of Medicine as "systematically developed statements to assist practitioner and patient decisions about appropriate care for specific clinical circumstances" [37]. These guideline aspire to improve the quality of care provided to patients, decrease health care costs, incorporate relevant research into clinical practice, and reduce the risk of legal liability to practitioners—all frequently cited goals of the increasing access to care movement in veterinary medicine. CPGs, while not a panacea, have been embraced in human medicine and have with rare exceptions, consistently been shown to improve clinical outcomes [38,39].

For physicians, CPGs produced by specialist associations, US government agencies, and health care organizations are collated by the National Guideline Clearinghouse to assist practitioners and patients in making decisions about appropriate health care in specific clinical circumstances. Although we all acknowledge the merits of randomized, placebo-controlled, double-blinded studies and systematic reviews, we should not suffer "paralysis by analysis". Waiting for such higher-level information on the evidence pyramid to be generated as an excuse not to act may give one the veneer of the intellectual high ground but does nothing to help the animals we need to treat now. Crosby, Stills, and Nash famously encouraged us to "love the one you're with". This classic folk-rock song makes for a good analogy for how we have to work with the evidence we currently have, not the evidence we wish we had. Creating a database of such white papers, consensus statements, practice guideline, position papers, and disease monographs promulgated by veterinary professionals and special interest organizations and combining it with a growing body of evidence-based research could serve as an excellent first step for our profession and provide a valuable resource for private practitioners (see Appendix 1 for such a compilation focused on companion animals). These resources will almost certainly provide more relevant and clinically useful information than veterinarians who practice by the previously noted unintentional credo of "your pet doesn't have what it has, it has what I know." One legitimate issue raised regarding specialty organization-produced resources usually created exclusively by board-certified specialists, is whether they are directly applicable to expectations of general practitioners. Although it is widely assumed that specialists are held to a higher medical standard than general practitioners, the author has been unable to find examples supporting this assumption in veterinary tort law. This would be particularly relevant to creation of CPGs if it is determined that CPGs for a generalist should be different than those for a board-certified specialist.

A full discussion of the limitations and controversies of using CPGs is beyond the scope of this article, but some of the most commonly reported barriers to why human doctors have not embraced CPGs include lack of awareness/familiarity, disagreement with the published CPG, and inability to overcome the inertia required to try something new [40]. Even a careful review of these shortcomings still leaves the reader to conclude that the veterinary profession's current lack of standardization and ambiguity creates a practical, philosophic, and jurisprudential obstacle to quality veterinary care [41]. That two veterinarians in the same clinic could create a vastly different Spectrum of Care for the same patient, crystallizes the potential benefits some form of veterinary CPGs could bring to our patients. If veterinarians are serious about using the Spectrum of Care to improve patient outcomes, then adopting some form of CPGs must be a priority for our profession. Perhaps focusing on some of the most commonly encountered conditions seen in clinical practice would be a reasonable and achievable initial goal and allow veterinarians to get exposed to CPGs in a way that is not overwhelming or intimidating.

Familiarity and utilization of veterinary CPGs will also avoid a legitimate criticism of Spectrum of Care medicine, which is its potential to condone an "anything goes" approach to veterinary medicine where clearly substandard care gets included on the spectrum. Practicing along the spectrum cannot and should not obviate the responsibility of incorporating EBM into the spectrum. EBM is traditionally defined as "the conscientious, explicit, and judicious use of current best evidence in making decisions about the care of individual patients" [42]. Acknowledging the central role of EBM in the Spectrum of Care should help prevent a medical "free-for-all" where veterinarians need to simply jot something in the pet's medical record that says they discussed options with the client and the client has elected to treat their pet's bleeding splenic mass with ground eye of newt! As one of the criteria that defines a profession is that it is self-regulating—CPGs will allow administrative and legal oversight of veterinarians to be based on broadly accepted, EBM [43]. It makes little sense that currently, determinations of acceptable or negligent care likely differ to varying degrees across the country. What might be considered acceptable care in one jurisdiction could be deemed to be malpractice in a neighboring jurisdiction. Even taking into account the need for flexibility in melding Spectrum of Care medicine with CPGs, would it not make more sense for state veterinary boards to utilize a similar set of resources when determining whether a veterinarian practiced below the standard of care? If the function of these boards includes safeguarding the welfare of animals and enforcing professional standards, using CPGs, white papers, disease monographs, and consensus statements will create a much more objective approach than the hodge-podge of medical resources that often includes the personal opinions a board member may happen to have with the medical condition before them when a veterinarian's license is on the line. Early steps are being taken toward achieving this goal with the launch of the "Evidence-Based Veterinary Medicine Manifesto." The stated goal of this initiative is to "drive best practice by helping veterinarians and veterinary nurses access, assess, and use the best evidence to treat and care for animals" [44]. The expected outcome of using the manifesto would be to "reduce unnecessary or harmful treatments, better educate clients on the best options for their animals, and inform policymakers on the best approach to advocate for policy changes;" in essence, mirroring many of the stated goals of CPGs and helping to further the incorporation of Spectrum of Care medicine throughout the profession.

Achieving this goal must be considered aspirational at this time. Acknowledgment of the utility of Spectrum of Care medicine has not yet filtered down through many of the educational, professional, and regulatory bodies of our profession, although the recently announced American Association of Veterinary Medical Colleges (AAVMC) Spectrum of Care initiative is encouraging [45]. In addition, and has been recognized in human medicine, incorporation of CPGs into daily clinical practice has sometimes proved challenging [40]. CPGs cannot become a "straight jacket" for practitioners and need to be created with enough flexibility to anticipate the wide range of clinical presentations and socioeconomic factors that must be incorporated into Spectrum of Care medicine. Given the triadic relationship between veterinarians, their clients, and their patients, combined with the fact that animals are still considered property in the eyes of the law, this is even more important and potentially creates a greater hurdle for the profession in creating CPGs. And in anticipation of criticism and accusations that CPGs will turn veterinarians into "cookie cutter" doctors who blindly follow a medical recipe, the author will reiterate that properly utilized, CPGs are not a *substitute* for clinical reasoning but a valuable adjunct.

In audiovisual presentations on the topic of increasing access to care, the author sometimes includes a slide of a despondent veterinarian, head in hands, titled "you'll know what the standard of care is when you're sitting in front of your state veterinary board after having been accused of malpractice." Adopting CPGs should have the additional benefit of alleviating some of the anxiety veterinarians experience when they are trying to determine whether the Spectrum of Care medicine they are proposing would potentially fall below the legal standard of care. In our increasingly litigious society, many veterinarians report that their concern about meeting the standard of care results in their practicing defensive medicine, unnecessarily increasing the cost of care. One study found that 35% of veterinarians "sometimes" or "often" performed unnecessary tests because they were worried about client complaints, being sued, or becoming subject to disciplinary action [46]. Removing ambiguity and providing greater consistency for veterinarians looking for practical clinical guidance will undoubtedly be more useful to clinicians than the current opaque standards that individual states use when evaluating cases of potential veterinary malpractice.

In veterinary medicine, CPGs or their closest equivalents, have already been put forth for disciplines including but not limited to anesthesia, dermatology, oncology, cardiology, and a variety of diseases (see Appendix 1). Despite their increasing numbers and

potential value, CPGs and other consensus statements have not been incorporated into veterinary definitions of the standard of care, rarely if ever are referenced in state practice acts, and have not been embraced by the American Association of Veterinary State Boards, and only a small fraction have been endorsed by the two largest veterinary professional organizations, the American Animal Hospital Association(AAHA) and the American Veterinary Medical Association(AVMA). One such example, the AVMA's "Guideline for the Euthanasia of Animals", is widely disseminated and often informs federal and state policy suggesting there is a role for these resources outside of just helping clinical practitioners. Whether CPGs become accepted and incorporated into daily veterinary practice will likely portend the role they may subsequently play in policy development and the legal system. Although CPGs do not have the force of law in human medicine, they are described as being "situated halfway between ethical rules and legal requirements" [47]. In human medicine, CPGs are often referenced to help determine whether a doctor breached the standard of care and also to provide an affirmative defense in cases where doctors are accused of malpractice [48]. And until veterinarians embrace and consciously commit to making EBM a foundational component of the practice of veterinary medicine, we will continue to be guilty of not honoring our veterinary oath which directs us to a "lifelong obligation [to] the continual improvement of my professional knowledge." More importantly, we will be failing our clients by presenting a Spectrum of Care that is variably divorced from the available evidence and relies on less robust sources of information.

Continuing to produce these resources and potentially synthesizing them into readily accessible and universally accepted veterinary CPGs make little sense if veterinarians are not going to use them to improve patient care, veterinary state boards are not going to reference them when complaints are made by the public, and the courts are not going to use them to assess whether veterinary practitioners are at least striving to provide EBM along the Spectrum of Care.

KEEPING CURRENT

Many have described the author's knowledge base as an internist as "an inch wide and a mile deep". Whether this is true or not, it does highlight the challenge that all veterinarians, and particularly those in general practice, have in keeping up with the literature. As many have noted, currently practicing veterinarians are fortunate to have access to an astounding amount of information provided in an ever-expanding panoply of delivery methods [49,50]. Although this is clearly preferable to what veterinarians previously had at their disposal, most veterinarians would readily acknowledge that they find it next to impossible to keep up with the exponential increase in the information they need to maintain currency in their particular practice type. As familiarity with this increasing body of knowledge is a prerequisite for practicing along the Spectrum of Care, we must find a way to make this information more accessible and more relevant to practicing clinicians. A number of publications have tried to shed light on this issue of "information overload" and also provided some resources to allow veterinarians to streamline their search methodology and to help them create and refine a clinical question [51]. Organizations such as the Evidence Based Veterinary Medical Association (https://www.ebvma.org), RCVS Knowledge (https://knowledge.rcvs.org.uk/home/), and the University of Nottingham's Center for Evidence-Based Veterinary Medicine (https://www.nottingham.ac.uk/cevm/evidence-synthesis/bestbets-for-vets/bestbets-for-vets.aspx) can provide valuable links and resources for veterinarians looking to practice EBM as part of their efforts to create the most useful and clinically relevant Spectrum of Care for their clients and patients.

Spectrum of Care in Action

Creating spectrum of diagnostic and treatment options can be variably complex depending on the disease process involved, the available evidence regarding diagnostics, treatment, and prognosis, client finances, and many of the psychosocial aspects related to the client's relationship with their pet. For example, only a small subset of veterinarians should be undertaking intervertebral disc disease surgery in dogs, but that should not preclude every small animal veterinarian from either knowing or easily accessing published statistics on the prognosis for typical thoracolumbar intervertebral disc disease (IVDD) dogs based on their neurologic presentation and whether medical or surgical intervention should be pursued [52]. This is critical information for any client weighing the risks, benefits, and costs of treating their pet with IVDD. Chronic renal failure (CRF) is one of the more common clinical conditions identified and managed in small animal veterinary practice and a good example of a disease with a lot of evidence-driven diagnostic and treatment guidance available. Veterinarians should ideally be using the International Renal Interest Society (IRIS) classification system that not only allows staging the renal failure but also provides diagnostic and treatment recommendations based on the stage of renal failure to which the pet is categorized [53]. In addition, and of great value to clients, is the published median survival data tied to a particular IRIS stage which may influence their decision regarding what type of workup and in what treatment options they may be interested.

The board of IRIS is made up of an international group of veterinarians with demonstrated interest, extensive research history, and experience managing renal disease in dogs and cats. What percentage of veterinarians—general practitioners and specialists alike—are aware of, let alone, utilize this valuable resource is unknown. In addition, there are numerous published journal article overviews, textbooks devoted to kidney disease, internal medicine textbooks with dedicated chapters summarizing the diagnosis and treatment of CRF, and even Veterinary Information Network (VIN)—often criticized for its excessive use of anecdotal recommendations—which do an excellent job of summarizing the workup and myriad treatment options associated with CRF.

The treatment options for managing dogs and cats with CRF are even more extensive than the diagnostic evaluation and veterinarians must not only be aware of to what IRIS stage their patient is classified but then use this information to sequentially initiate therapies as the disease process progresses. Treatments including diet changes, intravenous and/or subcutaneous fluid therapy, anti-hypertensives, phosphate binders, calcitriol, appetite stimulants, antacids, antiemetics, and fatty acids are just some of the therapies that are utilized for treating CRF. Aggressive therapies such as erythropoietic stimulants and even renal transplants might be considered to be on the far end of the spectrum. Whether one defines these latter options as "gold standard", extreme or futile may be in the eye of the beholder.

As an internist who routinely sees patients referred for CRF, the author can attest that many of the aforementioned resources, diagnostics, and treatments are not utilized with any regularity by referring veterinarians. By crude example, an informal survey of the six board-certified internists at my own practice estimated that less than 50% of animals referred for additional CRF care have ever had their blood pressure checked and in many of these patients, their CRF diagnosis had been made many weeks to months before referral. The fact that these general practitioners concluded the client would be willing to spend the money for referral, yet they still did not do any blood pressure monitoring, at minimum, argues against this omission being related to client finances. Knowing what *should* be part of the Spectrum of Care for renal failure and not doing it is probably more unpardonable than not knowing what should be included in the spectrum. The former suggests a lack of desire to practice quality medicine, and a lack of belief in EBM that clearly demonstrates the deleterious effects of uncontrolled hypertension, not having the technical ability to measure blood pressure, or trying to save the client money which, in this situation, is likely "penny wise and dollar foolish", whereas the latter is an issue of information management, continuing education, and access to EBM [54].

An example of veterinarians simply not having the knowledge and information to help them create the most cost-effective and evidence-based Spectrum of Care would be the use of antibiotics in cases of nasal disease in dogs. This is one of the more common referrals seen in the author's practice and despite ample evidence that primary bacterial infections in the noses of dogs are exceedingly rare, almost all dogs referred for workup of chronic nasal signs have been on antibiotics before referral, and in many cases, multiple courses of antibiotics. This not only increases the cost of care but usually delays the ultimate diagnosis and initiation of proper treatment. This clinical observation was confirmed by a large study that found not a single case of primary bacterial infection in the nasal cavity of dogs with nasal discharge, and in that study, 72% of the dogs had received prior antibiotic therapy [55]. Another illustration of this problem is when newer information does not get adequately disseminated which, in turn, results in veterinarians continuing to practice the way they were previously taught or older references recommended. For example, until recently, it was routinely recommended that animals treated for simple urinary tract infections have a recheck urine culture run after finishing their course of antibiotics to confirm infection resolution. Now, the International Society for Companion Animal Infectious Diseases (ISCAID) guideline recommend *not* performing urine culture for sporadic bacterial cystitis when clinical signs have resolved which represents a considerable time and financial saving for clients [56]. Despite the frequency with which veterinarians in every type of practice encounter this clinical scenario and its potential to save clients' money, this evidence-based recommendation has not been routinely adopted due to what is likely a combination of lack of awareness and our profession's general reluctance to challenge dogma.

WHEN TO HEAD "LEFT" ON THE SPECTRUM
Although the knowledge and experience required to fully and accurately understand the tradeoffs associated between a client's financial means and the likely outcome for the pet is admittedly a daunting task, there are innumerable examples where less expensive diagnostic and treatment options are associated with either comparable results or clinically insignificant differences. Failure to include these options on the "left side" of the spectrum is a failure of both knowledge and imagination. For example, veterinarians and veterinary technicians are well trained—or capable of being trained in 5 minutes—to estimate a platelet count on a blood smear, but most veterinarians send out a full complete blood count in animals they are treating for immune-mediated thrombocytopenia. In both cases, an accurate, actionable platelet count is possible but the send-out test is almost certainly more expensive to the pet owner than a simple in-house blood smear read by a veterinary technician. Other evidence-based examples of less expensive care providing comparable efficacy include identifying an individual dosing interval for dogs with Addison's disease on desoxycorticosterone pivalate as a way to save hundreds or even thousands of dollars over the life of the pet and using an immediate pre-Trilostane basal cortisol measurement to assess control of Cushing's disease in dogs instead of the more expensive adrenocorticotropic hormone (ACTH) stimulation test [57,58]. Listing other examples would be redundant, but as an internist, the author would be remiss if he did not reference the increasing body of research directing veterinarians to not only limit their antibiotic use for certain disease processes such as acute colitis, but also to decrease the duration of antibiotic therapy in many conditions—both of which will limit client expenses and side effects to the pet while enhancing antibiotic stewardship [59,60].

Other than striving to remain current, one sometimes neglected and simple way for general practitioners to save client money and thus increase access to care is to consider doing some of the initial diagnostics in-house because in some cases, the results may make referral practically and/or clinically unwarranted. Examples of this include obtaining thoracic radiographs on dogs with suspected cancer, because gross metastatic disease to the lungs would, in most of these cases, result in the client electing not to pursue what could be more expensive and invasive surgery and/or chemotherapy. Running basic lab work on older animals before referral to look for obvious metabolic or systemic disease that would impact significantly on the prognosis, the safety of anesthesia, and/or the owner's desire to pursue referral, is another example where general practitioners can help improve the referral process. Performing these diagnostics before referral has the added benefits of keeping this money in-house, saving the client money because the same diagnostics at tertiary care facilities are often more expensive, and of course, saving the client time and money for what sometimes ends up being a futile referral. With all veterinarians grappling with the increased demand for veterinary services, this will have the added benefit of freeing up referral appointment slots for other pets in need.

Veterinarians are naturally curious and understandably want to provide pet owners with the most information possible as part of helping them decide how they want to pursue treatment of their pet. Although admirable traits, this sometimes results in veterinarians forgetting one of the cardinal rules of the practice of medicine; one that the author would argue falls right behind "primum non nocerum" ("first, do no harm"); and that is "don't do tests if the results aren't going to change the way you treat your patient!" Too often veterinarians—and frequently recent graduates—fall victim to dogma or veterinary school lessons that stressed the importance of a thorough, systematic evaluation of every patient but failed to emphasize that testing for testing's sake rarely serves the client or the pet. Examples of this abound, and in the author's practice, with long-standing internship and residency programs, we constantly try to drive this point home to our young colleagues. Taking thoracic radiographs on a dog with a bleeding abdominal mass to check for metastatic disease only makes sense if you have confirmed with the client their interest in possibly pursuing abdominal surgery. For a dog with confirmed multicentric lymphoma, if the client is interested in an aggressive CHOP-type chemotherapy protocol, is immunophenotyping critical since at present, the evidence for treating B cell versus T cell multicentric large cell lymphoma in dogs differently is lacking [61]. Some oncologists even eschew thoracic radiographs and abdominal ultrasound if no clinical indications exist in these patients, and in particular, if this would financially hamstring the client's ability to optimally treat their pet [62]. Although Cushing's disease might appropriately be on the differential diagnosis list for a small-breed older dog with an elevated serum alkaline phosphatase, absent clinical signs of disease, why would (relatively expensive) testing for hyperadrenocorticism be undertaken as few if any internists would suggest treating a dog with Lysodren or Trilostane absent clinical signs of disease. Even

common procedures such as fecal exams should be re-evaluated with a more critical eye. Because fecal exams—and particularly those run in-house—do not uncommonly yield false negative results, veterinarians often empirically deworm animals knowing that the risks of untreated endoparasitism are potentially serious for both the patient and potentially as a zoonotic risk [63]. If a veterinarian knows they are going to use a broad-spectrum dewormer such as fenbendazole no matter the test result, this does beg the question about why the fecal exam was done in the first place! If practicing intelligently and effectively along the Spectrum of Care is going to include being cognizant and respectful of clients' finances, then this mantra must become internalized to the point that it becomes second nature.

If veterinarians are serious about incorporating the concept of Spectrum of Care into their daily practice, then there must be an acknowledgment of both its value and limitations. Fundamental to this effort will be trying to blend a more expansive and likely fluid definition of standard of care with a genuine effort to make EBM the foundation upon which diagnostic and treatment options are presented to pet owners. Lacking more robust sources of evidence, veterinarians could still create modified CPGs along the Spectrum of Care tailored to the unique triadic nature of veterinary practice that take advantage of pre-existing consensus statements, specialty organization disease monographs, and white papers. Such guideline would allow greater consistency and understanding of what is expected of veterinarians while also creating a more transparent and uniform reference when situations arise regarding a veterinarian's potential professional liability. Achieving these goals will require engaging with practitioners, veterinary professional associations, regulatory bodies, and the legal system.

DISCLOSURE

The author reports no conflicts of interests.

SUPPLEMENTARY DATA

Supplementary data related to this article can be found online at https://doi.org/10.1016/j.yasa.2023.04.003.

REFERENCES

[1] Vaughan v Menlove, Ct of Common Pleas, England (1837). 132 ER 490 (CP).
[2] Dyess v Caraway 190 So. 2d 666 (La. Ct. App. 1966).
[3] Hall v. Hilbun, 466 So. 2d 856, (1985).

[4] National Cancer Institute. Complementary and Alternative Medicine. Available at: https://www.cancer.gov/about-cancer/treatment/cam. Accessed December 15, 2022.

[5] Lulich JP, Osborne CA. Quantitative urolith analysis: a standard of practice? DVM360 2007; Dec 1.

[6] Godbold JC. CO2 laser surgery: standard of care. Vet Pract News 2012.

[7] McGraw-Hill Concise Dictionary of Modern Medicine. Available at: https://medical-dictionary.thefreedictionary.com/Managed+care+SOC Accessed March 12 2023.

[8] Boatright, K. What is the spectrum of care? AHAA NEW Stat®2022:11. Available at: https://www.aaha.org/publications/newstat/articles/2022-11/what-is-the-spectrum-of-care/#:~:text=Practicing%20a%20spectrum%20of%20care%20offers%20a%20way,set%20baseline%20or%20follow%20a%20prescribed%20"gold%20standard

[9] Evidence Based Practice in Health; University of Canberra Library; Available at: https://canberra.libguides.com/c.php?g=599346&p=4149721 Accessed March 4, 2023.

[10] Telford T. Walmart wants to fetch more business with in-store vet clinics and an online pet pharmacy. Washington Post. May 7, 2019.

[11] Available at https://www.shotvet.com/. Accessed December 4, 2022.

[12] Access to Veterinary Care Coalition. Access to veterinary care: barriers, current practices, and public policy. Available at: https://trace.tennessee.edu/utk_smalpubs/17/. Accessed Nov 19, 2022.

[13] Peterson NW, Boyd JW, Moses L. Medical Futility is commonly encountered in small animal practice. JAVMA 2022;260(12):1475–81.

[14] Morgan CA. Autonomy and paternalism in quality of life determinations in veterinary practice. Animal Welfare J 2007;16(Suppl 1):143–7.

[15] Brown CR, Garrett LD, Gilles WK, et al. Spectrum of care: more than treatment options. JAVMA 2021;259(7):712–7.

[16] Cornell KK, Kopcha M. Client-veterinarian communication: skills for client centered dialogue and shared decision making. Clin North Am Small Anim Pract 2007; 37(1):37–47.

[17] Miller J. More money, same results. Cambridge, MA: Harvard Gazzette; 2017.

[18] Nessler J, Flieshardt C, Tunsmeyer J, et al. Comparison of surgical and conservative treatment of hydrated nucleus pulposus extrusion in dogs. J Vet Intern Med 2018; 32(6):1989–95.

[19] Hamill LE, Smeak DD, Johnson VA, et al. Pretreatment aerobic bacterial swab cultures to predict infection in acute open traumatic wounds: A prospective clinical study of 64 dogs. Vet Surg 2020;49(5):914–22.

[20] BestBETs for Vets; Telmisartan versus benazepril in the treatment of proteinuria associated with feline CKD. Updated Oct 1 2020. Available at: https://bestbetsforvets.org/bet/389. Accessed Dec 9, 2022.

[21] Cyclophosphamide in dogs with IMHA; BestBETs for Vets; 2018. Available a:t https://bestbetsforvets.org/bet/178. Accessed Dec 9, 2022.

[22] Azathioprine in dogs with IMHA. BestBETs for Vets 2019. Available at: https://bestbetsforvets.org/bet/21. Accessed Dec 9, 2022.

[23] AlignCare Incremental Veterinary Care Guide. Available at: https://pphe.utk.edu/wp-content/uploads/2019/07/AlignCare-Incremental-Veterinary-Care-Guide-Narrative-1.pdf; Accessed March 3, 2023.

[24] Measure outcomes and costs for every patient; Harvard Business School, Institute for Strategy and Competitiveness. Available at: https://www.isc.hbs.edu/health-care/value-based-health-care/key-concepts/Pages/measure-outcomes-and-cost.aspx. Accessed Dec 17, 2022.

[25] Weiner E. Nobel Panel Urged to Rescind Prize for Lobotomies. From NPR Public Radio; August 10 2005. Available at: https://www.npr.org/templates/story/story.php?storyId=4794007 Accessed Nov 4, 2022.

[26] Moore PF. A review of histiocytic diseases of dogs and cats. Vet Pathol 2014;51(1):167–84.

[27] Keir S. Defensive medicine-A symptom of fear. Nov 10, 2020. Available at: https://jobs.vettimes.co.uk/article/defensive-medicine-a-symptom-of-fear. Accessed Sept 23, 2022.

[28] Miller S. Spectrum of care: How it is helping vets be their best and ensure optimal patient health. Vet Practice News 2022.

[29] Bridger H. The changing roles of pets in society. J Small Anim Pract 1976;17(1):1–8.

[30] Ouedraogo FB, Bain FB, Hansen C, et al. A census of veterinarians in the United States. JAVMA 2019;255(2):183–91.

[31] Access to Veterinary Care Coalition. Access to veterinary care: barriers, current practices, and public policy. Available at: https://trace.tennessee.edu/utk_smalpubs/17/. Accessed Nov 19, 202233.

[32] Cushing M. What are we doing about access to care? Today's Veterinary Business, Dec22/Jan23. Available at: https://todaysveterinarybusiness.com/policy-politics-access-1222/.

[33] Survey results: The spectrum of veterinary care. DVM360.com May 24, 2016. Available at: https://www.dvm360.com/view/survey-results-spectrum-veterinary-care. Accessed Oct 13, 2022.

[34] Christiansen SB, Kristensen AT, Lassen J, et al. Veterinarians' role in clients' decision-making regarding seriously ill companion animal patients. Acta Vet Scand 2016;58(1):30.

[35] Villalobos A. Quality Of Life Scale. Veterinary Practice News 2009.

[36] How do I know when it's time? The Ohio State University; Available at: vet.osu.edu/honoringthebond. Accessed Nov 7, 2022.

[37] Field MJ, Lohr KN. Institute of Medicine. Committee on Clinical Practice Guidelines. Division of Health Care Services. Guidelines for clinical practice: from development to use. Washington: National Academy Press; 1992.

[38] Bahtsevani C, Uden G, Willman A. Outcomes of evidence-based clinical practice guidelines: a systematic review. Technol Assess Health Care 2004;20(4):427–33.

[39] Murad HM. Clinical Practice Guidelines: A Primer on Development and Dissemination. Mayo Clin Proc 2017;92(3):423–33.

[40] Cabana MD, Rand CS, Powe NR, et al. Why don't physicians follow clinical practice guidelines? A framework for improvement. JAMA 1999;282(15):1458–65.

[41] Guerra-Farfan E, Garcia-Snachez Y, Jornet-Gilbert M, et al. Clinical practice guidelines: The good, the bad, and the ugly. Injury 2022 S0020-1383(22)00077-00078.

[42] Sackett DL, Rosenberg WM, Gray JA, et al. Evidence based medicine: what it is and what it isn't. BMJ 1996; 312(7023):71–2.

[43] Cruess SR, Cruess RL. The medical profession and self-regulation: A current challenge. Virtual Mentor 2005;7(4):320–4.

[44] Launching an evidence-based veterinary medicine manifesto to drive better practice. Vet Rec 2020;187(5):174–7.

[45] American Association of Veterinary Medical Colleges Receives $1. 3M grant from the stanton foundation for the development of spectrum of care initiative. Washington DC: AAVMC Newsletter; 2022.

[46] Bryce AR, Rossi TA, Tansey C, et al. Effects of client complaints on small animal veterinary internists. J Small Anim Pract 2019;60(3):167–72.

[47] Pugliese M, Voslarova E, Biondi V, et al. Clinical Practice Guidelines: An Opinion of the Legal Implication to Veterinary Medicine. Animals 2019;9(8):577.

[48] Mackey TK, Liang BA. The Role of Practice Guidelines in Medical Malpractice Litigation. AMA Journal of Ethics 2011;12(1):36–41.

[49] Grindlay DJC, Brennan L, Dean RS. Searching the veterinary literature: a comparison of the coverage of veterinary journals by nine bibliographic databases. Vet Med Educ 2012;39(4):404–12, Winter.

[50] Prior F. Dwindling support in the age of information overload(Editorial). Aust Prescr 2019;42(6):178–9.

[51] Robertson SR. Refining the clinical question: the first step in evidence-based veterinary medicine. Vet Clin North Am Small Anim Pract 2007;37(3):419–31.

[52] Pancotta T. Canine neck and back pain. Clinician's Brief; 2016.

[53] Available at: http://www.iris-kidney.com/guidelines/staging.html Accessed Sept 2022-Jan 2023.

[54] Acierno MJ, Brown S, Coleman AE, et al. ACVIM consensus statement: Guidelines for the identification, evaluation, and management of systemic hypertension in dogs and cats. J Vet Intern Med 2018;32(6):1803–22.

[55] Rösch S, Bomhard WV, Heilmann RM, et al. Nasal discharge in dogs - are microbiological and histopathological examinations clinically useful? Tierarztl Prax 2019;47(2):84–96.

[56] Weese JS, Blondeau J, Boothe D, et al. International Society for Companion Animal Infectious Diseases (ISCAID) guidelines for the diagnosis and management of bacterial urinary tract infections in dogs and cats. Vet J 2019;247:8–25.

[57] Jaffey JA, Nurre P, Cannon AB, et al. Desoxycorticosterone Pivalate Duration of Action and Individualized Dosing Intervals in Dogs with Primary Hypoadrenocorticism. J Vet Intern Med 2017;31(6):1649–57.

[58] Dechra UK Monograph; 2020 Available at: DVP1412-Vetoryl-PVC-Flowchart-AW.pdf. Accessed Nov 12, 2022.

[59] Shmalber J, Montalbano C, Morelli G, et al. A Randomized Double Blinded Placebo-Controlled Clinical Trial of a Probiotic or Metronidazole for Acute Canine Diarrhea. Front Vet Sci 2019;4(6):163.

[60] Lappin MR, Blondeau J, Boothe D, et al. Antimicrobial use Guidelines for Treatment of Respiratory Tract Disease in Dogs and Cats: Antimicrobial Guidelines Working Group of the International Society for Companion Animal Infectious Diseases. J Vet Intern Med 2017;31(2): 279–94.

[61] Angelo G, Cronin K, Keys D. Comparison of combination l-asparaginase plus CHOP or modified MOPP treatment protocols in dogs with multi-centric T-cell or hypercalcaemic lymphoma. J Small Anim Pract 2019; 60(7):430–7.

[62] Clifford C, Bergman P. What's New in Veterinary Oncology? VIN Rounds 2021.

[63] Starkey LA. Fecal diagnostics with new information on fecal AI technology. ACVIM Virtual Forum; 2021.

Advances in Small Animal Care 4 (2023) 171–183

ADVANCES IN SMALL ANIMAL CARE

Preparing Veterinarians to Practice Across the Spectrum of Care

An Integrated Educational Approach

Sheena M. Warman, BSc, BVMS, DSAM, DipECVIM(CA), EdD, SFHEA, FRCVS[a,*],
Elizabeth Armitage-Chan, VetMB, DipACVAA, PhD, MRCVS[b], Heidi Banse, DVM, PhD, DACVIM (LA)[c],
Deep K. Khosa, BSc, BVMS, MANZCVS (SAM), PhD[d], Julie A. Noyes, DVM, PhD, MS, MA[e],
Emma K. Read, DVM, MVSc, DACVS-LA[f]

[a]Bristol Veterinary School, University of Bristol, Langford House, Langford, Bristol BS40 5DU, UK; [b]LIVE Centre, Royal Veterinary College, Hawkshead Lane, North Mymms, Hatfield AL9 7TA, UK; [c]School of Veterinary Medicine, Louisiana State University, Skip Bertman Drive, Baton Rouge, LA 70803, USA; [d]Ontario Veterinary College, University of Guelph, 2 College Avenue West, Guelph, Ontario N1G 2W1, Canada; [e]American Association of Veterinary Medical Colleges, 655 K Street Northwest, Suite 725, Washington, DC 20001, USA; [f]The Ohio State University College of Veterinary Medicine, 1900 Coffey Road, Columbus, OH 43210, USA

KEYWORDS
• Spectrum of care   • Veterinary education   • Primary care

KEY POINTS
- Veterinary teaching settings are increasingly using approaches that support students' skill development in spectrum of care (SoC) practice.
- A combination of primary care and referral settings is likely to provide an optimal workplace-based training program for students.
- A collaborative approach to classroom and workplace learning, including both primary care and specialist clinicians, can help integrate SoC pedagogy within veterinary curricula.

INTRODUCTION

The phrase "Spectrum of Care" (SoC) has only recently emerged in the veterinary literature, defined as "…a wide spectrum of diagnostic and treatment options [that veterinarians] can provide for their patients" [1] (p 1386). Practicing across the spectrum involves providing "a continuum of acceptable care that considers available evidence-based medicine while remaining responsive to client expectations and financial limitations" [2] (p 464). Affordability is not the only consideration with options influenced by several factors, "including the knowledge and skills of the veterinarian; the current scientific evidence regarding the safety and efficacy of available treatments, recommendations, or best-practice guidelines; practice-specific goals, culture and available resources; the owner's goals, values and resources" [1] (p 1387). "Phrases such as "contextualized care" and "incremental care" have also emerged. Contextualised care can be considered synonymous with Spectrum of Care; incremental care refers to the use of a step-wise, sequential approach rather than immediately moving forward with the most expensive or most comprehensive option [3–5].

As veterinary teaching settings, it is our duty to educate future veterinarians who can thrive in the workplace and serve their communities and the animals

---

*Corresponding author, E-mail address: Sheena.Warman@bristol.ac.uk

https://doi.org/10.1016/j.yasa.2023.04.004

within them, through the provision of effective, safe, and economic care. The more broadly a student is trained to practice across the SoC, then the more likely they are to be able to provide SoC options [2]. We also have a duty to support the formation of our students' professional identities, such that the values and priorities they bring to their work are not dissonant to the decisions and actions they will be able to achieve [6,7]. This means equipping our graduates to offer (and value) a wide range of options that are appropriate for the patient, the client and their family, the veterinarian, and the practice. The combination of circumstances for any one patient will often mean that a "gold-standard" textbook approach is neither achievable nor appropriate; furthermore, it is argued that the term "gold standard" is unhelpful, as the "best" approach will be variable for each individual case [4]. In this regard, SoC can be considered a new framing of the age-old art of veterinary practice: making clinical decisions that meet the goals and resources of all involved, without engendering a sense of failure for either client or veterinarian if the textbook approach is not appropriate for the patient being treated [8]. SoC offers the opportunity to focus on more individualized care for all involved while also achieving other important outcomes such as financial sustainability of the practice and provision of service of a wide variety of clients with differing needs.

Traditional Educational Model: a Focus on Tertiary Referral Settings

Traditional models of veterinary education have relied heavily on clinical experience within tertiary referral hospitals. Here, students have worked alongside dedicated specialist teams, developing many core skills such as history-taking, clinical examination, performing and interpreting diagnostic tests, medicating patients, and communicating with owners and colleagues. Students have been likely to spend significant periods of time discussing diagnoses in a great deal of depth while also being challenged to apply their growing knowledge to a range of clinical scenarios that require students to navigate complex and intertwined aspects of clinical knowledge. Skilled clinical teachers work hard to draw out the day-one relevant primary care learning from their complex specialist caseload. However, it is increasingly recognized that a reliance on the referral hospital teaching environment alone may not effectively prepare students with the skills and confidence required to practice across the SoC [1,2,8–12]. Specialist veterinarians often work with a relatively narrow preselected and referred client population who have financial means

and who are seeking the most advanced diagnostic and care options that can be recommended to them. Clients who are referred to specialists to pursue these options also arguably represent a select population; their values and attitudes surrounding animals mean that they generally have a desire for these options, and they have already overcome some of the barriers that may prevent others from seeking this type of care, including animal factors (age, temperament, health condition, environment) and client factors (transportation, capabilities, preferences and circumstances of the client and referring clinic) [4]. Much of the problem-solving and negotiating of which approach within the full SoC options is the "best fit" is therefore absent, underplayed, or presumed within this referral environment, and consequently a relatively narrow spectrum of options is offered and emphasized in teaching.

In Box 1, we consider two examples that highlight some aspects of the importance of delivering effective SoC training to our students.

Both of these examples highlight challenges in delivering SoC training that emerge from traditional tertiary referral settings. A focus on referral teaching settings mean that veterinarians with limited personal experience in primary care practice are routinely asked to develop teaching resources and prepare our students for unfamiliar aspects of professional life. In addition, students may perceive a "hidden curriculum" message [13] that all but the most basic procedures need to be referred to specialists, creating an unintended impression that primary care practice is a lesser discipline.

Developing Models: Increased Use of Primary Care Training Environments

As a result of the limitations of the traditional approach and recognizing the benefits realized in a renewed approach, many veterinary teaching institutions are refocusing their clinical training. There is a shift to include more emphasis on the primary care environment, thereby improving the authenticity of the workplace and ensuring a caseload for training that is similar to that which will be experienced by most new graduates [9,14,15]. With careful selection of sites, students can have opportunities to work with a wider general demographic of clients (and their expectations) as well as historically underserved populations where multiple axes of disadvantage intersect [16]. Students can also gain experience of a "wait and see" approach for patients with ambiguous symptoms that may recover before a specific diagnosis can be determined or before a treatment can be prescribed [17]. Students rotating through these authentic environments are exposed to primary

---

BOX 1
Experiences of referral and primary care educators

Example 1: Marnie is a staff surgeon in a long-established veterinary college. She completed her surgical residency 2 years ago, having gone straight into internship and residency from veterinary school. She is an exceptional clinician, ambitious, caring, and hard-working. She wants the best for her students on surgical rotations, recognizes that most will likely work in primary care practice, and goes out of her way to spend time with them discussing cases and involving them in the often complex surgical procedures that make up the bulk of her caseload. She recognizes the privileged environment in which she is working, and frequently challenges her students to consider how they would approach a case if referral was not an option. She enjoys working through the challenges of developing less resource-intensive care plans, but feels slightly uncomfortable in doing so, as she has very little firsthand experience of that type of problem-solving. She loves teaching laboratory sessions focused on basic surgical skills, but is surprised when her teaching evaluations from students state that her lecture material is pitched above the level of what they will likely need in practice. Marnie recognizes that many of the things she knows and can teach students will be useful in practice even if the students are not specialists in the future.

Example 2: Dan has 20 years of experience in primary care practice and is an excellent veterinarian according to his peers and clients. He has grown his practice from two to ten full-time veterinarians and is very well respected by his clients and colleagues. He has invested in his own personal development and has a strong interest in orthopedics, frequently attending advanced courses and national conferences. He routinely performs advanced procedures, has frequent communication with specialists, and regularly audits his clinical outcomes (which are excellent). He is surprised when a veterinary student on placement at his practice expresses a strong opinion that he should not have undertaken a particular (and very familiar) procedure as "these cases require referral." He has also noticed an initial reluctance among the new graduates he hires to undertake routine surgeries such as cystotomies and enterotomies; however, under his mentorship and with a significant investment of his time, they soon develop their skills and confidence to perform several routine procedures.

---

care veterinarians as role models whose identity is constructed around the value of offering a range of options to clients across the SoC. Primary care clinicians are likely to role model a perspective that high-quality clinical practice means offering acceptable and appropriate, evidence-based alternatives that may differ from the perceived "gold standard." Students thus have the opportunity to also internalize these values as part of their professional identity and develop the confidence to provide such care without concerns of negligence or litigation. A focus on SoC rather than gold-standard care avoids the client, veterinarian, or veterinary team members feeling shame, guilt, dissatisfaction, or anger at providing what might otherwise be perceived as inadequate or lower quality care [4]. From a practical perspective, students can develop the skills required to manage 15 to 30 minute consultations, the quick decision-making required for a wide range of presenting problems and the sequential approach to care that is common and often required in primary care practice.

In the context of veterinary education, teaching for SoC means also providing new ways to help support learner well-being and help graduates transition into practice [7]. As most of the students can be expected to enter primary care practice (predominantly companion animal) [18–20], it is important that students are familiar with and confident in practicing across a spectrum at graduation. Being able to tolerate the

inherent uncertainty of SoC, and make SoC decisions with limited information, is challenging, but those clinicians who are able to do so tend to demonstrate higher levels of personal resilience and emotional well-being [21]. There is also evidence that a professional identity that aligns with an SoC approach confers well-being benefits; graduates demonstrating an identity that embraces SoC ("challenge-focused": relational elements focused on engaging the client in decision-making and problem-solving elements targeted at reasoning through a range of acceptable options) seem to have better well-being than those whose identity is more "academic-focused" (oriented toward the exclusive valuing of tertiary referral-type care) [17]. Supporting the construction of a "challenge-focused," SoC-oriented professional identity is multifaceted but includes institutional valuing of role models who practice the SoC approach, high-stakes assessments that reward SoC competences, clinical rounds that incorporate discussions across the SoC, and positive discourses surrounding clients whose values and needs range across the spectrum of clinical care options. Embracing the SoC approach may thus help ease the transition from veterinary school to that of a busy practice environment with more supporting evidence likely to be gathered in the future as schools increasingly embrace this pedagogical model.

The Importance of a Collaborative Approach

A combination of both primary care and referral settings, with experienced teachers in both, is likely to provide the optimum training environment for our clinical students, underpinned by exposure to a range of learning approaches earlier in the curriculum. Supporting our graduates to develop the skills essential to deliver as far across the SoC as they can is a truly collaborative endeavor. All veterinary clinicians practice across a spectrum in some form, balancing the needs and resources of the patient, client, and business with every decision they make. What varies with workplace context is the "home" point on the spectrum, and the range across the spectrum over which care is delivered. We need our graduates to be comfortable delivering care across as wide a range as is possible in the context of their workplace and skillset, such that creating innovative solutions to support a range of different clients is perceived to be as professionally valuable as delivering the type of care they may have experienced in tertiary referral hospitals. Clients equally deserve such expertise in all aspects of care.

Veterinary educators are starting to develop strategies to help us overcome these teaching challenges. Questions are being pondered, such as how can we educate students about the social context and the barriers that exist around providing veterinary care? How can we teach students to be respectful of one another's contributions and keep moving them further away from a competitive, judgmental mindset? How can we teach students to support each other in their decision-making and to share experiences so they can learn collectively to better help future patients and clients?

The following sections explore some potential strategies that might support colleagues to explicitly introduce SoC pedagogy within their curricula, whether within university teaching hospitals, partner practices, or during internships and externships. We have chosen to use a "bricks and mortar" analogy to support our discussions. We recognize that many teaching settings already embrace learning opportunities that support SoC learning, incorporating the essential building blocks (the "bricks": areas of competence that are critical to SoC) and that there are many examples of good practice. We will provide some examples of these focusing on two key "bricks": communication and clinical reasoning. For each, we will consider approaches in classroom and clinical workplace settings and draw on the work of the Association of American Veterinary Medical Colleges (AAVMCs) SoC Initiative in defining the competences. Next, we will consider the "mortar" that holds these bricks together. This includes a focus on a collaborative institutional culture, faculty development, and approaches to teaching that integrate the "bricks" and that allow students and educators alike to engage fully with these, internalize the values of SoC and practice effectively, with confidence and a sense of achievement, across a range of settings and with diverse clients. We have chosen small animal examples for this article due to the focus of the journal readership; however, the principles can be readily transferred across species.

"Brick" EXAMPLE: COMMUNICATION

The SoC approach requires empathic, effective communication with a focus on relationship building. Relationship-centered veterinary care implies a partnership between client and veterinarian, emphasizing shared input in the decisions that are best for the patient [22–24]. Encouraging sharing requires that students understand their own biases and their role in filtering their view of the world. Inclusive teaching practices are important to model the skills that we are trying to instill [25].

If we consider that approaches to clinical decision-making can range from paternalistic, veterinarian-directed approaches at one extreme to client-directed at the other, then the SoC approach can encompass both extremes, but will often sit somewhere in the middle as a negotiated, relationship-centered approach. During the initiation of consultation, a veterinarian should ensure communication is structured to elicit a client's perspective on their concerns for their pet, goals for their pet's outcome, cost range they are willing and able to invest into their pet, values and beliefs surrounding pet care, and schedule and ability to administer different treatments or management options [22] (p 192). The use of inclusive language may help facilitate the shared perspective (eg, using "we" or "us" rather than "I," "me," or "you"). Furthermore, ensuring options are presented in a balanced way, identifying potential risks and benefits, rather than presenting an option as the "gold standard" is important to ensure continued owner engagement and support of the veterinary team in the decision-making process [4]. As stated by Brown and colleagues, "…Veterinarians should empower owners to choose the care option that best fits their expectations and financial considerations, without making them feel they are failing their pet if the most intensive, most expensive, or most technologically advanced option is not chosen" [8] (p 712).

Classroom Instruction and Assessment

Students in the preclinical classroom need to learn core communication skills to improve the client experience and to allow more effective transfer of information between parties as decisions are made [8]. Alongside communication training, it is critical that students are taught a wide variety of options for care of different diseases. Communicating the risk, cost, and likely outcomes of care options requires the underpinning knowledge of available options as well as the identification of client perspective. In the classroom, teaching approaches may include the provision of video or written examples of simulated client/veterinarian interaction, whereby students can compare and contrast different approaches to patient care. The inclusion of humanities education, such as exercises in the creative arts (poetry or song writing) or interpretation of art and literature, may improve empathy [26–28]. Assessment may include reflections following a video-recorded client interaction or written scenario or objective-structured clinical skills examinations with clients with a variety of financial and socioeconomic situations and different values and beliefs surrounding pet care in a simulated client environment [29–32].

In Box 2, we suggest an example approach for classroom-based communication teaching. These could be video or paper-based cases where students watch the videos or read through the case scenarios, then debrief in small groups.

This scenario could also be used as the basis for a simulated client role play exercise (laboratory session) with a postexercise debrief session.

Workplace Instruction and Assessment

The workplace provides an opportunity for role modeling SoC conversations with clients and an opportunity to assess and coach students in their client interactions. The workplace opportunity does not need to be solely isolated to the latter part of training, and near-peer observation can provide meaningful learning to learners starting to consider why learning effective communication is important. To achieve a meaningful SoC communication skill learning environment, it is helpful to ensure students are evaluated in different practice contexts, such as shelter/charity, primary care, and referral settings. Assessment in the workplace environment may include reflections on interactions (including recorded interactions) or the use of other workplace-based assessments such as mini-clinical exercises or the use of entrustment-supervision scales in assessment of entrustable professional activities (EPAs) [31–33]. In Box 3, we suggest an approach to workplace-based communication training.

"Brick" EXAMPLE: CLINICAL REASONING: INTEGRATING CONTEXT WITH DIAGNOSTIC AND TREATMENT PLANNING

Veterinarians have access to a wide range of diagnostic and treatment options, and care options rarely (if ever) fall into the two extremes of either costly, invasive, and technological advanced options or those that are less costly, less invasive, and requiring less technology. Integrating all of the considerations important for SoC provision to create a care plan is challenging, particularly if students' prior experience of clinical decision-making has focused on relatively more linear text book approaches. The use of a professional reasoning framework [34], which positions clinical reasoning as one of many "stakeholders" alongside the client, business, human–animal bond, public health, regulations, welfare, colleagues and self, can provide students with a structure to ensure that all perspectives are considered when creating a clinical plan.

It is also important to train students to practice a "sequential approach" to patient care [8]. Compared with referral practice, where patients often have complex, long-standing conditions that may or may not have already undergone a range of diagnostic tests

---

BOX 2
An approach to classroom-based communication teaching

Scenario for classroom-based teaching: Jo, a new client to the practice, presents with their dog Jensen for preventative health care. They have owned Jensen for 3 years. Jensen has been vaccinated annually but has not been on a heartworm preventative. At this visit, Jo consents to heartworm testing; Jensen tests positive. The veterinarian discusses melarsomine as the "gold standard" for treatment, which Jo declines due to concerns surrounding costs. The veterinarian proceeds to discuss euthanasia as the next viable option. Jo becomes visibly upset and storms out of the examination room.

After being presented with this scenario, students work in small groups to discuss the meaning of "gold standard," why the client might have been angry and what other approaches may have led to an improved client and patient outcome; groups also investigate other potential options of diagnostic investigations and associated treatments, including risks and relative costs. At the end of the session, each group presents their alternative scenario of treatment options and approaches.

BOX 3
An approach to workplace-based communication training

Primary care practice rotation: Ali, a long-standing client at the veterinary clinic, presents with their older dog Ferdie for head shaking and ear scratching. Cytology of a swab taken from the external ear canal reveals a mixed yeast and bacterial infection. Ali is anxious to treat Ferdie. The veterinary student initially suggests daily eardrops as part of the treatment plan. Ali notes that Ferdie has always had sensitive ears, and they are not sure they can consistently administer daily drops. Considering Ferdie's sensitivity to touch, the veterinary student pivots to provide options of daily eardrops or a single-dose option, discussing the risks of long-acting medications and the benefits of ensuring medication is consistently achieving concentrations that are effective for treatment.

In this example, the veterinary student demonstrates the ability to operate across the SoC, adjusting the treatment plan based on client abilities and patient compliance. Additional preparation for the appointment by reviewing the medical record and/or gathering this information during history-taking would have enabled a broader discussion of treatment options earlier in the client interaction.

---

and treatment options, and where clients are often prepared to pay for a wide range of tests at an initial visit, patients in primary care practice often benefit from diagnostic testing and treatment options provided in a sequential manner. Baseline or minimal diagnostics coupled with empirical treatments are used first, and further diagnostics coupled with more advanced treatment plans are decided on based on the patient's response and in specific consideration of clients' resources and desired goals of outcome.

As the concept of SoC can be overwhelming to students (especially when compared with learning a single "gold-standard" approach), framing potential clinical solutions according to the limited range of options below can be helpful [35].

- Do everything (carry out as much diagnostics and treatment as possible to achieve the greatest certainty of disease resolution)
- Stage/prioritize diagnostics and/or treatments (incremental or sequential approach)
  - Prioritizing selected tests based on the likelihood of diagnostic yield (increasing uncertainty in some cases but reducing cost)
  - Treatment trials (that may palliate or provide short-term therapy rather than long-term prognostic benefit)
- Do nothing (wait and see)
- Euthanasia/surrender

Many of these solutions are less financially costly, but also less interventional, so may have animal welfare benefits and/or provide pet owners with some valuable time to make difficult decisions relating to cost, invasiveness, or euthanasia or come to terms with severe illness.

Although the practice of SoC in the context of diagnostic and treatment planning has the potential for clear benefits for all stakeholders, there are challenges and

barriers to consider, particularly in the context of teaching. For educators in veterinary medicine, deliberately prompting and purposefully unpacking the nuances of clinical decision making may be one way to provide instruction in SoC. It is also important to consider the use of educational strategies to develop students' confidence with decision-making in the face of uncertainty (eg, lack of diagnostic test results or limited availability of evidence). Some potential approaches are outlined below.

Classroom Instruction and Assessment

Exposure to a wide variety of case presentations and disease processes is essential for students to develop context for the wide array of diagnostic tools and treatment options. Case-based learning (CBL) provides an opportunity to do this from early in curricula. CBL encompasses a broad range of teaching approaches, from curricula that are built around CBL pedagogy [36,37], to those that use small- or large-group CBL to contextualize and apply theoretical learning [38,39]. Whatever the extent of the approach, using case examples as educational prompts provides the opportunity to contextualize learning and provide opportunities for students to develop skills in decision-making across the SoC. Increasing the complexity of cases as the students' progress through their preclinical years is a practical way to build confidence and competence in applying SoC considerations in the face of ambiguity and uncertainty. Existing CBL scenarios can be easily adapted to require students to develop skills in sequential, prioritized approaches to case management, and incorporating SoC considerations that require a range of approaches to be considered and justified. One simple approach is to add "what-if" questions within existing approaches. For example, what if the client has financial limitations? What if the client is unable to pill their cat? What if the client is ethically opposed to euthanasia?

Another approach is to draw on the concept of a professional reasoning framework to build student confidence in contextual decision-making and offering care across a spectrum [34]. Students can be given a case scenario, and asked to consider the needs of all stakeholders and how these may influence care decisions. Box 4 provides an example approach to a classroom session using the professional reasoning approach.

The assessment of clinical reasoning can be achieved in a variety of ways, and it is often more authentic to integrate this with a clinical problem. Examples include carefully written clinical vignettes as a basis for single-best answer multiple-choice questions, encouraging students to prioritize tests within budget or other limitations. However, single-best answer formats can perpetuate a hidden curriculum that there is only one "best" answer to a given situation. Other formats such as script concordance tests or situational judgment tests may also have value (albeit with significant resource implications in the design phase) [31,32]. As students progress through their curriculum, the assessment of clinical reasoning can move from being a "desk-based" method, such as an essay, clinical case report, or set of short answers to a more authentic approach, such as

integrating clinical and professional dilemmas within an objective structured clinical examination. Effective assessment relies on provision of authentic, highly valid scenarios with careful use of marking rubrics to enhance reliability of assessment when there are multiple possible "correct" ways of resolving the scenario. Assessment rubrics therefore need to focus on rewarding students for their powers of analysis and ability to engage with the complexity of the scenario, rather than exclusively examining students' knowledge of disease or theories of communication.

Workplace/clinical instruction

Interacting, engaging, and making decisions with clinicians and clients in a wide variety of clinical settings (eg, primary, outreach, shelter, and referral) expose students to a wide range of contextual factors and provide opportunities to work with clinicians using a variety of clinical decision-making processes appropriate to different settings. These rich learning environments not only provide students with a range of contexts for clinical decision-making but can also be used to reinforce the importance of explicit consideration of SoC approaches to clinical reasoning.

Case exposure is critical; it can be tempting to assume that a good teaching case is one in which there is a

---

BOX 4
An approach to classroom-based training in professional reasoning

Classroom scenario (written or video prompt): Sam is a new client of the practice who lives alone and with limited financial resources. His cat Tom, a castrated male, has developed acute signs of urethral obstruction.

Students can be asked to identify the immediate and essential needs of the cat, which may include ensuring prompt management of pain and addressing imminent threat to life from urinary obstruction. They can then be asked to explore the long-term needs of the cat, which may include preventing future recurrences that are painful and dangerous, and require multiple stressful veterinary visits. Immediate and longer term needs of the client can be similarly explored; the immediate needs are not only financial, but also related to the bond with the cat, and the many emotions arising from making decisions about treating or euthanizing a pet. In the longer term, the costs (both emotional and financial) need to be weighed against the emotional and companionship benefits provided pet ownership, particularly for this client. The business is another stakeholder, and the students can be asked to consider financial and economic considerations alongside issues such as local reputation as a caring and compassionate provider of veterinary care. The veterinarians and their colleagues (such as the veterinary technicians and reception staff) are also important stakeholders, and the veterinarian's needs may include (depending on their identity and values surrounding their work) care of the client, avoiding distressing or highly inflammatory client interactions, feeling they have done a good job for the cat, and clinical interest (for academic and intellectual reasons, most veterinarians would like to treat as many patients as we can). Immediate needs may be those more focused on engaging constructively and feeling a sense of satisfaction from this case (client and patient); in the longer term, the veterinarian's needs may additionally incorporate feeling supported by their team and perceiving that, in general, they achieve sufficient clinical interest from their work.

After this approach to stakeholder analysis, students can then be asked to develop a range of care plans for both the short and long terms that take into account the different needs of all parties. These plans incorporate cost and other logistical considerations as well as incorporating prioritized, sequential approaches to diagnosis and treatment.

complete set of diagnostic information or a relatively simple set of client needs. However, this hides from students the complexity of clinical cases and implies that the only "good" cases are those where finances, values, and logistics do not complicate decision-making, and the only "good" veterinarians are those who carry out a "gold-standard" approach to veterinary care; this hidden curriculum can have significant impacts on students as they progress through their careers [40]. It is also important not to assume that a good teaching case is one in which there is a defined beginning and end with complete diagnostic testing and a definitive diagnosis. Cases that are ambiguous or mostly symptomatic and somewhat ill-defined are common in primary care practice and often make good teaching material. Box 5 provides an example.

The assessment of clinical reasoning in the workplace can be both formative (low stakes) and summative (high stakes) and informal and formal. More formalized assessments, grading students on clinical activities using a rubric, could include mini-clinical examinations (mini-CEX) and entrustable professional activities (EPAs), which include assessment of skills related to sequential approaches to care and consideration and integration of the needs of all stakeholders [31–33]. During informal assessment opportunities (such as case rounds or review sessions, when asking students to speak about their cases and patients), it is important that students' efforts to engage with the wider complexities of cases and their initiative in discussing a spectrum of management approaches are recognized and rewarded equally alongside their disease-specific knowledge.

THE MORTAR

The examples above provide a flavor of the competences and curriculum activities that can support SoC outcomes in the modern veterinary curriculum. As important as these "bricks" is the "mortar" that holds them together. Major curriculum redesign is a significant undertaking,

---

BOX 5
An approach to workplace-based training in professional reasoning

Primary care rotation: Omar has just started their first week of small animal primary care rotation, having spent the last 2 weeks with the referral internal medicine service. Their first consultation is Sonic, an 18-month old male neutered German Shepherd cross with a 4-day duration of watery diarrhea. Omar takes the history from the client noting that they have less time on this rotation to collect a history and establishes that Sonic is not vomiting but is eating less than usual and is less active. Sonic was recently in a boarding facility, where his owners were moving (relocating). Sonic's owners are very concerned but declare that they currently do not have a lot of money to spend. Physical examination does not show any significant abnormalities.

Dr Smith is supervising Omar and asks what their diagnostic and/or treatment plan is for this case. Omar saw several cases of diarrhea on their medicine rotation—those all had fecal tests, bloodwork, abdominal ultrasound, and endoscopy with biopsies. Omar is finding it difficult to adjust their clinical reasoning to this common primary care scenario. Dr Smith asks Omar to consider the following:

- How unwell is Sonic? How urgent is the problem? Is a sequential approach appropriate?
- If so, what is the first intervention (if any) that you want to suggest? Take into account both patient and client factors.
- Would you plan for a follow-up visit? If so, what is your follow-up plan?

Omar quickly recognizes that the situation is not urgent and suggests a diet change to an alternative that is easily digestible. Omar checks that Sonic is vaccinated and up-to-date with deworming and ensures that the clients understand the importance of good fecal hygiene for Sonic and good hand hygiene for the owners. Omar asks to see Sonic in the clinic again if he deteriorates, or is no better in 48 hours, and asks the owners to bring a fecal sample with them at that stage. Dr Smith is happy with that plan, and Omar communicates it to the client. Later that day, during a break in consultations, Dr Smith could ask Omar to reflect on some/all of the following:

- What is the full spectrum of diagnostic tests and treatments that could be offered in this instance? What other client and patient factors do you need to consider in offering the full spectrum?
- Why did you select the plan that you chose? What was the range of considerations that influenced your decision? What were the pros and cons of each possible plan in reference to, for example, cost or likelihood to provide actionable diagnostic information?
- If Sonic comes back for a follow-up appointment, what will you consider in that appointment? For example, what clinical indicators (and client indicators) will you look for if you are to decide that there has been response to treatment? What diagnostic and/or treatment options might you present in that next appointment?

and whereas some institutions have embraced SoC within this context [2], this may not be an option for all schools for a variety of reasons. Below we suggest some different approaches to creating this "mortar" that we hope will help colleagues and leadership teams identify ways in which they can best support the development of SoC skills in their students.

Faculty Collaboration

Bringing specialists and primary care clinicians together is powerful. All clinicians work across the SoC, and it is important that students are aware of this and recognize the full range of options available within different contexts. What is likely to differ between the specialist and primary care settings is the location and range across the spectrum over which an individual practices. It is also important to recognize that the spectrum may vary for an individual for different areas of clinical interest. Many primary care veterinarians have areas of particular interest where they wish to be able to offer more advanced procedures. Although specialists have a relatively filtered caseload, they still routinely adapt plans to specific situations and some specialties (eg, emergency and critical care) by routinely working across a very broad spectrum. It is the responsibility of educators to ensure that students understand what procedures might reasonably be expected to be undertaken in primary care settings, and emphasis should be placed on this care being performed by suitably qualified and/or experienced veterinarians who are confident in their approach.

An institutional culture that facilitates open and respectful collaboration among colleagues from a wide range of workplace contexts can support transformative change. Primary care clinicians, particularly those that are relatively recently graduates, can work collaboratively with specialists to develop and refine teaching and assessment materials, ensuring that the focus is on the aspects of clinical care that are most important for new graduates; several authors of this article have witnessed firsthand the success of this team approach. The team-based delivery of case-based classroom sessions by primary care and specialist clinicians can provide multiple perspectives for students, encouraging constructive and authentic discussions around the options available for different scenarios, and the relative merits and disadvantages of each. In the clinical workplace, where a program may be heavily reliant on tertiary referral settings, primary care and specialist clinical educators can "team-teach" within referral settings to support student learning: at one of the authors' institutions (SW), the introduction of

"veterinary clinical demonstrators" has transformed the student and faculty experience within the referral hospital [41]. The clinical demonstrators are primary care clinicians who work with referral teams in clinical rotations and have responsibility for ensuring that student learning is focused on the important day one competences, through involvement in a range of activities such as case discussions, rounds, and drop-in sessions. The clinical demonstrators do not have case responsibility within the referral clinic, enabling them to focus on teaching and student experience and enabling referral clinicians to better balance their clinical work and teaching responsibilities. Initiatives such as this require that the faculty involved authentically role model respect and openness to the varied perspectives and experiences of others, genuinely valuing one another's expertise and recognizing that the different and complementary expertise embodied by both primary care and specialist clinicians [17].

Curricular Innovation

There are many aspects of the curriculum that can be leveraged to support SoC education. Careful choice and structure of case exemplars for CBL activities can ensure that students become familiar with a range of approaches for common conditions. Using an outcome-based approach (eg, Competency-Based Veterinary Education https://cbve.org) helps focus faculty on the important skills and knowledge required in both clinical and basic science subjects. Techniques such as "think-aloud" can be used in both classroom and workplace settings, opening the "black-box" of clinical reasoning for both the student (who otherwise is not aware of the often tacit thought processes of the veterinarian) and for faculty (for whom many aspects of clinical reasoning may have become habitual and tacit) [42]. Teaching and reflective activities that draw students' attention to context, the diversity of client values, resources, experiences and expectations, and how these relate to clinical decision-making, can be instrumental in encouraging students to think beyond the relative simplicity and comfort of the textbook approach. Embracing concepts such as the professional reasoning framework [34] throughout the curriculum can ensure faculty and students are familiar with the concepts and approach, framing clinical reasoning as just one part of the professional reasoning. Extensive use of facilitated small group collaborative CBL requires students to work together and share their knowledge, developing respect for one another's contributions and perspectives [43]. Where feasible, early clinical exposure within primary care workplaces can help students conceptualize the SoC early in their training, observing the barriers that clients experience, and developing realistic understanding of the goals of care [2]. Intertwining case material between that experienced in the clinic setting and that explored in the classroom creates a powerful spiral curriculum experience [2].

Assessment strategies can consider how best to support the development of learning across the spectrum. Are assessments testing knowledge, application of knowledge, or more advanced skills such as decision-making? Is there a reliance on single-best answer multiple-choice questions? Multiple-choice style questions may generate the "hidden curriculum" message that there is only one solution to a problem, irrespective of wider context and considerations. How many times have you, as an experienced clinician, read an multiple choice questions (MCQ) and thought…"it depends…"? Are students supported to learn the basics across the breadth of subjects, but given permission, through strategic assessment, to focus their areas of depth on subjects that are of particular interest to them? Are faculty focusing on authentic day one competences? Enthusiastic specialist teachers may be tempted to teach (and assess) at a level beyond that strictly necessary for day one competence; faculty want to inspire our students to stretch themselves, but we need to reflect on where, when, and how we most effectively do this. Consideration can also be given to the overall assessment strategy; there is evidence that moving from a grade-based strategy to a pass/fail strategy improves student well-being and constructive collaboration, reducing the competitiveness that can foster an inappropriately judgmental culture [44,45].

Faculty Training

Embracing SoC education within an institution requires that colleagues have a shared understanding of what is meant by SoC and the purpose and values of such an approach. Faculty training is critical to support any degree of curriculum change [46]. Stepping away from a focus on concepts of "gold-standard" care toward more contextualized approaches to SoC can be challenging, particularly for clinicians who have worked only in referral settings. Faculty may experience this shift as sitting quite uncomfortably with their own professional identity and values; it can be helpful to train faculty not just in the principles of SoC and any related tools being embraced by the curriculum, but also to highlight work around professional identity [7,40], in which a distinction can be made between an academic-focused identity (prioritizing definitive clinical reasoning and best-evidence treatment), compared

with a challenge-focused identity with an emphasis on broader consideration of client and contextual needs when reasoning across a range of valid options. Many specialist clinicians might recognize themselves as more academic-oriented in their clinical priorities and career goals and may not naturally role model the challenge-focused identity which can help veterinarians thrive in the primary care setting.

The American Association of Veterinary Medical Colleges SoC initiative Task Force was established in 2021 and consists of private practitioners as well as primary care and specialist educators currently collaborating to create resources to assist programs interested in integrating new approaches and enhancing existing approaches to SoC training (The Spectrum of Care Initiative: AAVMC). The outputs of this initiative include the SoC education model composed of specific curricular elements that prepare graduates for SoC practice. These curricular elements are: SoC-specific sub-competencies aligned with the competency-based veterinary education (CBVE) competency framework; examples of assessments that can be used to provide evidence of students' achievement of SoC learning outcomes; and specific learning activities and instructional strategies for courses, laboratories, and clinical experiences scaffolded throughout the curriculum that can prepare students for SoC practice. In addition, the SoC initiative will develop implementation guidelines that provide essential tools for integrating the SoC education model into veterinary teaching institutions and wider settings, such as curricular and cultural change management strategies and faculty support resources. Ultimately, the AAVMC SoC initiative aims to provide programs with strategies and resources developed by both primary care and specialist educators that support an integrated educational approach to preparing graduates for SoC practice.

The Transition to Practice

How do we best support our graduates to build on their competence and confidence in practice? We are privileged as veterinary professionals in the breadth and variety of our daily practice, whether that is in primary care or referral settings. How can we encourage our graduates to embrace that diversity and develop their skills across a wide range of the spectrum? They need to feel empowered to try new procedures and approaches; skills such as cystotomy, routine orthopedic procedures, and management of complex comorbid medical conditions have, for many years, been part of daily practice in primary care. If we view the transition to practice as a shared endeavor between schools and the profession, then we can combine the basic training provided during veterinary school (in classes, laboratories, and a variety of workplace contexts) with an expectation that, appropriately mentored, graduates will routinely challenge themselves to develop new skills throughout their professional careers, extending the spectrum over which they can offer care to their clients. They may choose to do this within a particular sphere of interest, with appropriate postgraduate training and continuing professional development, but there needs to be a degree of comfort and support with stepping out of the immediate comfort zone. This is as true for a specialty resident undertaking a specialist procedure for the first time under the watchful eye of their supervisor as it is for their colleague in primary care practice undertaking their first cystotomy, supported by experienced technicians and colleagues. Many corporate practices have introduced graduate schemes, which provide a framework to scaffold the development of newly-graduated veterinarians, with carefully planned induction periods, the support of a trained mentor within the practice and bespoke continuing professional development events for the newly-graduated cohort.

Also of note is the recently updated Veterinary Graduate Development Programme (VetGDP) run by the Royal College of Veterinary Surgeons in the United Kingdom. Completion of this program is a requirement for all recently graduated veterinary surgeons working in the United Kingdom (rcvs.org.uk). The VetGDP aims to ensure that all graduates have a structure in place for effective support as they gain experience and confidence, on which to build a fulfilling career. Any practice using a recent graduate must become an RCVS Approved Graduate Development Practice and have a dedicated and trained VetGDP mentor to support the graduate as they develop their skills through regular discussion, observation, and feedback. EPAs are used to frame an e-portfolio, with the graduate and their advisor agreeing which are relevant to their role and with the aim that by completion of the VetGDP graduates will have reached the point across all relevant EPAs where both they and their adviser agree that additional support is no longer required.

SUMMARY

The SoC options for any given patient will be influenced by many factors such as owner goals, values, and resources; available evidence for treatments; and clinic capabilities as well as veterinarian competence and confidence. Veterinary education programs are uniquely positioned to directly impact the veterinarian factors that affect the range of high-quality affordable care options they make available to patients. To achieve this goal, veterinary programs are shifting toward outcome-based curricula focused on preparing graduates for day one practice. SoC pedagogy includes approaches that help graduates achieve day one outcomes by refocusing clinical training to embrace a combination of both primary care and referral learning environments. Although there are specific areas of competence that programs can focus on to help graduates prepare for SoC practice (eg, communication and clinical reasoning), these are by no means new elements for curricula to consider. Instead, the educational innovation of SoC pedagogy challenges programs to develop clinical preparation strategies through the collaboration of both primary care and specialist educators. The input of faculty from all areas of clinical practice is essential to support the transformational change required to broaden the SoC where graduates are confident and competent to practice. Ultimately, a fundamental step toward this integrated educational approach to SoC pedagogy is establishing an institutional culture that encourages collaboration among educators from a wide range of clinical environments.

As veterinary educators strive toward enhancing SoC preparedness for graduates, the veterinary education community must remain cognizant of how to track the success of these efforts. This requires yet another collaborative approach that entails partnering with the workforce and potential employers of new graduates. Work that identifies specific knowledge, skills, and attributes of a confident and competent SoC practitioner cannot be performed in an academic vacuum but instead should be conducted by teams comprising educators and a variety of members from the workforce (eg, primary care clinicians, specialist practitioners, veterinary nurses/technicians). Developing outcomes through these collaborations will help to establish workplace-based metrics that can be instrumental in tracking the success of SoC-focused training programs. Ultimately, how successful veterinary education is at preparing graduates for SoC practice will rely on interprofessional collaborations and strategies to support and evaluate graduates as they transition to the workforce.

CONFLICTS OF INTEREST

None of the authors has any commercial or financial conflicts of interest. The drafting of this article was not supported by any specific funding.

REFERENCES

[1] Stull JW, Shelby JA, Bonnett BN, et al. Barriers and next steps to providing a spectrum of effective health care to companion animals. J Am Vet Med Assoc 2018; 253(11):1386–9.

[2] Fingland RB, Stone LR, Read EK, et al. Preparing veterinary students for excellence in general practice: building confidence and competence by focusing on spectrum of care. J Am Vet Med Assoc 2021;259(5): 463–70.

[3] Evason MD, Stein MR, Stull JW. Impact of a Spectrum of Care Elective Course on Third-Year Veterinary Students' Self-Reported Knowledge, Attitudes, and Competencies. J Vet Med Educ 2022;e20220010.

[4] Skipper A, Gray C, Serlin R, et al. Gold standard care' is an unhelpful term. Vet Rec 2021;189(8):331.

[5] Wiltzius AJ, Blackwell MJ, Krebsbach SB, et al. Access to veterinary care: barriers, current practices, and public policy. Access to Veterinary Care Coalition; 2018.

[6] Cruess RL, Cruess SR, Boudreau JD, et al. Reframing medical education to support professional identity formation. Acad Med 2014;89(11):1446–51.

[7] Armitage-Chan E, May SA. Identity, environment and mental wellbeing in the veterinary profession. Vet Rec 2018;183(2):68.

[8] Brown CR, Garrett LD, Gilles WK, et al. Spectrum of care: more than treatment options. J Am Vet Med Assoc 2021; 259(7):712–7.

[9] Meindl AG, Roth IG, Gonzalez SE. Never apologize for wanting to be "just" a general practitioner. J Am Vet Med Assoc 2019;255(8):891–3.

[10] Bachynsky EA, Dale VH, Kinnison T, et al. A survey of the opinions of recent veterinary graduates and employers regarding early career business skills. Vet Rec 2013; 172(23):604.

[11] Brown CM. The future of the North American Veterinary Teaching Hospital. J Vet Med Educ 2003;30(3): 197–202.

[12] Routly JE, Taylor IR, Turner R, et al. Support needs of veterinary surgeons during the first few years of practice: perceptions of recent graduates and senior partners. Vet Rec 2002;150(6):167–71.

[13] Roder CA, May SA. The Hidden Curriculum of Veterinary Education: Mediators and Moderators of Its Effects. J Vet Med Educ 2017;44(3):542–51.

[14] Alvarez EE, Gilles WK, Lygo-Baker S, et al. Teaching Cultural Humility and Implicit Bias to Veterinary Medical Students: A Review and Recommendation for Best Practices. J Vet Med Educ 2020;47(1):2–7.

[15] McCobb E, Rozanski EA, Malcolm EL, et al. A Novel Model for Teaching Primary Care in a Community Practice Setting: Tufts at Tech Community Veterinary Clinic. J Vet Med Educ 2017;45(1):99–107.

[16] Patterson D, Blane DN. Training for purpose - a blueprint for social accountability and health equity focused GP training. Educ Prim Care 2021;32(6):318–21.

[17] May S. Towards a scholarship of primary health care. Vet Rec 2015;176(26):677–82.

[18] Bain B, Hansen C, Ouedraogo FB, et al. AVMA Report on the economic state of the veterinary profession. Illinois: American Veterinary Medical Association; 2022.

[19] Robinson D, Edwards M, Mason B, et al. The 2019 survey of the veterinary profession. London, UK: Royal College of Veterinary Surgeons; 2019.

[20] AVA. Australian Veterinary Association Veterinary Workforce Survey 2021: Analysis Report. 2021.

[21] Strout TD, Hillen M, Gutheil C, et al. Tolerance of uncertainty: A systematic review of health and healthcare-related outcomes. Patient Educ Couns 2018;101(9): 1518–37.

[22] Englar R. A guide to oral communication in veterinary medicine. Sheffield, UK: 5M Publishing; 2020.

[23] Kedrowicz AA. Clients and Veterinarians as Partners in Problem Solving during Cancer Management: Implications for Veterinary Education. J Vet Med Educ 2015; 42(4):373–81.

[24] Kanji N, Coe JB, Adams CL, et al. Effect of veterinarian-client-patient interactions on client adherence to dentistry and surgery recommendations in companion-animal practice. J Am Vet Med Assoc 2012;240(4): 427–36.

[25] Dewsbury B, Brame CJ. Inclusive Teaching. CBE-Life Sci Educ 2019;18(2):fe2.

[26] Batt-Rawden SA, Chisolm MS, Anton B, et al. Teaching empathy to medical students: an updated, systematic review. Acad Med 2013;88(8):1171–7.

[27] Graham J, Benson LM, Swanson J, et al. Medical Humanities Coursework Is Associated with Greater Measured Empathy in Medical Students. Am J Med 2016; 129(12):1334–7.

[28] Cao EL, Blinderman CD, Cross I. Reconsidering Empathy: An Interpersonal Approach and Participatory Arts in the Medical Humanities. J Med Humanit 2021; 42(4):627–40.

[29] Adams CL, Nestel D, Wolf P. Reflection: a critical proficiency essential to the effective development of a high competence in communication. J Vet Med Educ 2006; 33(1):58–64.

[30] Hecker KG, Adams CL, Coe JB. Assessment of first-year veterinary students' communication skills using an objective structured clinical examination: the importance of context. J Vet Med Educ 2012;39(3):304–10.

[31] Foreman JH, Danielson JA, Fogelberg K, et al. Competency Based Veterinary Education (CBVE) Assessment Toolkit. 2022.

[32] Baillie S, Warman SM, Rhind S. A guide to assessment in veterinary medical education. 3rd edition. https://doi.org/ 10.35542/osf.io/kectf.

[33] Molgaard LK, Chaney KP, Bok HGJ, et al. Development of core entrustable professional activities linked to a competency-based veterinary education framework. Med Teach 2019;41(12):1404–10.

[34] Armitage-Chan E. Best Practice in Supporting Professional Identity Formation: Use of a Professional Reasoning Framework. J Vet Med Educ 2020;47(2):125–36.

[35] Armitage-Chan E. Principles of professional reasoning and decision-making. In: Maddison JE, Volk HA, Church DB, editors. Clinical reasoning in veterinary practice: problem solved!. 2nd edition. Oxford, UK: Wiley Blackwell; 2022. p. 391–406.

[36] Thistlethwaite JE, Davies D, Ekeocha S, et al. The effectiveness of case-based learning in health professional education. A BEME systematic review: BEME Guide No. 23. Med Teach 2012;34(6):e421–44.

[37] Burgess A, Matar E, Roberts C, et al. Scaffolding medical student knowledge and skills: team-based learning (TBL) and case-based learning (CBL). BMC Med Educ 2021; 21(1):238.

[38] Crowther E, Baillie S. A method of developing and introducing case-based learning to a preclinical veterinary curriculum. Anat Sci Educ 2016;9(1):80–9.

[39] Gold JM, Collazo RA, Athauda G, et al. Taking CBL to the Lecture Hall: a Comparison of Outcomes Between Traditional Small Group CBL and a Novel Large Group Team-Based CBL Teaching Method. Med Sci Educ 2020;30(1): 227–33.

[40] Armitage-Chan E'. I wish I was someone else': complexities in identity formation and professional wellbeing in veterinary surgeons. Vet Rec 2020;187(3):113.

[41] O'Shaughnessy S, Bates L, Gould L, et al. Enhancing Primary Care Learning in a Referral Hospital Setting: Introducing Veterinary Clinical Demostrators. J Vet Med Educ 2023;20220143. https://doi.org/10.3138/jvme-2022-0143.

[42] Delany C, Golding C. Teaching clinical reasoning by making thinking visible: an action research project with allied health clinical educators. BMC Med Educ 2014; 14:20.

[43] Khosa DK, Volet SE. Productive group engagement in cognitive activity and metacognitive regulation during collaborative learning: Can it explain differences in students' conceptual understanding. Metacogn Learn 2014; 9(3):287–307.

[44] Frank N, Sutherland-Smith J. Evidence-Based Approach to Switching to a Pass-Fail System for Clinical Year Veterinary Student Grading. J Vet Med Educ 2021;48(4): 503–10.

[45] Royal K, Hedgpeth M-W, Flammer K. Veterinary medical students' perspectives on traditional and pass-fail grading models in preclinical training. Education in the Health Professions 2020;3:116–20.

[46] Warman S, Pritchard J, Baillie S. Faculty Development for a New Curriculum: implementing a strategy for veterinary teachers within the wider University context. J Vet Med Educ 2016;42(3):346–52.

Moving?

Make sure your subscription moves with you!

To notify us of your new address, find your **Clinics Account Number** (located on your mailing label above your name), and contact customer service at:

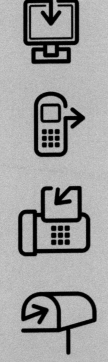

Email: journalscustomerservice-usa@elsevier.com

800-654-2452 (subscribers in the U.S. & Canada)
314-447-8871 (subscribers outside of the U.S. & Canada)

Fax number: 314-447-8029

Elsevier Health Sciences Division
Subscription Customer Service
3251 Riverport Lane
Maryland Heights, MO 63043

*To ensure uninterrupted delivery of your subscription, please notify us at least 4 weeks in advance of move.